McGraw-Hill Series in Health Science
AMOS CHRISTIE, M.D., *Consulting Editor*

HEALTH SERVICES FOR THE CHILD

McGraw-Hill Series in Health Science
AMOS CHRISTIE, M.D., *Consulting Editor*

HEALTH SERVICES

FOR THE CHILD

Edward R. Schlesinger, M.D., M.P.H.

Associate Director of Medical Services,
formerly Director of Maternal and Child Health Services,
New York State Department of Health;
Associate in Pediatrics,
Albany Medical College, Union University

foreword by
Herman E. Hilleboe, M.D.

McGraw-Hill Book Company, Inc.
New York   Toronto   London
1953

THE MAPLE PRESS COMPANY, YORK, PA.

To SYLVIA

EDITOR'S FOREWORD

The ideal of preventive pediatrics is the complete prevention of disease, and the need for treatment is an admission of failure. Yet the means of accomplishing the ideal is very much a part of the history of human relationships within the community. Many entirely non-medical factors such as social and economic forces are constantly operating and actually influence preventive medicine. As a matter of fact, one of the basic tasks consciously or unconsciously of statesmanship or democratic government has been and probably always will be the creation of an environment in which there will be no human suffering or premature deaths.

Our current concept of pediatrics has broadened tremendously in the past twenty-five years. The specialty now deals with the child not only in disease but in health. It is cognizant of and responsible for his health requirements as well as the causes of premature death and crippling disease. The medical historian will find the history of preventive pediatrics exactly parallel to the history of the whole child welfare movement. Child welfare is nothing more or less than the public acceptance and practice of good preventive pediatrics by the individual.

In order to do this, the community must have a child health program. This is the subject of this book, and in so far as I am aware it is unique in that it is the only one to attempt to define and to cover the field of a child health program.

When one asks the question, "Does our community have a child health program," he really means, "Is our community a safe place in which to have and to raise children." The answer to this question inevitably involves a correlation of social and economic forces working in the community with the medical care facilities. Only through such understanding can the individual physician, mother, or father, aid in creating an environment in which it is safe to have and to raise children.

So I hope it will be clear why I as a professor of pediatrics am so enthusiastic about this volume. It correlates in separate chapters all the factors which go to make up a child health program in its broadest and idealistic sense.

Furthermore, it demonstrates that this environment is purchasable— purchasable as a clean water supply or adequate sewage disposal is purchasable in a community educated to accept its responsibility by voting tax funds to bring these desirable things about. And these facilities must be available to all. Communicable or crippling disease has no regard for the railroad tracks.

Although this book was written primarily for the busy practicing physician, it was also written for everyone interested in child health services. Citizens anticipating a project of developing a convalescent home or other rehabilitation facilities will find it useful. Teachers and students in public health and schools of social work and nurses will find it indispensable. As a member of the faculty at one time or another of each of these ancillaries I have repeatedly felt the need of reference material of exactly this kind. The author is to be congratulated on bringing together so beautifully and for the first time a book outlining the ideals and objectives of preventive pediatrics and indicating how we as citizens may attain them. The late great Professor Rosenau must have had something like this effort by Dr. Schlesinger in mind when he wrote, "Preventive medicine dreams of these things, not with the hope that we, individually, may participate in them, but with the joy that we may aid in their coming to those who shall live after us. When young men have vision, the dreams of old men come true."

AMOS CHRISTIE, M.D.

FOREWORD

In the forefront of the consciousness of responsible parents is the desire to have healthy children and to bring them up in an emotional and physical environment that will aid them to grow up to be happy and productive citizens. To reach these attainable goals requires not only the care and devotion of the parents, but the total child health services of the community as well.

In the social and emotional complex that we call modern society, the practicing physicians must help parents find the guideposts through the intricate network of winding trails of babyhood, childhood, and adolescence. There are so many blind endings and hairpin curves that one easily can get off the road never to get on again. Out of this maze of medical and social problems confronting family physicians and the parents and children under their care, the author has skillfully brought forth some fundamental concepts for the provision of adequate child health services in any community, large or small. Drawing upon his training as a pediatrician and a public health physician, and his seasoned experience as Director of Maternal and Child Health Services in the New York State Health Department during the last decade, he has clarified the main issues and developed patterns for the strengthening and improvement of the health and well-being of children.

The author points out that public health programs for maternal and child health have been accepted and supported by the American people as a community responsibility. The New York State Citizens' Committee of One Hundred for Children and Youth in 1950 was of the opinion that no public health activity is more important than that affecting the lives and health of children. The report based on the work of this group and on the New York State Study of Child Health Services of 1946 and 1947, endorsed by the medical profession of the State, concluded that child health is everybody's business.

Much has been accomplished in the second quarter of the twentieth century, but still more remains to be done. Too many deaths still occur from prematurity, rheumatic fever, diarrhea of the newborn, accidents, and needless infections. Many of the early deaths and disabling diseases of adulthood need never occur if we but seek out their real origins in childhood illnesses.

It is amply evident that child health, school health, and community health are interdependent social enterprises. To meet their challenges, it is essential that basic considerations must include a concept of total child health services on a broad scale. We cannot wait until critical illness or severe disability brings the child and his parents into the doctor's office for belated diagnosis and treatment. It is essential to provide services in the home and the school and the clinic that will detect early disease and hidden disability in time for the physician to preserve function and prevent unnecessary death and incapacity. Expert care in later years can never make up fully for the lost opportunities in the infant and preschool years.

The author has ably interwoven preventive mental health knowledge into the fabric of child health services. The application of this knowledge to the social and emotional problems of parents and children offers strong hope of easing the stresses and strains of modern living. The causes of mental illness remain largely obscure, but exhaustive studies have indicated that much mental illness in adult life derives from emotional disturbances and personality quirks acquired in early childhood. It follows that the greatest potential for the promotion of positive mental health in adulthood lies in the field of maternal and child health services.

Child health, the author aptly remarks, is inseparable from maternal health. Even before conception occurs, the attitudes of the parents toward marriage, parenthood, pregnancy, and labor are of vital concern. The health of the mother during pregnancy and labor is reflected in the health and vigor of the newborn child. The critical neonatal period requires all the maternal and medical skills at one's command to avoid infection and afford proper nutrition for growth and development. When the newborn enters life as a premature infant, the high level of anticipated mortality can be appreciably reduced by applying recent advances in medical science on a community-wide basis. Expert care and well-equipped nurseries for premature babies offer the best chance to transform the tragedy of a premature death into the triumph of a new life.

It is in the preschool age that community health services come into their own as lifesaving and life-preserving measures on a grand scale. Public health nursing services, child health conferences, and health education services of local health departments reach out into the rural and urban homes in the community to provide preventive services so important in the formative years. The school health services, the mental health and dental clinics, the clinics for handicapped children of all types—these are the facilities that enable the family physician and his host of consultants and other health teammates to utilize their professional skills where they will do the most good. Once good health habits are established for the children in a family, they are more than likely to continue on through adolescence and into adult life. Health supervision requires the combined efforts of the parents, the physician and his cohorts, and all health facilities in the community skillfully blended into the most effective combination, depending upon the age of the child, his physical, mental, and emotional status.

The integration of these multiple services and skills that vary with time and place has been accomplished by the author with the realism that comes only from long experience with children in the home, the school, the clinic, and the hospital.

In the development of community programs to meet the needs of children of all ages, the public health physician and his colleague the family physician are beset by many special problems. Not the least of these are the special-interest groups whose personal experiences with handicapped children in their own homes compel them to demand special consideration for their particular problems. Cerebral palsy, mental retardation, muscular dystrophy, epilepsy—these are just a few of the special problems that must be faced by those persons responsible for the wise use of limited resources in the community, the city, the county, and the state. Unsolved health problems exist because of lack of recognition of the problem, lack of resources, or an inability to develop a balanced health program based upon sound knowledge of the extent of the problems and their relative importance in community health. It is essential to measure these problems as separate entities and in relation to one another, before steps are taken to meet the community needs, within the limits of available resources at a particular time and a particular place. An important resource that is often overlooked is the attitude of the people themselves toward health problems. With knowledge comes understanding; with recognition comes acceptance and support.

In the interplay of community forces, there is need for guidance so that professional skills and costly facilities will not be wasted or misused. There is need for strong minds and firm hands in the planning and execution of community health services for children. The author has presented a comprehensive approach to the social and emotional problems of children as well as the medical ones associated with growth and development. He has brought together for the family physician, the pediatrician, and the public worker current knowledge on total child health services. This knowledge should help these individuals to solve their problems of child health more easily and to aid them in providing the children under their care the best services modern medical science can offer.

HERMAN E. HILLEBOE, M.D.
Commissioner of Health,
State of New York

PREFACE

The physician has always been regarded as a leading citizen in his community, and his influence on community affairs has extended far beyond the bounds of his medical background. This informal type of leadership based on professional prestige is being replaced increasingly by more specific responsibilities. Many physicians serve on boards of governmental or voluntary health agencies, or their advice is otherwise sought when health services are planned or reviewed. Others devote a proportion of their time to health services in clinics, schools, and in other activities outside their private practices. Physicians are often called upon to discuss health problems before citizen groups. Within their own medical organizations special committees are formed to define the relationships of the local medical profession to community health services. As stated in an editorial comment in the *Journal of the American Medical Association*,[1] "Unless practicing physicians are closely identified with (local health) programs at all stages, they run the risk of being overlooked when the time comes to decide how a given health unit shall function best at the local level."

In no field are greater demands made upon the physician's time and energy than in relation to community services on behalf of mothers and children. To meet these broadening demands, the physician must view the entire community as his patient, using techniques that differ markedly from traditional care of the individual patient. "Health Services for the Child" is an attempt to interpret to the practicing physician this approach to health problems in the community—methods of analyzing the problems involved, of planning, supervising, and evaluating needed services, and other aspects of a well-rounded health program.

At the same time, this book attempts to set forth the common goals

[1] Vol. 147, p. 328, Sept. 22, 1951.

and the complementary activities of the physician in private practice and the health worker in a community agency. By increasing the mutual respect and understanding of all members of the health professions, a team approach to the health problems of the community may be fostered.

What has been sought in the main has been the interpretation of a viewpoint. Material of a factual nature is given mainly to illustrate or clarify points being discussed, rather than as an end in itself. Wherever possible, the book is a distillation of the current opinions and practices of acknowledged leaders in the field of maternal and child health. Whatever opinions and interpretations deviate from this endeavor, especially on still controversial topics, must obviously be the full responsibility of the author.

The purpose of the book is to give an integrated picture of health services for mothers and children. To accomplish this, it has been necessary to treat the same subject material from different viewpoints as the book progresses. For example, the subject of communicable diseases is discussed incidental to general considerations at the start. The control of communicable diseases is then treated as a specific health service. This service is then included with proper emphasis in the provision of health supervision during the maternity cycle and successive periods of infancy and childhood. Finally, attention is given to the role of communicable diseases in respect to special health problems. While a certain amount of duplication is unavoidable, every effort has been made to reduce it to a minimum. The index has been prepared with this in mind.

References have been selected on the basis of their accessibility and timeliness. Recent review articles have been chosen in preference to the articles of the original investigators, since the former lead to the earlier references about the subject under discussion, thus eliminating unwieldy bibliographies. Editorials in readily accessible periodicals have been frequently cited for the same reason. Exceptions have naturally been made to this rule in order to give proper credit for earlier work quoted or cited directly without actual quotation.

"Health Services for the Child" is a reflection of the progressive leadership of Dr. Herman E. Hilleboe and of my daily stimulating contacts with members of the staff of the New York State Department of

Health, especially those now or formerly with the Bureau of Maternal and Child Health. I cannot allow this opportunity to pass without expressing my gratitude to the late Dr. Clinton P. McCord, who helped me find the inner resources to conceive and complete the project. Above all, words cannot express my heartfelt thanks to my wife—and truly co-author—who typed the successive drafts of the manuscript, insisting upon clarity of thought in the process, and who, at sacrifice of vacations and social life, encouraged me to carry the book through to completion.

EDWARD R. SCHLESINGER

Albany, New York
May, 1953

CONTENTS

PART IV. *Special Problems*

Part I

BASIC CONSIDERATIONS

1 THE COMMUNITY CHILD HEALTH PROGRAM

The health of the child in his family and in his community—this is the focus, near or distant, of all health services for children. The provision of adequate health services in the locality in which the child lives is one of a host of community services designed to assist the family in achieving this goal. Services promoted or financed by Federal or state agencies, both governmental and voluntary, have no reality unless they ultimately bear upon the health of children in their communities. Planning in all spheres of health activity for children must keep this focus clearly in mind.

Health is defined by the World Health Organization as a state of complete physical, mental, and social well-being and not merely the absence of disease or infirmity. "The enjoyment of the highest attainable standard of health is one of the fundamental rights of every human being." (1) According to this positive concept, an individual is not considered healthy simply because a physical examination discloses no demonstrable defects and a psychiatric interview reveals no clear-cut mental illness. Optimal health in this sense is achieved when the individual has developed to the fullest extent within the limits set by his hereditary endowment.

Definition of Program. Development of a well-rounded child health program presupposes this positive definition of health. A complete community child health program, in a broad sense, may therefore be defined as *the application of current knowledge through available techniques for the attainment of the greatest possible physical, mental, and social well-being of all children, within the limits set by their inherited capabilities. This involves the use or development, in a coordinated man-*

ner, of existing or potential resources and services in the community, whether under voluntary or governmental auspices. The condition of the child at birth is determined by his inherited traits, his fetal environment, and the course of his delivery. What happens to the woman during pregnancy and delivery is of the greatest importance to the health of her offspring. Maternal health services must therefore be included within the broad definition of the child health program. The terms *maternal and child health services* or simply *child health services* will therefore be used interchangeably.

The goal of optimal health set by such a definition admittedly can never be fully attained. Yet, if the course is not set toward this distant goal, complacency with lesser achievements may be the result. The fullest mental and social well-being of individuals can be attained only in a democracy, in which government represents the needs and wishes of an educated and alert citizenry. Government is not a machine for the people to serve blindly, nor is it a paternalistic structure, which ultimately has an equally destructive effect upon the individual. Within this setting, physical, mental, and social health is a dynamic concept. It implies a reciprocal relationship between the individual citizen and his government—local, state, and national. The healthy, self-reliant citizen finds fulfillment in socially useful channels which contribute to his own welfare and to the welfare of his family and community. Community resources and services should be used only to help him attain self-reliance in so far as possible, with state and Federal assistance provided to supplement and reinforce community efforts.

Coverage of Program. A child health program has the interests of all children in the community at heart. It does not restrict itself to families of certain income levels, nor does it restrict its services to any one social group. Health education, for example, must reach parents in all segments of the population, to motivate them to obtain medical supervision for their children during periods of presumably good health as well as to seek medical care during illness. Otherwise, many parents who can meet the costs of health supervision for their children without community assistance will fail to do so because of ignorance or indifference. Other families, outwardly independent, may actually be developing serious difficulties which might be averted through the temporary assistance of a local governmental or voluntary agency. For such families community support expresses itself through family guidance and educational services, rather than financial assistance. Whatever form community assistance may take, the objective remains the same. Such support, whether of a financial or educational nature, should encourage rather than destroy the self-reliance of the child and his family.

Role of the Family Physician. Medical and other health services initiated and financed entirely by the family are implicit in the broad definition of health services for children. The nationwide study of child health services conducted by the American Academy of Pediatrics disclosed that about 95 per cent of the care given children outside hospitals was rendered in the offices of physicians or in the homes of the children; the greater part of this care was financed by the families concerned. There is good reason to believe that the proportion of care paid for privately will not change significantly even if there should be a marked increase in other types of services. "It has been demonstrated time and time again that when public health services are brought into a community, there is a concomitant increase in the demand for private care. As a community learns the value of diphtheria immunization, more patients request it of their own physicians." (2)

The family physician and his counterpart in allied professions are at the hub of the community health program, and they will remain in this relationship to the majority of families in spite of, or perhaps even because of, the growing complexity of medical practice. Under favorable circumstances, he knows the families of his child patients intimately and can therefore suspect deviations from normal physical and emotional states at an early stage of development. Whatever services may be provided for special problems, it is the family physician who must provide continuing medical care for the child in his home.

An organized public health program, when properly conducted, does not displace the family physician from this central role in any way. On the contrary, it supplements and reinforces the position of the family physician in many ways. It often helps him keep children under his care when this might not otherwise be possible. For example, specific services may be provided through the program which are beyond the resources of the family physician. When such services are made available locally, the child can continue under the family physician's general care and not have to be transported to another community for the purpose. Through certain mass screening procedures, abnormalities may be suspected and children brought under the family physician's care for further diagnosis and for treatment. Through participation in clinic services with consultation from medical specialists, the general practitioner has an opportunity to round out his experience for the benefit of other children in the community. The family physician also benefits from postgraduate medical education programs which are often conducted as joint enterprises of medical societies and official and voluntary health agencies.

Even though medical care initiated and financed entirely by the child's family is the largest single element in community health services, it is not within the realm of this book to discuss this phase of the child health program as such. Emphasis throughout the discussion that follows will be placed upon those services provided or promoted through the organized program which supplement and reinforce services privately initiated and financed. These aspects of the community health program will be considered in some detail as they mesh with private services.

Preventive and Curative Health Services. Prevention and treatment overlap, so that a fine line cannot be drawn between preventive and curative health services. In a sense all health services are preventive, in that they aim to prevent death before the end of the natural life span. Indeed, one of the earliest public health efforts was a program for the discovery and treatment of infants with "summer complaint" to prevent their death. Patients with communicable diseases have been segregated and treated by governmental agencies for centuries in an effort to prevent further spread of infection. More recently, children with potentially handicapping conditions, such as poliomyelitis and rheumatic fever, have been included in the community health program in an effort to prevent or minimize resulting disability. For children already disabled to a greater or lesser degree, rehabilitation programs have been instituted to reduce the extent of their handicaps and to help them use their remaining abilities effectively. In spite of the impossibility of splitting off the purely preventive aspects of care, the statement is still frequently heard that prevention should be the only concern of the organized public health program and treatment entirely the family's responsibility.

Even though it must deal with existing abnormal conditions, the objective of the child health program remains positive. The successive phases of health services for children may be looked upon as an attempt to prevent further damage and to make the most of the child's remaining abilities. Since the final objective of complete physical and mental well-being of a child is so rarely attainable, the program then strives to prevent as great a degree of ill health or disability as possible. Faced with unprevented or unpreventable ill health, it then seeks through community effort to minimize the deleterious effects. If irreversible physical or mental changes have occurred, it tries to assist in the rehabilitation of the affected child to the greatest degree of personal and social usefulness attainable and to prevent him from becoming a drain upon his family and community. Approached from one viewpoint, increasingly complicated curative services are needed to prevent more serious or permanent disturbances of health. Seen from the opposite viewpoint, preventive services such as immunization procedures are often referred to as treatments.

The question of the preventive versus the curative nature of the services required is largely immaterial in determining whether a given problem is of public health importance. Appendicitis, for example, was formerly accepted as a serious public health problem. Yet the chief attack on disability and death from appendicitis in childhood before the advent of antibiotic drugs was education of the public in the need for early medical attention and avoidance of laxatives in the event of abdominal pain. This was a public health approach to the problem even though obtaining the needed medical services remained the responsibility of the child's family. Judgment as to what constitutes a public health problem is based on either one of two considerations other than the type of services needed. First, the problem must be of such magnitude as to require community effort, even though adequate control measures are difficult to apply. Second, the problem must be of such nature, even though not necessarily of great size, that readily available techniques can bring it under control as part of an organized community program.

Coordination of Program. "The ideal of community health organization is nothing less than the mobilization of all the rich and varied forces within an American community in free and friendly association to combat a common enemy and to strive for the common heritage of health and longevity." (3) Health services for children, no matter how extensive, cannot be considered an organized program unless an attempt is made to tie them together. To make each service a source of strength to the others rather than a jealously guarded prerogative of one agency or group, to avoid unnecessary duplication of services in one field and lack of coverage in others—these activities constitute coordination. Though much overworked as a word, coordination still remains the high-road to a successful child health program. This does not mean the services of each agency can be fitted neatly into an assigned niche. A certain degree of overlap is unavoidable and is bound to engender irritation and antagonism. When agencies are aware of this, it may pave the way for careful review of the situation and lead to further progress.

Communities vary markedly in the ability or willingness of their local organizations to get together for joint planning. Some communities are organizationally minded, and the flimsiest pretext is an excuse for another coordinating committee. In such communities the danger exists that so much time and energy will be spent in conferences that little remain for implementing any decisions reached. In other communities civic-mindedness may be practically nonexistent, requiring dramatic approaches to arouse a flicker of interest. In such communities coordination is only a theoretical consideration.

Community Health Councils. In the more highly organized communities, efforts are usually made to channel varying interests into a health council. There are more than 1,200 health councils covering state or local areas in the nation (4). To a large extent the success of a health council is dependent upon the active participation of the medical profession. The American Medical Association has urged state and local medical societies to take the lead in organizing and working with health councils (5). Most community health councils have several physicians as members, either as representatives of the local medical society or health agencies or as individual citizens. From their personal knowledge of health problems and with their prestige in the community, physicians active in health councils can be most influential in promoting better understanding among the various agencies.

A health council, with subgroups concerned with different aspects of child health, may even be part of a broad council of all social agencies. These bring together not only those agencies and individuals whose primary interest is in health, but also many agencies whose first concern is in fields having only indirect implications in regard to health. In the poorly organized community, on the other hand, it may be possible to arouse interest in health in general by focusing on a restricted field such as health services for children of school age or children with one type of physically handicapping condition. Such limited approaches can be broadened in time to include more comprehensive consideration of the health needs of all children and ultimately of the total health needs of the community. The emotional appeal of the helpless infant and the handicapped child is often the wedge to crack the shell of community indifference to its own health problems.

Eligibility for Services. Careful attention must be paid to the eligibility of children for admission to services provided through the public health program in its more limited sense. This question of eligibility must be resolved into two distinct parts to avoid confusion. These are, first, the admission of children for care altogether and, second, the extent of financial participation required of the family to cover the costs of care.

A broad rule to be followed is that a child should be admitted for specific types of care if the service involved is not otherwise readily available to the family. Adherence to this rule will avoid duplication of service and will encourage families to assume full responsibility for care of their children whenever possible. Certainly no child already under regular health supervision should be admitted to a child health (well-child) conference simply because the parents wish a second medical opinion. On the other hand, specific services such as speech therapy or psychiatric care may be available only through the organized public health program. In general, also, services primarily of an educational nature should be available to all children and parents in the community.

When a family of borderline income is faced with the need to pay for all or part of the costs of care, all the financial circumstances of the family should be weighed to avoid destroying the family's independence. If such a family is required to pay for the prolonged and expensive care of a child with cerebral palsy, for example, it may impoverish the family to the detriment of other members of the household and ultimately harm the physically handicapped child himself.

CITED REFERENCES

1. Constitution of World Health Organization, quoted by Brock Chisholm, International Health: 2. The Role of WHO, Past, Present, and Future, *Am. J. Pub. Health,* Vol. 41, pp. 1460–1463, December, 1951.
2. "Child Health Services and Pediatric Education, Report of the Committee for the Study of Child Health Services," American Academy of Pediatrics, Commonwealth Fund, Harvard University Press, Cambridge, Mass., 1949.
3. SCHEELE, LEONARD A., Public Health Statesmanship, *Pub. Health Rep.,* Vol. 68, pp. 1–11, January, 1953.

4. "Directory of Community Health Planning Councils—1950," National Health Council, New York, 1951.
5. "The Community Health Council: Its Organization, Its Functions, and a Few Suggested Projects," Council on Medical Services and Committee on Rural Health, American Medical Association, Chicago, 1949.

ADDITIONAL REFERENCES

1. STEVENSON, GEORGE S., Dynamic Considerations in Community Functions, *Ment. Hyg.,* Vol. 34, pp. 531–546, October, 1950.
2. BUCK, CARL E., BRADLEY BUELL, and ROSCOE P. KANDLE, Family Health in Tomorrow's Community, *Am. J. Pub. Health,* Vol. 41, pp. 1258–1262, October, 1951.
3. BACHMAN, GEORGE W., and ASSOCIATES, "Health Resources in the United States: Personnel, Facilities, and Services," The Brookings Institution, Washington, D.C., 1952.

2 PLANNING AND EVALUATION OF CHILD HEALTH SERVICES

In providing medical care to individual patients, the practicing physician goes through certain steps in gathering information to arrive at a diagnosis, to select the proper type of treatment, and to do what he can to ensure that needed procedures are carried out. The steps are performed so rapidly in most cases that they are not readily identified as such; in others, delineation of the diagnostic problem and treatment are drawn out and complicated. Whatever the degree of complexity of the clinical situation, these steps are so much a part of the physician's day-to-day functioning that he goes through the process almost without realizing that he is following a well-established pattern.

The approach to public health problems involves steps that correspond to diagnosis, determination and provision of treatment needed, and return appointments to be sure that recommended treatment is carried out. The difference is that the entire community or groups within the community, rather than the individual patient, are the objects of attention. Analysis of the problem corresponds roughly to diagnosis, the facilities and services in a community to treatment, and evaluation and follow-up services to return appointments for the patient of the practicing physician.

Planning of Programs. Planning is basic to the development of sound programs. The stages of planning may be presented as a series of questions.

1. What is the objective of the program and what services are needed to reach this objective?
2. What is the extent of the problem?

3. What scientific and administrative tools are available to attack the problem and how readily may they be applied?

4. How do community attitudes influence the possibility of attacking the problem effectively? If these attitudes are unfavorable, what are the chances of altering them?

5. What financial support is available immediately, or is being anticipated over a longer period? What are the possible sources of such support?

6. What services are already being provided to meet the problem?

7. What are the gaps between needs and services?

8. How much can better use of existing services achieve in narrowing the gap?

9. What additional services are needed to achieve a reasonable goal in further narrowing the gap?

10. How may these services be introduced so as to provide a sound foundation for a broad program?

Some health problems in children lend themselves fairly readily to quantitative answers to these questions. Notable examples are dental caries and certain communicable diseases against which effective immunizing agents are available. Quantitative answers may also be obtained about some aspects of the problem of premature birth. In other programs, as in the promotion of mental health and the care of emotionally disturbed children, only informed opinions are possible. This may detract to only a small degree from the value of the planning process and certainly does not reduce the need for such planning.

Planning requires a clear understanding of the ultimate objectives to be achieved and of the more immediate goals to be reached at set intervals. Setting goals that can be attained within a period of a year or two helps to maintain community interest. Achieving these immediate goals, and moving on to new ones at the same time, promotes the interest and morale of participants in the program.

Numbers Served. Program planning requires first an idea of the number of mothers and children in different age groups in the community. The decennial Federal census provides information on the number of women of childbearing age, according to race, and the number of children according to age, sex, and race, in each political subdivision. As the interval of years following a census lengthens, these figures become less reliable, especially in relation to the count of young children. The past several decades of industrialization, wars, depression, and prosperity have been characterized by rapid population changes due to internal migration. In addition, sharp fluctuations in the number of births from year to year have resulted in rapid changes in the size of the younger age groups.

Sources of information other than the Federal census are available to provide a more adequate estimation of numbers. Registration of births through the filing of birth certificates is almost complete in large areas of the country; in 1950, birth certificates were filed for all but 2.2 per cent of the live births in the United States (1). To estimate the number of children under six years of age, it is therefore often advisable to use birth-registration data for the previous five years, subtracting the number of deaths occurring at each year of life in this age group. Correction will still have to be made in this estimate for the effects of migration.

School registration may be used to ascertain the number of children of school age, provided corrections are made for children who have left school or who are not attending schools in the community for other reasons. There is an added drawback, in that school districts may overlap health jurisdictions. A school census at the beginning of each academic year is a legal requirement in some areas. Children under five or six years of age, as well as those of school age, may be registered. The school census is unreliable in many areas, although it may be of some help in locating individual children with handicapping conditions.

The need for an accurate estimate of the number of children in each age group varies with the adequacy of the local program. When services do not begin to meet the local need, it makes little difference if a large number of children enter or leave the community; a more adequate program would be thrown seriously out of gear by changes of smaller magnitude. Administrators of health services for children of school age were forewarned well in advance of the unprecedentedly heavy elementary school enrollment of recent years, since they were aware of the record number of births in the preceding period.

Rates Used in Maternal and Child Health. Knowledge of the number of illnesses or deaths in a given area from any cause does not permit measurement of the size of any problem for comparative purposes over a period of time or in relation to other areas. Rates of morbidity and mortality provide convenient tools for these purposes. A rate is the ratio of one happening to another. Some of the more frequently used rates in the field of maternal and child health, usually expressed on an annual basis, are the following:

1. The *birth rate* is the number of live births per 1,000 total population. A live birth is defined as an infant showing any sign of life (heart beat, respiration, or muscular movements) after complete separation from the mother, even though the uncut umbilical cord may still be attached to an undelivered placenta.

2. The *crude death or mortality rate* from all causes is the number of deaths per 1,000 total population. The crude death rate is affected strongly by differences in the age distribution of the population, especially in a period of increasing longevity and rapid shifts in the birth rate. When the rates for a single cause or a group of causes of death are calculated, a denominator of 100,000 is generally used. These rates have meaning on an annual basis only in areas or states with large populations. Otherwise, an average annual rate for a period of five years or more must be used, even though recent changes may be thereby obscured.

3. An *age-specific mortality rate* from all causes is usually expressed as the number of deaths in a given age group per 1,000 persons in that age group. For age-specific rates for individual causes, as in the rates for the total population, a denominator of 100,000 is used. Calculation of rates for the total population adjusted for differences in age distribution is based on the rates found in each age group.

4. The *infant mortality rate* is the number of deaths of infants under one year of age per 1,000 live births. The infant mortality rate is an age-specific mortality rate in which the denominator is the number of births, rather than the enumerated or estimated number of infants under one year of age, because of the greater accuracy of the former. It is usually calculated from the births and deaths occurring during the same calendar year, even though the same infants may not be counted in both the numerator and denominator of the ratio. During periods of rapidly changing birth rates, correction must be made for the fluctuations. In presenting the individual causes or groups of causes of death under one year of age, the base of 1,000 live births is retained; the number of deaths in each group is still large enough to avoid rates which are small fractions of one.

5. The *neonatal (newborn) mortality rate* is the number of deaths under one month (or twenty-eight days) of age per 1,000 live births. To

study factors related to conditions of pregnancy and delivery, the mortality rates for infants under one hour of age, one day of age, and one week of age are also used frequently. The rate during later infancy, or from one month to one year of age, is presented separately.

Certain of the rates most useful in guiding the child health program are also considered to be reliable indices of the health status of the entire population. This is particularly true of the mortality rate among infants from one month to one year of age. It is during this short age period that the effects of poor sanitation, inadequate housing, and a generally low standard of living are felt most keenly. It has been a common experience to have excessively high rates drop perceptibly soon after the introduction of even limited health services on an organized basis.

6. The *fetal mortality rate* is generally defined as the number of deaths occurring at any time during fetal life per 1,000 live births, although this is really a ratio in which the numerator is not directly related to the denominator. Fetal deaths include all products of gestation which do not terminate as live-born infants as defined previously. In a few areas, the base of the fetal mortality rate is calculated as the total of live births and fetal deaths. While this is theoretically more accurate, the inclusion of fetal deaths in the base affects the rate only slightly and the marked discrepancies in methods and completeness of reporting of fetal deaths in different areas nullify the theoretical advantages.

The Third World Health Assembly, held in 1950, recommended that fetal deaths be classified in four groups according to period of gestation (2). Period of gestation is calculated from the first day of the last menstrual cycle before the beginning of pregnancy.

  I. Early fetal deaths, or those occurring at less than twenty completed weeks of gestation
 II. Intermediate fetal deaths, occurring at twenty or more completed weeks of gestation but before twenty-eight
III. Late fetal deaths, occurring at twenty-eight or more completed weeks of gestation, and
 IV. Fetal deaths not classifiable in the first three groups

The Assembly also recommended that live births be tabulated by the same four groups by gestation, as well as by birth weight groups of not less than 250 gm. (about ½ lb.). Tabulation of live births in this manner makes unnecessary any consideration of "viability" of the fetus in deciding whether a very small live birth should be reported as a fetal or a neonatal death. It also eliminates the manifest incongruity of reports of the survival of a certain proportion of "nonviable" infants. A standard method of reporting and tabulating live births, fetal deaths, and infant deaths makes possible better planning and evaluation of child health programs (3).

The use of the recommended groups of fetal deaths should supplant the terms *abortion, miscarriage,* and *stillbirth.* While these three terms, when used in clinical practice, correspond roughly to early, intermediate, and late fetal deaths, respectively, there is no general agreement on their definition. Stillbirths are variously defined in different areas as fetal deaths occurring after twenty weeks, after five months, or even after twenty-eight weeks. Miscarriage is a clinical term rarely used in recording vital statistics. Abortion is a term which should be applied only to the mother; it suffers from the added disadvantage of being commonly used as synonymous with induced abortion.

To gain a clearer picture of the size and nature of the problem of mortality before and soon after birth, increasing use is being made of a *perinatal mortality rate.* This is usually calculated as the total of intermediate and late fetal deaths and neonatal deaths, or all deaths occurring between twenty weeks of gestation and the end of the first month after birth, per 1,000 live births. Narrower limits may be used to study specific problems. Use of a perinatal mortality rate eliminates the variations in fetal and neonatal mortality rates resulting from the not uncommon practice of counting deaths of liveborn infants immediately after birth as fetal deaths.

7. The *maternal mortality rate* is the number of deaths from conditions related to pregnancy, childbirth, and the puerperium per 10,000 live births. The denominator of 10,000 is preferable to 1,000 because the rate has reached such low levels that the rate would otherwise be expressed as a fraction of one in most areas. A theoretically more accurate rate used in a few places is the number of maternal deaths per 10,000 live births and fetal deaths. The discussion on this point in connection with the fetal mortality rate is entirely applicable to the maternal mortality rate as well.

Prior to 1948, many deaths from unrelated causes which occurred during pregnancy or the postpartum period were counted as maternal deaths. This source of error was eliminated in the 1948 revision of the

"International Classification" (4). The change in classification is responsible for about a 9 per cent decrease in the maternal mortality rate (5).

Breakdown of Rates. Additional information about births and deaths should be available in the analysis of maternal and child health problems. The place of birth or death must be known by the usual residence of the parents or child. For larger areas the urban or rural character of residence should be stated. For births, the place of occurrence, whether hospital or home, and the type of attendant, whether physician, midwife, nurse-midwife, or none, should also be known. In large cities breakdown of this information by census tract is highly informative, especially in the years close to a decennial Federal census. The relationship between these facts and the social, economic, and educational status of the population studied can then be readily determined through use of the census data for each tract. Breakdown of the data by race and, in some areas, by nationality further delineates the problems.

Indices of Nonfatal Conditions. Information on deaths alone is a crude index of the health status of a community, especially when the death rates from specific causes have fallen to low levels. Information should also be available on the frequency of illness, accidents, and other conditions detrimental to health, and on the length and extent of ill health attributable to these causes. The 1948 revision of the "International Classification" included for the first time specific categories for nonfatal diseases and injuries, so that statistics on both mortality and morbidity are more comparable (4).

The frequency of any event during a given period is known as its *incidence.* The number of persons affected by any condition at a given time is stated as its *prevalence.* Knowledge of the frequency or incidence of a communicable disease over a period of time, for example, may be used as a measure of the efficacy of a specific immunizing procedure. Planning services for handicapped children requires knowledge of the number of affected children in the area at a given time as well, in other words, the prevalence of the conditions. The impact of a disease in a community may also be gauged by the duration of illnesses and the extent of absenteeism from education or employment it causes.

Reporting of Morbidity. Morbidity data may be obtained, among other ways, through routine reporting, through special surveys, or from birth certificates and hospital records. Compulsory reporting of selected communicable diseases to governmental health agencies was one of the earliest public health procedures. In some areas noncommunicable diseases have also been added. Rheumatic fever, premature birth, cerebral palsy, cancer, epilepsy, and blindness and deafness in children must each be reported by law in at least one health jurisdiction in the United States. Some health departments may require reporting by physicians only, whereas in others any person knowing of such conditions in any capacity must complete and forward a report to the local or state department of health (6). Morbidity reporting on a national basis is becoming more standardized and simplified (7).

The benefits of compulsory reporting of each disease or condition, especially those of a noncommunicable nature, must be weighed against the effort and expense of the procedure. Such reports can rarely be used to give an accurate measure of these conditions. This is especially true in diseases, such as rheumatic fever, which frequently present diagnostic difficulties. Gross underreporting is common unless the physician sees some tangible benefit to his patient or to himself from the reporting procedure.

Special Surveys. Surveys are often used to obtain a picture of health conditions in the community. Surveys may serve the dual function of obtaining information and of stimulating the interest of the community through the participation of volunteers and through the attendant publicity. A simple example of this type of survey is one conducted by trained volunteers to ascertain the extent of health supervision of young children in the community, before deciding on the need for new or expanded services. The possibility of using volunteers altogether and the amount of training needed by the volunteers are determined by the complexity and the nature of the information to be gathered. Even a comparatively simple survey requires careful preparation, to be sure the right questions are asked in a manner leading to an unbiased answer.

The objectives of a given survey should determine how extensive a sampling is needed. As many homes as possible in the community should be visited, if promotion of health services is accepted as one function of the survey. If gathering of information is the sole objective, only enough homes should be sampled to obtain the desired data. The nationwide survey of child health services conducted by the American Academy of Pediatrics in 1946 was one of the most ambitious surveys of any type ever conducted. In planning for this survey, the sampling method was deliberately rejected since it was the desire of the Academy to have the broadest participation possible in carrying out the survey. Sampling was used later in smaller surveys to check on the validity of the results obtained in the original survey.

Maternal and child health services lend themselves readily to survey through mail questionnaires, with follow-up of unanswered letters by telephone calls and personal visits. Although the validity of mail surveys has been seriously questioned in some quarters, several factors are operative in maternal and child health which tend to make surveys in this field more reliable. Many of the services surveyed are fresh in the minds of the parents, since the mothers and children can be located through recently filed birth certificates or through school registration. Since the health of their children is often a matter of more immediate concern and of a less personal nature to parents than the state of their own health, the questionnaires attract the interest of a large proportion of parents. Mail questionnaires elicit an especially good response from parents when they are related to special health problems which their own children have faced; advantage may be taken of this in obtaining information on the health of children who were born prematurely or in determining the use of services by children with various types of handicapping conditions.

Birth-certificate Data. The value of information obtained from birth certificates and infant death certificates is greatly enhanced by matching birth and death certificates in each infant death. From the death certificate can be obtained the reported cause of death, the place of residence, the sex, and the age of the infant at death. The birth certificate provides information on the age and previous obstetrical history of the mother, the period of gestation, the place of birth, and the attendant at delivery. Fetal death (stillbirth) certificates are actually birth and death certificates combined, since they carry both types of information. Studying these factors in relation to each other does much to clarify the problem of fetal, neonatal, and later infant mortality in any area.

Since 1939, many state and city health departments have requested physicians to supply supplementary information, generally on the reverse of the birth certificate. Accurate reporting of this information by the physician filing the certificate makes possible many studies of great interest to the medical profession itself. The desired information usually covers weight of the infant at birth, conditions of pregnancy and labor, operative or instrumental procedures used, and congenital mal-formations or birth injury in the infant. The item on birth weight was transferred in 1949 to the face of the standard birth certificate issued by the National Office of Vital Statistics and in the following year was adopted as a required item for completion throughout the country, with the exception of only one state.

Prior to inclusion of the item on birth weight on the birth certificate, the only sources of information on prematurity were either the diagnosis of prematurity or the length of gestation as reported by the person com-pleting the certificates. These reports were highly unreliable because dif-ferent criteria of prematurity were used and there was a tendency to lump an undue number of infants as term unless they were markedly pre-mature. Knowledge of birth weight of all infants in itself has greatly increased the value of the data obtained by matching birth and infant death certificates. For statistical purposes, there is general agreement on the definition of a premature infant as one weighing 2,500 gm. or $5\frac{1}{2}$ lb. or less at birth. Even though birth weight should be used as the basic criterion of prematurity, it is still desirable to obtain as accurate informa-tion as possible on length of gestation for additional analysis.

The medical data on complications of pregnancy and delivery and condition of the offspring, like other types of morbidity information, are generally underreported. The information given usually corresponds with the actual statements to be found on the hospital records, as was the case in a study of the validity of such reporting on birth certificates, when these reports were checked against hospital records (8). More complete reporting may be encouraged by substituting check lists of con-ditions for the general items to be completed by physicians on the re-verse of the birth certificates. Separate lists of types of conditions of pregnancy and delivery and of operative procedures may be used with the request that the attending physician check the pertinent items (Fig-ure 1).

The information may also be used as a base line against which to measure the frequency of abnormalities during pregnancy and the new-born period, in spite of the manifest underreporting. Such a base line is especially useful in studying the relation of conditions such as cerebral palsy and mental deficiency in the child to complications of pregnancy and delivery in the mother. The data on birth certificates for children

COMPLICATIONS OF PREGNANCY AND LABOR (*Check at least one item in each column*)

Related to Pregnancy	Not Related to Pregnancy	Labor	Operative Procedures
0 ☐ None	0 ☐ None	0 ☐ None	0 ☐ None
1 ☐ Pre-eclampsia	1 ☐ Heart Disease	1 ☐ Placenta Previa	1 ☐ Low forceps
2 ☐ Eclampsia	2 ☐ Diabetes	2 ☐ Premature separation of placenta	2 ☐ Midforceps
3 ☐ Hypertensive disease	3 ☐ Syphilis	3 ☐ Prolapse of cord	3 ☐ High forceps
4 ☐ Nephritis	4 ☐ Tuberculosis	4 ☐ Anomaly of cord	5 ☐ Cesarean section
5 ☐ Pernicious vomiting	x ☐ Other—specify	5 ☐ Breech presentation	6 ☐ Breech extraction
6 ☐ Pyelitis		6 ☐ Other malpresentations	7 ☐ Internal version and extraction
7 ☐ Anemia		7 ☐ Contracted pelvis	x ☐ Other—specify
x ☐ Other—specify		8 ☐ Other dystocia	
		9 ☐ Postpartum hemorrhage	
		x ☐ Other—specify	

Was mother's blood tested for Rh factor?
No ☐   Yes, Rh + ☐   Yes, Rh − ☐

Birth injury to infant: No ☐   Yes ☐   If yes, describe

Congenital malformation of infant: No ☐   Yes ☐   If yes, describe

Figure 1. Confidential medical report on reverse of New York State birth certificate. (*Reproduced with permission of the New York State Department of Health.*)

with these conditions may be compared with the data from all births during the same period, since there is no reason to believe that the information is provided more completely in the case of children who later develop these conditions.

Mortality Surveys and Conferences. Special studies of the causes of individual maternal, fetal, and infant deaths have been carried out in many communities throughout the country. Most of these have been confined to a review by the medical staff of the deaths occurring in a given hospital. Some have covered all deaths at home and in the various hospitals of the community. The broader type of survey is far more productive, since the staffs of those hospitals having the poorest type of maternity and newborn services rarely conduct such studies themselves. In addition, local medical organizations usually work closely with the health department in the community-wide survey in gathering the social as well as the medical data needed to give an adequate picture of the possible causative factors in each case.

The results of the study of individual deaths are generally used as the basis for a thoroughgoing analysis of the management of each case at a subsequent mortality conference. The physicians whose cases are being discussed are urged to attend, even though the identity of the physician and the patient concerned is not revealed. The frank criticism of unacceptable medical practices and the debate about questionable procedures that may have been responsible for a preventable death are intended only as a step toward improved management of similar problems in the future. This type of conference has been used most extensively in relation to maternal deaths. At maternal mortality conferences, every maternal death is usually investigated and reviewed. At fetal or neonatal conferences, or at combined or perinatal mortality conferences, the number of deaths to be covered is too great for detailed individual review. A sampling of such deaths, preferably those which illustrate some preventable factor, must therefore be selected.

Evaluation of Community Programs. Evaluation of existing services is basic to planning a more adequate program. As the new program develops, periodic evaluation of its accomplishments makes possible sound planning of the ongoing program. Unless the maternal and child health program is adapted to changed conditions and needs, using new tools as they become available, it may lose out in competition with new types

1. Name of Infant
2. Date of Death
3. Cause of Death
4. Physician Signing Death Certificate
   Address
   Staff Position
5. Death Registration Number
   (Filled by Division of Vital
   Statistics)
6. Place of Death
7. Sex: M F
8. Race: W N Other
9. Birthdate
10. Age at Death Days Hrs. Mins.
    (Hrs. and mins. when less than 48 hrs.)
11. Place of Birth
12. Autopsy: Yes No If No, Why
    (If copy not attached, send later)
13. Birth Registration Number
    (Filled by Division of Vital
    Statistics)
14. Attendant at Birth { M.D.
                        { Other
    Address
    Staff Position
15. Age of Mother
16. Length of Pregnancy Wks.
17. This Birth: Single 1st Twin
    2nd Triplet
18. Previous
    { A. Term   —Living Dead
    {   Stillborn
    { B. Premature—Living Dead
    {   Stillborn
    { C. Abortions—
19. Prenatal Care: Adequate Inadequate
    None
20. Hospital Status: Private Semipri.
    Ward (Pay Free)
21. Pregnancy (Complications): None
    or Specify

22. Labor (Complications): None or
    Specify
23. Puerperium (Complications): None
    or Specify
24. Cord, Placenta, Amnion (Complications): None or Specify
25. Analgesia: None or Specify (Amt. &
    Time)
26. Anesthesia: None or Specify
27. Type of Delivery: Spontaneous Forceps Cesarean Breech Version
    Other
28. Labor Induced: Yes No
    If Yes, Why
29. Rh: Pos. Neg. Not Taken Other
30. Serol. Test for Syphilis: Pos. Neg.
    Not Taken
31. Birth Wt. Condition
32. Resuscitation: None or Specify
33. Congenital Malformations: None or
    Specify
34. Birth Injury: None or Specify
35. Feeding (When Started, How Taken)
36. Check Any of the Following That
    Were Important Factors in the
    Death:
    A. No Medical Care Available
    B. Lack of Expert Consultation
    C. Lack of Proper Hospital
       Facilities
    D. Patient's or Family's Ignorance
       or Neglect
    E. Inability of Family to Pay for
       Proper Care
    F. Other Factors
37. Name and Address of Physician
    Responsible for Infant
38. Report Filled out by
    Mailing Address Date
39. Case Discussed at Staff Meeting: Yes
    (Ped. Obs.) No
40. Staff Opinion

Figure 2. Suggested data for study of neonatal deaths. (*Adapted from revised form used in Philadelphia Neonatal Mortality Study, 1952. Reproduced with permission of the Study.*)

of health services which may not necessarily give equal returns in health for the funds and energy expended.

The intensity of efforts to evaluate child health services should be in accordance with local facilities. Local health services may be evaluated by comparing them with some accepted standards. This type of evaluation may be purely qualitative, in that it is concerned only with the provision of certain services considered necessary according to the guideposts used. It may go a little further and measure the amount of each type of service per unit of population against an amount set up as desirable in the standards used. Use of accepted standards for purposes of evaluation does help to disclose gaps or deficiencies in a local program, but this approach fails to relate these deficiencies to general conditions in the community or to the relative urgency of various problems. It also has limited value in measuring progress over a period of time.

Services may also be evaluated in relation to broader predetermined objectives or to changes in mortality or morbidity rates. This is justifiable so long as those performing the evaluation are aware of certain pitfalls. The mortality rate from a particular communicable disease may have been falling throughout the country at the same rate as in the area being studied, as a result of indefinable factors which may be of greater relative importance than the services being evaluated. Within the community itself, other factors may have started to operate at the same time the particular health service was initiated, as is often the case when community interest has been aroused. The group performing the evaluation should avoid the temptation of claiming sole or major credit for improvement in the health status of the community as measured by available indices.

Determination of the quantitative results of the services studied is the most difficult type of evaluation. Such evaluative studies require careful advance planning to ensure selection of an adequate control group as similar as possible to the group being studied except for the service or group of services in the program being evaluated. This form of applied research is similar to well-conducted studies in clinical practice for determining the efficacy of a new form of treatment. Federal and state health agencies are devoting increasing attention to studies of this nature in an effort to obtain reliable information to guide expenditures of funds. While only the strongest and largest local health agencies can conduct such studies successfully by themselves, many smaller health agencies are glad to participate in them as a stimulus to their staffs and as a means of gaining basic information not otherwise obtainable.

Practical Uses of Evaluation. Evaluation of services has many values beyond the guidance it offers in determining the future direction of the program. By bringing groups of professional persons together, and even extending participation to community groups such as women's clubs and parent-teacher organizations for joint consideration of what the community is doing for its children, it promotes coordination of services and helps place emphasis on those services which are most needed rather than those having the greatest dramatic appeal. Participation of the staffs of health agencies in the evaluative process gives them an opportunity through frank discussion to understand the strengths and weaknesses of their own services and gives them a feeling of being part of a dynamic organization. Above all, judicious use of the findings creates favorable publicity for health services and is helpful in securing public support for additional services which may be needed.

CITED REFERENCES

1. Shapiro, Sam, and Joseph Schachter, Birth Registration Completeness: United States, 1950, *Pub. Health Rep.,* Vol. 67, pp. 513–524, June, 1952.
2. "International Recommendations on Definitions of Live Birth and Fetal Death," Public Health Service Publication No. 39, National Office of Vital Statistics, Washington, D.C., October, 1950.
3. Parkhurst, Elizabeth, and Edward R. Schlesinger, Basic Data Needed in Planning Programs for the Care of Premature Infants, *Am. J. Pub. Health,* Vol. 41, pp. 712–715, June, 1951.
4. "Manual of the International Statistical Classification of Diseases, Injuries and Causes of Death. Sixth Revision of the International Lists of Diseases and Causes of Death," Bulletin of the World Health Organization, Supplement, World Health Organization, Geneva, Switzerland, 1948.
5. "The Effect of the Sixth Revision of the International Lists of Diseases and Causes of Death upon Comparability of Mortality Trends," Vital Statistics—Special Reports, Vol. 36, pp. 153–168, National Office of Vital Statistics, Dec. 3, 1951.
6. West, Margaret D., Morbidity Reporting in Local Areas, I. Patterns of Reporting, *Pub. Health Rep.,* Vol. 63, pp. 329–346, Mar. 12, 1948; II. Problem of Measuring the Completeness of Reporting, *Pub. Health Rep.,* Vol. 63, pp. 1187–1202, Sept. 10, 1948.

7. DAUER, C. C., National Morbidity Reporting: Revised System, *Pub. Health Rep.,* Vol. 67, pp. 21–25, January, 1952.
8. LILIENFELD, A. M., E. PARKHURST, R. PATTON, and E. R. SCHLESINGER, Accuracy of Supplemental Medical Information on Birth Certificates, *Pub. Health Rep.,* Vol. 66, pp. 191–198, Feb. 16, 1951.

ADDITIONAL REFERENCES

1. PUFFER, RUTH RICE, "Practical Statistics in Health and Medical Work," McGraw-Hill Book Company, Inc., New York, 1950 (see pp. 80–88 for method of calculating rates).
2. KANDLE, ROSCOE P., and HENRY GOETZ, A Method to Determine Levels of Immunizations, Medical, and Nursing Services in Prenatal and Infant Care, *Pub. Health Rep.,* Vol. 65, pp. 315–330, Mar. 10, 1950.
3. DORN, HAROLD F., Methods of Measuring Incidence and Prevalence of Disease, *Am. J. Pub. Health,* Vol. 41, pp. 271–278, March, 1951.
4. (*a*) "Evaluation Schedule for Use in the Study and Appraisal of Community Health Programs," Committee on Administrative Practice, American Public Health Association, New York, 1947; (*b*) "Guide to the Evaluation Schedule," *ibid.,* about 1950; (*c*) "What's the Score? Evaluation of Local Public Health Services," *ibid.,* 1950.
5. "Planning for Health Services: A Guide for States and Communities," Public Health Bulletin No. 304, Public Health Service, Washington, D.C., 1950.
6. Methods in Public Health Research, Special Supplement, *Am. J. Pub. Health,* Vol. 41, pp. 1–117, August, 1951.
7. VAN VOLKENBURGH, V. A., Public Health in the United States—Appraisal of Local Health Services, *Am. J. Pub. Health,* Vol. 42, pp. 49–55, January, 1952.
8. DUNN, HALBERT L., The Survey Approach to Morbidity and Health Data, *Pub. Health Rep.,* Vol. 67, pp. 998–1002, October, 1952.
9. MATTISON, BERWYN F., The Administrative Value of Statistics to a Local Health Officer, *Pub. Health Rep.,* Vol. 67, pp. 747–754, August, 1952.
10. HAENZEL, WILLIAM, Birth Statistics in Maternal and Child Health Programs, *Pub. Health Rep.,* Vol. 68, pp. 71–80, January, 1953.
11. SPIEGELMAN, MORTIMER, Population Implications for the Public Health Department, *Am. J. Pub. Health,* Vol. 43, pp. 460–465, April, 1953.
12. ERHARDT, CARL L., Reporting of Fetal Deaths in New York City, *Pub. Health Rep.,* Vol. 67, pp. 1161–1167, December, 1952.

3 TRENDS IN MORBIDITY AND MORTALITY

The physician in private practice bears as his primary responsibility the treatment of patients under his immediate care. Unless he participates actively in a wide variety of community activities, he may have a somewhat distorted picture of the character and extent of the health problems even within a limited geographic area. It is worth while, therefore, to review briefly some of the major problems in maternal and child health, so that local problems may be seen in the broader context of the nation as a whole over a period of time. Physicians and health workers in every field, in their concern for individual problems that are still insoluble, often forget the massive progress made during the past half century in the conquest of ill health and death in infancy and childhood and during the maternity cycle. The overwhelmingly favorable long-term trend encourages the hope that solutions of outstanding problems will also be found and applied in the not too distant future.

TRENDS IN MORTALITY

The saving of lives of children has been spectacular in all age groups from birth through adolescence.[1] In actual number of children saved, the greatest gains have been among infants under one year of age. Because of the high level of infant mortality at the start of the century, the reduction in infant deaths has been the greatest single factor in increasing the expectancy of life in the United States. The hypothetical average male infant born alive in 1900 could expect to live to the age of forty-

[1] Additional data on mortality and morbidity will be found in the chapters on specific subjects such as communicable diseases, accidents, and handicapping conditions.

eight years; if he survived the hazards of the first year of life, he could expect to live to fifty-five years of age. In contrast, his life expectancy at birth in 1949 had increased by eighteen years to sixty-six years; the same hypothetical infant surviving to his first birthday in 1949 could look forward to only thirteen years of life beyond that of his age peer in 1900, or to an age of sixty-eight years.

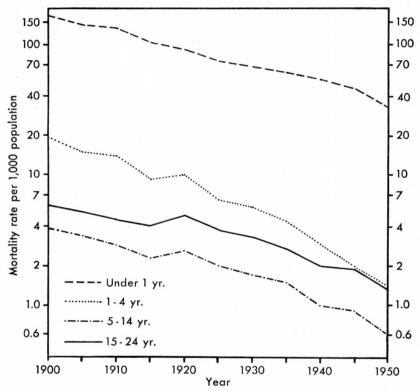

Figure 3. Mortality rates in various age groups from birth through twenty-four years, United States, 1900–1950. (*Data provided by National Office of Vital Statistics.*)

Even greater proportional reduction of mortality has been registered at later periods of childhood than in infancy. The mortality rate in 1950 among children of school age (five through fourteen years of age) was 15 per cent of the 1900 rate, while the infant mortality rate in 1950 was 20 per cent of the 1900 level. The greatest proportional improvement

Table 1. LEADING CAUSES OF DEATH AMONG CHILDREN IN THE UNITED STATES, 1900–1950

Age	1900	1920	1940	1950
1–4 years	1. Pneumonia and influenza 2. Diarrhea and enteritis 3. Diphtheria 4. Tuberculosis 5. Measles	1. Pneumonia and influenza 2. Diarrhea and enteritis 3. Diphtheria 4. All accidents 5. Whooping cough	1. Pneumonia and influenza 2. All accidents 3. Diarrhea and enteritis 4. Tuberculosis 5. Congenital malformations	1. All accidents 2. Pneumonia and influenza 3. Malignant neoplasms 4. Congenital malformations 5. Tuberculosis
5–14 years	1. Diphtheria 2. All accidents 3. Pneumonia and influenza 4. Tuberculosis 5. Diseases of the heart	1. Pneumonia and influenza 2. All accidents 3. Diphtheria 4. Tuberculosis 5. Diseases of the heart	1. All accidents* 2. Pneumonia and influenza 3. Diseases of the heart 4. Appendicitis 5. Tuberculosis	1. All accidents* 2. Malignant neoplasms 3. Pneumonia and influenza 4. Acute poliomyelitis 5. Congenital malformations
15–24 years	1. Tuberculosis 2. All accidents 3. Typhoid and paratyphoid fevers 4. Pneumonia and influenza 5. Diseases of the heart	1. Tuberculosis 2. Pneumonia and influenza 3. All accidents 4. Diseases of pregnancy, childbirth, and the puerperium 5. Diseases of the heart	1. All accidents 2. Tuberculosis 3. Diseases of the heart 4. Diseases of pregnancy, childbirth, and the puerperium 5. Pneumonia and influenza	1. All accidents* 2. Tuberculosis 3. Malignant neoplasms 4. Diseases of the heart 5. Homicide

* Motor-vehicle accidents alone and all other accidents alone lead all other causes of death.
Data provided by National Office of Vital Statistics.

occurred in the preschool group (one through four years) in which the rate was only 7 per cent of that of 1900. The saving in human lives can be visualized more clearly in another manner. If the mortality rates of 1900 still prevailed in 1949, 812,400 children under fifteen years of age would have died in the United States during that year instead of 145,935.

While the death rates from all major causes of death except malignant conditions have declined steadily and significantly among children over one year of age, the rates of decline have differed markedly. This has brought about a shifting of the order of the leading causes of death during childhood and early adult life (Table 1). In each of the age groups, accidents have become relatively more important as a cause of death. The exceedingly rapid decline in deaths from both the acute and chronic communicable diseases has resulted in the elevation of the essentially static rate from malignant diseases to a higher position.

Infant Mortality. The rate of decline in infant mortality for the country as a whole has been fairly constant. From time to time the suggestion has been offered that the infant mortality rate could not be reduced below an "irreducible minimum." Each "irreducible minimum rate" suggested had to be revised downward periodically as the goal previously set was reached and passed. As recently as 1940, a student of the problem of infant mortality stated, "It must be realized that the achievement of a rate below a certain point is, in all probability, impossible. Not only that, but any further considerable reduction of the rate in areas where it is now relatively low is not likely to be realized even with our newly acquired knowledge." (1) Since this statement was published, the infant mortality rate for the United States has decreased by more than a third, and the decline in areas initially having the lowest rates has as a rule proceeded even more rapidly than in other areas. It is obviously foolhardy, therefore, to suggest a minimum rate attainable even with present knowledge, apart from the effects of new scientific developments and their application.

The two most important groups of causes of infant deaths at the start of the century were diarrheal conditions and infections of the respiratory tract, exerting their force mainly after the neonatal period. Each group consisted of a number of different conditions not clearly understood at the time. The concentration of deaths from diarrheal conditions in the late summer and early fall and of deaths due to respiratory infections in the winter and early spring produced two sharp peaks in the graph of infant mortality plotted by calendar months. The peak in the late summer was by far the higher of the two. The passage of years has seen these peaks diminish like the erosion of a mountain range. By 1930 the rate of diarrheal deaths had fallen below the level of respiratory infections. In areas in which the greatest progress has been made, the seasonal curve

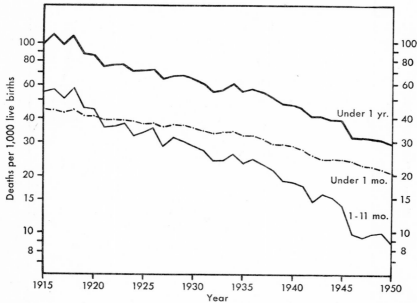

Figure 4. Infant mortality rates by age, birth-registration states of the United States, 1915–1950. The birth-registration states increased in number from 10 states and the District of Columbia in 1915 to the entire continental United States in 1933. Starting in 1949, deaths were recorded as under 28 days and 28 days—11 months. (*Data provided by National Office of Vital Statistics.*)

of infant mortality has become flat, and for the country as a whole, there is only a slight rise to mark the sites of the former peaks (Figure 5).

Later Infant Mortality. Infant mortality after the first month of life is no longer a universal public health problem. Further significant gains can still be made by concentration on those geographic areas and those groups within the population having higher rates. The excessively high rates prevailing in some of the Southwestern and Rocky Mountain states are due mainly to the mortality among the Spanish-speaking and Indian

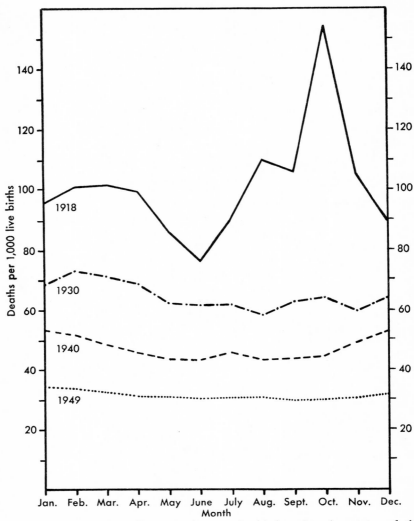

Figure 5. Infant mortality rates by month, birth-registration states of the United States, 1918, 1930, 1940, and 1949. (*Data provided by National Office of Vital Statistics.*)

groups. Within large cities, the highest residual concentration of infant mortality is found in the districts having the lowest socioeconomic status. Improved housing alone may set off a favorable chain reaction among the families concerned, which results in greater interest in health matters and a saving of infant lives (2).

For the nation as a whole, pneumonia and other acute respiratory diseases and gastrointestinal infections still cause more than two-thirds of all deaths in later infancy, with the respiratory diseases leading diarrheal disorders in a ratio of two to one. Congenital malformations cause the bulk of the remainder. The role of premature birth as a predisposing factor in deaths after one month of age is lost in the groups of causes immediately responsible for the death (Table 2).

Table 2. INFANT MORTALITY RATES UNDER 28 DAYS AND FROM 28 DAYS TO 1 YEAR, AND PERCENTAGE DISTRIBUTION FOR SELECTED CAUSES, UNITED STATES, 1950

	Under 28 *days*		28 *days to* 1 *year*	
	Rate	*Percentage*	*Rate*	*Percentage*
All causes..............................	20.5	100.0	8.7	100.0
Influenza and pneumonia, except pneumonia of newborn..........................	0.0*	0.1	2.4	27.0
Gastritis, duodenitis, enteritis, and colitis, except diarrhea of newborn................	0.2	0.8	0.1	1.3
Congenital malformations..................	2.5	12.3	1.4	16.4
Certain diseases of early infancy............	16.5	80.7	0.6	6.9
Birth injuries.........................	3.3	16.1	0.0*	0.4
Postnatal asphyxia and atelectasis........	3.6	17.7	0.1	0.9
Pneumonia of newborn.................	0.8	3.8	0.0*	0.0
Diarrhea of newborn..................	0.2	1.0	0.0*	0.1
Immaturity unqualified.................	6.2	30.4	0.1	0.9
All other diseases of early infancy........	2.4	11.7	0.4	4.7
Accidents........................	0.2	0.9	0.8	9.5
All other causes (residual).................	1.1	5.1	3.4	38.9

* Very small numbers involved.
Data provided by National Office of Vital Statistics.

Neonatal Mortality. The trend in the decline of the death rate in later infancy has not been paralleled among infants less than one month of age. The shorter the interval after birth, the less marked has been the rate of decline. For the twenty years preceding 1935, the death rate under one day of age remained at the same level. The slow decline in the death

rate among very young infants starting about 1935 occurred simultaneously with the onset of the dramatic decline in maternal mortality.
Presumably the factors in improved obstetrical care which saved the lives
of the mothers were reflected to a lesser extent in the survival of infants
in the early newborn period. For infants between one day and one month
the decline has been fairly steady since 1915, with a drop of about 80
per cent in the death rate among the infants surviving the first week of
life (Figure 6).

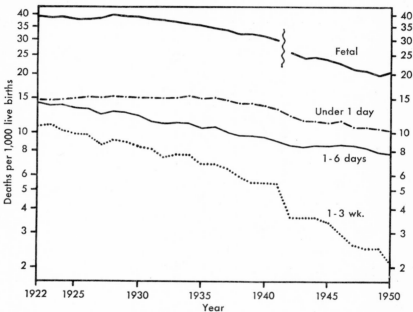

Figure 6. Neonatal mortality rates for specified ages and fetal death ratios,
birth-registration states of the United States, 1922–1950. The birth-registration states increased in number from 30 states and the District of Columbia
in 1922 to the entire continental United States in 1933. Fetal death ratios
through 1941 include all fetal deaths reported regardless of stated period
of gestation; after 1941, only those with stated period of gestation of 20
weeks (or 5 months) or more, or not stated at all. (*Data provided by
National Office of Vital Statistics.*)

The causes of death in the newborn period are far more poorly defined than in later infancy. Premature birth is stated as the cause of about
half of all neonatal deaths although, strictly speaking, it should not be
listed by itself at all (Table 2). The full force of mortality and mor-

bidity from premature birth is discussed later in relation to the problem of prematurity. Birth injury, the second ranking stated cause of death during the first month of life, will probably soon fall below the essentially unchanging rate for congenital malformations.

Fetal Mortality. Information on the extent of fetal mortality is very inadequate. Even late fetal deaths, for which fetal death (stillbirth) certificates must be filed, are incompletely reported (3). The reported fetal mortality rates are probably well below the true level, despite the reporting as fetal deaths of some infant deaths occurring soon after birth. The stillbirth rate for the country as a whole, comprising in general the total reported intermediate and late fetal mortality, declined only about 10 per cent between 1922, the year when such data first became available, and 1935, whereas a decline of 40 per cent has occurred subsequent to the latter date. In New York State, the almost flat line of the curve of fetal mortality extended back to 1910, when fetal mortality certificates were first required by law. Knowledge of early fetal deaths is even less complete, and no evidence bearing on trends in the early fetal mortality rate is available. Study of several series of pregnant women seen in both clinics and private offices of physicians has pointed to an early fetal loss rate of about 10 per cent. Whether this figure is applicable to the country as a whole can only be conjectured.

The causes of death as given on fetal death certificates are generally considered highly unreliable. New York State data for 1949 reveal that 43 per cent of fetal deaths are reported to be associated with abnormal conditions of the placenta and cord, 11 per cent with congenital malformations, 6 per cent with toxemia, 4 per cent with erythroblastosis fetalis, and 15 per cent with miscellaneous conditions. In 21 per cent of the fetal deaths, no attempt was made to report the possible cause (4).

More reliable information may be obtained from hospitals in which careful postmortem examinations are performed. In a series of fetal deaths studied at the Chicago Lying-In Hospital from 1941 to 1946, it was found that 38 per cent were due to anoxia, mainly from premature separation of the placenta and obstruction of the umbilical cord (5). Ten per cent were caused by congenital malformations and 8 per cent by erythroblastosis fetalis. Even in this carefully studied group, no abnormality could be discovered in the fetus in almost 40 per cent of the cases. Reproductive failure early in pregnancy, in so far as it is understood, presents a somewhat different type of problem from intermediate and late fetal loss. Studies of early fetal deaths have shown that more than one-half are due to some defect in the ovum or embryo or to a significant abnormality of the placenta (6). In most instances, death occurs in the earliest stages of embryonic development so that the embryo appears to be doomed from the start.

Maternal Mortality. During the first three decades of the century, the contrast was drawn frequently between the consistently high mortality rate in the United States and the lower rates in other countries and to the rates in the Scandinavian countries in particular. Until 1934, the rate in the United States remained above 60 deaths per 10,000 live births, whereas the mortality rate in Sweden was only half as high. The decline in maternal mortality in the United States, setting in slowly in 1934, accelerated rapidly. As a result, the rate has fallen far below that of other nations which previously fared better in this regard. "The fact that the chances of an expectant mother surviving the diseases of pregnancy, childbirth and the puerperium are . . . better than 999 out of 1000 is truly a story of human and social progress." (7)

The three major groups of causes of death during the maternity cycle are those related to puerperal infection, to the toxemias of pregnancy, and to hemorrhage. The death rates from all three causes have decreased markedly and to about the same extent (Figure 7). In some areas having the lowest maternal mortality rates, deaths from hemorrhage, whether associated with antepartal conditions such as placenta previa or premature separation of the placenta, or occurring in the post-partum period, have shown the least relative decline, especially when it is realized that hemorrhage is the primary factor in some of the deaths reported as due to infection.

Concentration of Mortality. Mention has been made of the higher infant mortality rates prevailing among the nonwhite portion of the population and in the poorer areas of large metropolitan centers. A concentration of other health problems of all sorts generally is found along with the higher infant mortality rates. A complex of social and economic conditions, with the relative weight of its interrelated components difficult to gauge, affects fetal and maternal mortality and mortality in later childhood as well. Great strides have been made in reducing mortality rates among Negroes, other nonwhite and Spanish-speaking groups; nevertheless, the mortality among these groups remains considerably higher than in the population as a whole.

Not only is the risk of an unfortunate outcome of pregnancy greater in certain broad groups of the population, but there is a further increased risk once a previous pregnancy has terminated in a fetal or neonatal death. A study of vital statistics records of over a quarter of a million de-

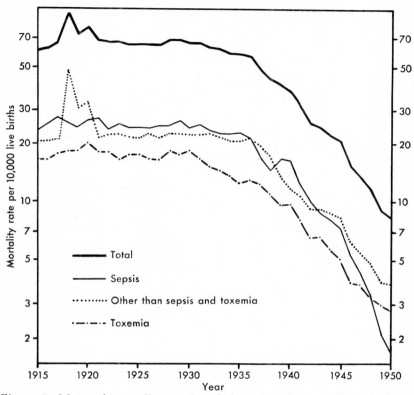

Figure 7. Maternal mortality, total and for selected causes, United States, 1915–1950. (*Data provided by National Office of Vital Statistics.*)

liveries has shown this risk to be about two and one-half times greater for fetal and neonatal deaths in subsequent deliveries (8). How much of this increased hazard is due to readily definable conditions, such as erythroblastosis fetalis, is a matter for further investigation. There is ground for belief that, as mortality rates for the population as a whole continue to decline, the residue tends to become more highly concentrated in an increasingly smaller segment of the population.

TRENDS IN MORBIDITY

The most comprehensive picture of the extent of nonfatal illness in children in the United States was obtained in the National Health Survey of 1935 and 1936 (9). Even this survey was limited in that the only illnesses covered were those causing disability for a minimum of seven days in the urban children studied. It was found that childhood is characteristically a period of high incidence of illness. After one year of age, the force of the high morbidity rate is more than offset by the comparatively short duration of individual illnesses and the great proportion of complete recoveries. These three characteristics—frequent illness, short duration of illness, and high recovery rate—were most evident in the group five through nine years of age. Acute communicable or respiratory diseases constituted 80 per cent of the total number of incapacitating illnesses and caused half the total days of disability in children under fifteen years of age.

Special surveys of local areas, providing data on illnesses of less than a week in duration, have confirmed the general findings of the national survey. In one survey carried out over a period of six years, the highest illness rate was found in children under five years of age, with a decrease in the rate in succeeding age periods (10). With increasing age above five years of age, girls had progressively higher morbidity rates relative to boys.

Apart from some specific communicable diseases, there is no evidence to indicate that a decline in the over-all morbidity rate in childhood has accompanied the decline in mortality. The study of absenteeism due to illness among school children is the most convenient method of obtaining information on this score. A report from New England, confirming earlier Maryland investigations, actually disclosed an increased number of illnesses and days of absence because of illness in the 1948–1949 academic year compared with a similar period eleven years earlier (11). The number of absences from school caused by illnesses of all kinds increased nearly 50 per cent, with the greater increase in absences the result of respiratory illness. At the same time, the average number of days of absence by individual illnesses decreased about one-third in all categories. It may be that children are kept home more frequently at early signs of illness. It would also be of interest to know if the presumed increase in relatively minor illness in children of school age represents in some measure a shift of illness occurring with greater frequency in former years in the preschool group.

CITED REFERENCES

1. SEIBERT, HENRI, The Progress of Ideas Regarding the Causation and Control of Infant Mortality, Bulletin, Institute of History of Medicine, Vol. 8, pp. 546–598, April, 1940.
2. FUERST, J. S., and ROSALYN KAPLAN, Chicago's Public Housing Program Helps to Save Babies' Lives, *Child,* Vol. 15, pp. 178–181, June–July, 1951.
3. YERUSHALMY, J., and JESSIE M. BIERMAN, Major Problems in Fetal Mortality, *Obst. & Gynec. Surv.,* Vol. 7, pp. 1–34, February, 1952.
4. Unpublished data, Office of Vital Statistics, New York State Department of Health, Albany, N.Y.
5. POTTER, EDITH L., and FRED L. ADAIR, "Fetal and Neonatal Death," 2d ed., University of Chicago Press, Chicago, 1949.
6. HERTIG, ARTHUR T., and JOHN ROCK, Series of Potentially Abortive Ova Recovered from Fertile Women prior to the First Missed Menstrual Period, *Am. J. Obst. & Gynec.,* Vol. 58, pp. 968–993, November, 1949.
7. Maternal Deaths—One in a Thousand, editorial, *J.A.M.A.,* Vol. 144, pp. 1096–1097, Nov. 25, 1950.
8. YERUSHALMY, JACOB, ELIZABETH M. GARDINER, and CARROLL E. PALMER, Studies in Childbirth Mortality, III. Puerperal Fatality in Relation to Mother's Previous Infant Losses, *Pub. Health Rep.,* Vol. 56, pp. 1463–1481, July 18, 1941.
9. HOLLAND, DOROTHY F., The Disabling Diseases of Childhood: 1. Characteristics and Leading Causes, *Pub. Health Rep.,* Vol. 55, pp. 135–156, Jan. 26, 1940.
10. COLLINS, SELWYN D., RUTH PHILLIPS, and DOROTHY S. OLIVER, Disabling Illness from Specific Causes among Males and Females of Various Ages: Samples of White Families Canvassed at Monthly Intervals in the Eastern Health District of Baltimore, 1938–43, *Pub. Health Rep.* Vol. 66, pp. 1649–1671, Dec. 14, 1951.
11. LINDE, JOSEPH I., ABRAHAM GELPERIN, and MORRIS A. GRANOFF, Causes of Absenteeism in New Haven Schools—Follow-up after 21 Years, *Pub. Health Rep.,* Vol. 65, pp. 1737–1744, Dec. 29, 1950.

ADDITIONAL REFERENCES

1. FERGUSON, JAMES H., Maternal Death in the Rural South: A Study of Forty-seven Consecutive Cases, *J.A.M.A.,* Vol. 146, pp. 1388–1393, Aug. 11, 1951.

2. CALKINS, L. A., Fetal Mortality, *Am. J. Obst. & Gynec.,* Vol. 60, pp. 1000–1005, November, 1950.
3. COLLINS, JASON H., Abortions—A Study Based on 1,304 Cases, *Am. J. Obst. & Gynec.,* Vol. 62, pp. 548–558, September, 1951.
4. BUNDESEN, HERMAN N., EDITH L. POTTER, WILLIAM I. FISHBEIN, FRANK C. BAUER, and GERTRUDE V. PLOTZKE, Progress in Reduction of Needless Neonatal Deaths: Challenge to the Health Officer and the Medical Profession, *J.A.M.A.,* Vol. 148, pp. 907–917, Mar. 15, 1952.
5. SMITH, CLEMENT A., The Valley of the Shadow of Birth, *Am. J. Dis. Child.,* Vol. 82, pp. 171–201, August, 1951.
6. AREY, JAMES B., and JOHN DENT, Causes of Fetal and Neonatal Death with Special Reference to Pulmonary and Inflammatory Lesions, *J. Pediat.,* Vol. 42, pp. 1–25, 205–227, January and February, 1953.
7. GRAHAM, STANLEY, Infant Mortality and the Social Services, *Canad. M.A.J.,* Vol. 67, pp. 323–326, October, 1952.
8. BAUMGARTNER, LEONA, Public Health Aspects of Problems of Current Interest in Neonatal Pediatrics, *Pediatrics,* Vol. 11, pp. 489–501, May, 1953.

4 BACKGROUND OF CHILD HEALTH SERVICES IN THE UNITED STATES

The present century has been called the century of the child. This statement is true if only in contrast to the almost complete lack of public concern for children before the United States reached its maturity as a nation. It is hard to realize that the highly developed health services for children on the contemporary scene, unevenly distributed as they still are, have been almost entirely a product of the twentieth century. Until the First World War, the United States lagged far behind a number of other nations in measures for the protection of the health of its mothers and children. Human as well as natural resources seemed to be limitless in supply; the growing nation was too busy developing its resources to take any steps for their conservation.

Though the deaths of infants and young children caused sorrow to their parents, the community as a whole was unconcerned. The public was unaware of the full extent of the losses and felt little could be done in any case to prevent them. The attitude prevailed widely that it was unwise to attempt to save the lives of the infants since it would somehow interfere with "natural" processes. Even the meager efforts to aid orphaned or abandoned children usually proved harmful; in foundling institutions it was common for more than half the infants to die before they reached their first birthday.

Early community efforts were devoted mainly to the treatment of far-advanced medical conditions or to ameliorating the effects of gross social neglect in children. The new hospitals of the first half of the nineteenth century rarely admitted children. Small special hospitals for children, the first in Philadelphia in 1855, were therefore established to help fill this gap in several cities before the Civil War. The Society for the Prevention of Cruelty to Children, founded in 1875, was concerned mainly with instances of maltreatment of children. Even this degree of protection came only as a belated offshoot of the work of a parent organization for the prevention of cruelty to animals which had its inception in a local organization in Philadelphia almost fifty years earlier.

The first real public health activity specifically for children came in 1879. In that year the New York State Legislature passed a law requiring New York City to appropriate $10,000 for child health work each year. With this modest sum the municipal health department employed physicians and nurses in an effort to save some of the thousands of infants dying of diarrheal illness every summer in the swarming tenements. Although no attempt was made to study and eradicate the causes of diarrheal disease among infants, the effort did create a precedent in that the sick infants were sought out and treated in their homes (1).

Of more far-reaching effect was the program of convalescent care for infants and children which was developed at the New York Postgraduate Hospital. Volunteers were secured in 1890 "to visit children in their homes, to report on conditions and interpret (the physician's) instructions to the mother." (2) A few years later, a woman physician replaced the volunteers, only to be succeeded shortly afterward by a nurse. This led in turn to convalescent care of children in foster homes.

Early Developments in Medical Profession. Interest was naturally focused on the treatment of disease among the first groups of medical specialists devoting their attention to the care of mothers and children. A section on obstetrics and diseases of women and children was formed within the American Medical Association in 1873. From this the section on diseases of children was split off six years later. The American Pediatric Society, an independent group formed in 1888 for the scientific study of diseases of children, was one of the first of the independent organizations of medical specialists.

The slowly broadening interests of the pediatric group were exemplified by the action of the pediatric section of the American Medical Association in devoting a special session of the annual meeting in 1909 to the subject of infant mortality. Speakers at this session pointed out that half the infant deaths of that day could be prevented by general application of medical knowledge then available. Cognizance was taken of the social as well as medical factors playing a role in the production of infant deaths. The growth of pediatrics as a specialty remained comparatively slow until the First World War. It was only in 1912 that the first clinic in the country devoted exclusively to children was opened at Johns Hopkins Hospital in Baltimore (3).

The American Medical Association was interested from the start in raising the standards of medical education and practice. This activity reached a climax following the formation of the Council on Medical Education and Hospitals in 1902. One of the first chairmen of the new Council stated, "If its creation is to result in good, it must be the means of obtaining cooperation between the medical profession, the medical schools, the colleges of arts, the state examining boards, the government services and all groups which are interested in elevating and regulating medical education." (4) The work of this group led to the study of medical education financed by the Carnegie Foundation, embodied in the Flexner report in 1910. Publication of this report resulted within a few years in the closing of many grossly inadequate medical schools and the merging of others. This laid the foundations for the present level of medical pediatric education, making possible the later development of broad health services of good quality for children.

Development of Governmental (Official) Health Services. The staggering loss of infant lives, particularly in the large cities, was the impetus to increasingly broad public health measures before 1900. Supported by private philanthropy under Nathan Strauss, the first stations for free distribution of pasteurized milk for the children of the poor were established in New York City in 1893.

The direct results of the quantity of milk actually dispensed were never through the years very marked, but the principles on which this movement were based—the value of milk depots in the feeding of infants and the education of the mother, and the necessity of pasteurization have been most potent in bringing not only the industry, but the medical profession and the public, to a recognition of the vital importance of safe milk for infant feeding. (5)

Within a few years it was realized that cow's milk had to be modified to meet the needs of the individual infant. The services of physicians and nurses were added later at the milk stations. A gradual evolution followed, culminating in the modern child health conference or well-child clinic in which health supervision of presumably normal infants and preschool children is provided.

The last decade of the nineteenth century also saw the beginnings of health services for school children in several large cities on the Eastern Seaboard. Epidemics of diphtheria, scarlet fever, and other serious communicable diseases, coupled with excessive absenteeism because of minor conditions like scabies and head lice, provided the stimulus to this development. The first systematic inspection of school children for evidence of communicable disease came in 1894 in Boston with the appointment of a part-time physician in each school district of the city. A few years later Connecticut took a further step by requiring testing of vision of each school child at the start of the school year by the teacher or school authorities. A crude follow-up system was instituted by written notification of the parents of the results of the tests.

With the passage of time, a gradual change of emphasis was to be noted in health services for school children. First came the addition of public health nursing services in the schools. This was followed shortly by the introduction of medical examinations and follow-up procedures for the correction of physical defects found. The school-lunch movement had its inception in New York in 1908 as an effort to supplement the diet of undernourished children. Only much later was any interest shown in the mental and emotional health of the school child. These developments were slow and spotty and confined for the most part to the large cities.

Local and State Health Services. By 1908 several unrelated units within the New York City Department of Health were carrying out different types of child health services. The communicable disease unit, for example, was responsible for administration of the program of medical inspection of school children. In that year these various activities for children were brought together under a new Bureau of Child Hygiene, the first full-time unit for child health in any official health agency in the country, under the brilliant and fearless leadership of Dr. Josephine Baker (6). The principles and the practical workaday methods which Dr. Baker developed set the pattern for the nationwide attack on child health problems that followed shortly afterward.

Health services for children were being incorporated at the same time in the work of state departments of health. In 1912 the Louisiana State Board of Health created a bureau of child hygiene "concerned primarily with health education and education of school children for defects," but this unit was discontinued for a period of seven years after 1929 (7).

In 1912 a pediatric consultant was appointed by the New York State Department of Health. A full-time division of child hygiene, created in this department two years later, was the first to function on a continuing basis to the present time. Both units, followed by others soon after, devoted their initial efforts to educating parents in child care.

Federal Health Services. Interest in child health also developed in the Federal government in the early years of the century. In 1902 the collection and publication of birth and death statistics by the Bureau of the Census was authorized by Congress. Four years later, the publication of mortality statistics for 1900–1904 provided the first clear picture of the staggering number of deaths of infants and young children occurring in the United States each year.

About this time, influential individuals and groups began to bring pressure on Congress to authorize an agency in the Federal government to be concerned exclusively with the health and welfare of mothers and children. The first draft of a bill for the creation of such a governmental unit was prepared in 1906, and introduction of a bill followed three years later. After prolonged hearings and acrimonious debate each year, the Children's Bureau was finally created by Act of Congress in 1912 and placed in the Department of Labor. Under the terms of the Act, the Children's Bureau was established primarily as an investigatory and reporting agency on "all matters pertaining to the welfare and child life among all classes of the people." It soon displayed a crusading zeal which made its influence widely felt in carrying out the mandates of its charter (8). The Bureau was transferred to the Federal Security Agency in 1946 as a separate unit maintaining its interest in the promotion of the well-being of the children of the nation. It retained its identity when the Federal Security Agency was transformed into the Department of Health, Education, and Welfare in 1953, with the department head having cabinet status.

The Public Health Service and the Children's Bureau conducted a number of noteworthy investigations into the causes of infant and child mortality throughout the nation, looking to possible measures for its reduction. These studies were hampered by the inadequacy of birth registration and the lack of uniformity in reporting of births and deaths. The establishment of the birth registration area by Federal law in 1915 under the Bureau of the Census removed many of these difficulties. For a state to be admitted into the birth registration area, the Bureau of the Census had to be satisfied that the registration of births in the state was at least 90 per cent complete. Initially only 10 states and the District of Columbia could meet this standard of completeness, but within eighteen years all the states were included in the registration area. In general, the first states admitted had the lowest infant and other mortality rates. The states admitted later, with the higher rates, tended to retard the reported decline in the mortality rates, but even this could not offset the rapid drop in the remainder of the expanding birth registration area.

Growth of Voluntary Health Agencies. Following the lead of the Strauss Milk Charity in New York, local philanthropic agencies developed new types of health services for mothers and children in widely scattered parts of the country. For example, The Association of Collegiate Alumnae in San Francisco, dismayed to learn that half the infants in a foundling hospital had died before their first birthday, experimented with placement of the infants in foster homes. Foster-home care resulted in a rapid drop in infant mortality to a small fraction of its former level. The first organized program of health care during the prenatal period was provided in 1908 by the pediatric department of the New York Outdoor Medical Clinic. Visiting nurse service for pregnant women in their homes followed a year later when a nurse was employed by the Committee on Infant Social Service of the Women's Municipal League of Boston.

Meeting the problem of infant mortality and the health needs of school children were the initial objectives of national organizations of private citizens interested in child health, just as they were the immediate concern of the first official health services for children. Spurred by the disclosures of the studies by the Bureau of the Census, a conference was called at Yale University in 1909 to investigate the factors responsible for the high death rate in infants. The conference resulted in the organization of the American Association for Study and Prevention of Infant Mortality. From its headquarters in Baltimore, the Association conducted a vigorous campaign to arouse the conscience of the nation to the need for active measures to save the lives of infants and children.

A clear example of the way voluntary agencies demonstrated the way to meet health needs which were not yet recognized by the official agency is seen in the combatting of infant mortality. While in 1910 voluntary agencies were carrying the entire responsibility for definite preventive programs in

26 out of 28 cities having a population of 20,000 or more, today it is the exception to find such activities carried by voluntary agencies. (9)

A group of public-spirited citizens in New York City, disturbed about the poor nutritional status of school children, banded together some years later to form the Child Health Organization in 1917. The main purpose of the new organization was to provide hot lunches to children in the schools. They soon felt the need to evaluate the results of their program, and they resorted to periodic measurement of the weight and height of children for this purpose. They broadened their activities further by including health education by the use of such devices as health clowns to gain the interest of school children.

The two major voluntary child health organizations merged in 1922 to form the American Child Health Association. In cooperation with the Commonwealth Fund, the enlarged organization embarked on a series of studies, at first concerned mainly with health problems of maternity, infancy, and the preschool period, and later with health services for children of school age. The Association worked closely with the Children's Bureau in Washington and with state and local departments of health until its dissolution in 1935.

White House Conferences. The early years of the twentieth century saw another manifestation of concern for the conservation of the nation's leading human resource, its children. It was fitting that President Theodore Roosevelt, a leader in the movement for the conservation of natural resources, should convene the first White House Conference on the Care of Dependent Children. This conference, a gathering of only 200 persons, deliberated on the need to strengthen care of children in their own homes or, as second choice, in properly run foster homes, rather than in the characteristically bleak child-caring institutions of the period. Following the precedent set by the first conference, an unofficial custom was followed by the President of the United States in office at the time to issue the call for a White House Conference at intervals of about ten years. Succeeding conferences focused professional and popular attention on problems of childhood and contributed in no small measure to the rapid advances in child health services.

The Children's Year, led by the Women's Committee of the Council of National Defense in conjunction with the Children's Bureau, preceded the White House Conference on Child Welfare Standards in 1919. One of the four major objectives of this campaign was the public

THE CHILDREN'S CHARTER

*President Hoover's White House Conference on Child Health
and Protection, recognizing the rights of the child
as the first rights of citizenship, pledges
itself to these aims for the
Children of America*

FOR every child spiritual and moral training to help him to stand firm under the pressure of life.

II. For every child understanding and the guarding of his personality as his most precious right.

III. For every child a home and that love and security which a home provides; and for that child who must receive foster care, the nearest substitute for his own home.

IV. For every child full preparation for his birth, his mother receiving prenatal, natal, and postnatal care; and the establishment of such protective measures as will make childbearing safer.

V. For every child health protection from birth through adolescence, including: periodical health examinations and, where needed, care of specialists and hospital treatment; regular dental examinations and care of the teeth; protective and preventive measures against communicable diseases; the insuring of pure food, pure milk, and pure water.

VI. For every child from birth through adolescence, promotion of health, including health instruction and a health program, wholesome physical and mental recreation, with teachers and leaders adequately trained.

VII. For every child a dwelling place safe, sanitary, and wholesome, with reasonable provisions for privacy, free from conditions which tend to thwart his development; and a home environment harmonious and enriching.

VIII. For every child a school which is safe from hazards, sanitary, properly equipped, lighted, and ventilated. For younger children nursery schools and kindergartens to supplement home care.

IX. For every child a community which recognizes and plans for his needs, protects him against physical dangers, moral hazards, and disease; provides him with safe and wholesome places for play and recreation; and makes provision for his cultural and social needs.

X. For every child an education which, through the discovery and development of his individual abilities, prepares him for life; and through training and vocational guidance prepares him for a living which will yield him the maximum of satisfaction.

XI. For every child such teaching and training as will prepare him for successful parenthood, homemaking, and the rights of citizenship; and, for parents, supplementary training to fit them to deal wisely with the problems of parenthood.

XII. For every child education for safety and protection against accidents to which modern conditions subject him—those to which he is directly exposed and those which, through loss or maiming of his parents, affect him indirectly.

XIII. For every child who is blind, deaf, crippled, or otherwise physically handicapped, and for the child who is mentally handicapped, such measures as will early discover and diagnose his handicap, provide care and treatment, and so train him that he may become an asset to society rather than a liability. Expenses of these services should be borne publicly where they cannot be privately met.

XIV. For every child who is in conflict with society the right to be dealt with intelligently as society's charge, not society's outcast; with the home, the school, the church, the court and the institution when needed, shaped to return him whenever possible to the normal stream of life.

XV. For every child the right to grow up in a family with an adequate standard of living and the security of a stable income as the surest safeguard against social handicaps.

XVI. For every child protection against labor that stunts growth, either physical or mental, that limits education, that deprives children of the right of comradeship, of play, and of joy.

XVII. For every rural child as satisfactory schooling and health services as for the city child, and an extension to rural families of social, recreational, and cultural facilities.

XVIII. To supplement the home and the school in the training of youth, and to return to them those interests of which modern life tends to cheat children, every stimulation and encouragement should be given to the extension and development of the voluntary youth organizations.

XIX. To make everywhere available these minimum protections of the health and welfare of children, there should be a district, county, or community organization for health, education, and welfare, with full-time officials, coordinating with a state-wide program which will be responsive to a nation-wide service of general information, statistics, and scientific research. This should include:

(*a*) Trained, full-time public health officials, with public health nurses, sanitary inspection, and laboratory workers.

(*b*) Available hospital beds.

(*c*) Full-time public welfare service for the relief, aid, and guidance of children in special need due to poverty, misfortune, or behavior difficulties, and for the protection of children from abuse, neglect, exploitation, or moral hazard.

For every child these rights, regardless of race, or color, or situation, wherever he may live under the protection of the American Flag.

protection of maternity and infancy. Many new activities took place in communities throughout the nation, such as the widespread promotion of medical examinations of preschool children.

The Conference on Child Health and Protection in 1930 represented the high water mark of White House Conferences in specific concern for health services for mothers and children. The stated purpose of the 1930 conference was "to study the present status of the health and well-being of the children of the United States and its possessions; to report what is being done; to recommend what ought to be done and how to do it." A monumental job of fact-finding was performed preceding the Conference, and some of the 32 volumes embodying the results are still used for reference purposes. The principles embodied in the Children's Charter issued by the Conference can well be used as a guide by the development of health services for children today. The 1930 Conference promoted general understanding of child growth and development and did much to advance pediatric education and the status of pediatrics as a specialty.

The White House Conference of 1940 on Children in a Democracy was held in the midst of a world at war, although the United States was not yet involved. The promise of follow-up action for children by the National Citizens' Committee was lost in the all-important defense effort when the country actually entered the war. The National Commission on Children in Wartime attempted to carry on in the face of difficulties and to prepare for opportunities in a postwar period.

Federal Grants-in-aid for Child Health Services. Probably the most significant single step in the development of public health services for children in the United States was the passage by Congress in 1921 of the Sheppard-Towner Act for the Promotion of the Welfare and Hygiene of Maternity and Infancy. For the first time during peacetime, Federal funds were made available to the states for health services based on the principle of grants-in-aid under which the states are required to appropriate funds to match in part those provided by the Federal government. The grants-in-aid for health services during the maternity cycle and infancy were extended once beyond the original period. However, a storm of opposition to the Act was instrumental in preventing its extension beyond 1929.

The Sheppard-Towner Act set a precedent for the many Federal grants-in-aid for specialized health services for children and adults which have been established by Congress in increasing numbers since 1935. It bestowed a new and potent responsibility on the Children's Bureau as the administrator of an annual appropriation of $1,200,000. The Act was the immediate stimulus to the development of full-time units for the administration of maternal and child health services in state departments of health. By the time the Act expired in 1929, full-time maternal and child health units had been formed in the health departments of all but one of the states.

Immediately after the termination of Sheppard-Towner funds, the legislatures in about half the states appropriated funds equal to the amounts previously available in the Federal grants-in-aid. With continuance of the depression, however, the amount of funds appropriated by the states dropped within four years to half the 1930 level. The lost ground was soon regained after the passage of the Social Security Act in 1935. Title V of the Social Security Act extended the principle of grants-in-aid to the states. It not only provided funds for maternal and infant care, but it raised the age limit to twenty-one years for children receiving health services through Federal or matching funds. It also provided financial assistance to the states for locating and treating handicapped or potentially handicapped children. Emphasis was placed in the Act on the provision of services in areas of economic distress and in rural areas.

The initial appropriation called for $5,820,000 for maternal and child health services and $3,870,000 for services for physically handicapped children. Unlike the short life of the Sheppard-Towner Act, the ceilings set for child health services under the Social Security Act have been increased by Congress on several occasions. The Social Security Act Amendments of 1950 finally raised the ceiling on funds for 1951 for general maternal and child health services to $16,500,000 and for services for crippled children to $15,000,000. However, in the face of a determined economy drive in Congress affecting all services not of an immediate defense nature, the actual appropriations subsequently made by Congress fell considerably below the ceiling for the first time since passage of the Social Security Act.

The provision of categorical grants-in-aid programs under the Public Health Service promoted improved generalized public health services which benefited children as well as adults. In some instances, direct services for children were included in the programs carried out with the help of the grants-in-aid funds. The Mental Health Act and the Hospital

Survey and Construction Act, both passed in 1946, were followed two years later by legislation providing for dental research and heart disease programs.

Attack on Maternal Mortality. The continuing high maternal mortality rate was disregarded by the medical profession and public alike until it was called to the attention of the nation by a few significant studies started in the late 1920's. Two of the studies, conducted by the Children's Bureau (10) and the New York Academy of Medicine (11), attracted the most attention. The latter, coming from the medical profession itself and pointing out that two-thirds of deaths associated with childbearing could be prevented by available means, aroused intense controversy in medical and lay circles.

Publication of these reports led to the formation of maternal mortality committees in local medical groups and hospitals throughout the nation. These committees studied the local problems and held maternal mortality conferences to review possible preventable causes in every maternal death. This activity on the part of the medical profession is the major factor to account for the sudden decline in maternal mortality. The emergence of other factors including the increased rate of hospitalization, the availability of chemotherapeutic agents and antibiotics, improved prenatal care through public and private sources, the increasing proportion of maternal care given by obstetrical specialists, and the wider use of blood and its derivatives undoubtedly accelerated the rate of decline, but these new elements cannot account for the initial dramatic break in the mortality rate. As one of the leaders in the battle against maternal mortality stated in reviewing its history, "It is less than twenty years since the shortcomings of American obstetrics were paraded in the public press, and it is much less than that since victory over maternal death statistics was won—if it has been won, yet the impact of the conquest has been so slight that they who have been responsible for the victory hardly know that there was a battle." (12)

Recent Developments Among Professional Organizations. Long active in promoting higher standards of public health practice, the American Public Health Association gave more specific attention to child health services with the formation of the Maternal and Child Health Section. Formed in 1921, when interest in child health services was high, the new section contributed significantly to solution of technical and administrative problems arising with the new programs. A separate

Section on School Health was established in 1942 to give more concentrated attention to health problems of school-age children and to attract to the Association professional persons interested in this field. Joint programs are frequently presented by these sections, along with the nutrition, dental, and other sections, for discussion of the many phases of health work as they relate to child health.

Formation of the American Public Health Association Committee on Child Health in 1947 helped bring the total health needs of the child back into focus. The Committee, with representation from various sections, has been interested in promoting standards for community child health programs. It has also been developing authoritative statements on health supervision of the young child, with special reference to the child health conference, and on programs for children with various types of handicapping conditions (13).

Since 1910 the American Medical Association has engaged in increasingly broad activities in child health. An early effort was the founding of a joint committee with the National Education Association on health problems in education. Although its major emphasis has been upon health education, it has also been concerned with health services for school children. A set of standards developed jointly by the two organizations has been of assistance to physicians rendering medical services in the schools and has otherwise contributed to the understanding of physicians in their relationships with school health services (14). Biennial conferences on school health have been held under the auspices of the American Medical Association since 1948. Conferences on rural health called by the Association have pointed to the need for special provisions for the child in rural areas. The Maternal and Child Health Committee of the Association's Council on Medical Service was formed in 1950 to act in a liaison capacity with other organizations in matters relating to the health of mothers and children.

Since the appearance of pediatrics as a medical specialty, pediatricians have pushed forward the frontiers of preventive care in its broadest aspects. The interest of this group of specialists was epitomized in the organization of the American Academy of Pediatrics in 1931. "It was made clear at that time that pediatricians were now convinced that a society was needed whose principal objective would be not solely to promote social and scientific needs of its members, but which would exist primarily to promote child welfare." (15)

Constantly recurring in the discussions of the Academy during its formative years was the idea of a nationwide survey of child health services. The Academy decided to embark on the project in 1944. The objective of the study was

to bring to the attention of the medical profession and to all those interested in the health of our children the deficiencies in our existing services for children in order that these deficiencies may be corrected. With these data at hand, it is hoped that the pegs of progress can be moved forward in an orderly, intelligent manner, and that all children will have fuller advantage of medical knowledge. (16)

The ambitious project was completed during the following two years. In addition to the national report, most states have completed their own surveys and have issued their own reports. In many states the pediatric groups have been active in promoting correction of the deficiencies disclosed in their own findings.

The American Academy of Pediatrics continues to be active in all phases of health services for children on the national, state, and local scenes. Standing committees are interested in specific problems such as emotional health, rheumatic fever, and accident prevention. The Academy's committee on fetus and newborn has done outstanding work in developing recommended standards for care of the newborn infant in hospital nurseries. The round-table and panel discussions at national and area meetings of the Academy have gone far beyond the clinical aspects of the subjects presented.

Action in relation to community health problems on the part of obstetrical specialists on a national scale has been slower to develop. As early as 1919, an influential group of obstetricians formed the American Committee on Maternal Welfare to awaken and stimulate the interest of members of the medical profession in cooperating with public and private agencies for the protection of the health of mothers and their offspring (17). A federation of local obstetrical societies was established about 1944. It was only in 1951, however, that the American Academy of Obstetrics and Gynecology was formed from the previously existing organization, giving individual membership to obstetricians in a national society of specialists. The objectives of the Academy are broad, including all aspects of the work for the welfare of women which properly come within the scope of obstetrics and gynecology (18).

Emergency Maternity and Infant Care (EMIC). Problems of maternity care from concentration of families of military personnel in the vicinity of training camps was the immediate reason for the development of the Federal Emergency Maternity and Infant Care program (EMIC). Coupled with this was the desire of Congress to maintain the morale of members of the armed forces. Payment for complete maternity care for the wives of enlisted men in the four lowest pay grades of the armed forces and of aviation cadets and medical, nursing, and hospital care for their infants from birth to one year of age were provided under the program.

The EMIC program had its real inception in the state of Washington when the Children's Bureau approved use of unexpended Federal maternal and child health funds by the state to provide care for servicemen's wives. No specific legislation was ever passed covering EMIC, but deficiency appropriations by Congress of increasing size, the first in 1943, confirmed the legality of this use of Federal funds to meet the emergency situation under the general provisions of the Social Security Act. EMIC rapidly became the most extensive and expensive public maternity and infant-care program in the history of the United States. By its termination in the middle of 1949, care had been authorized for 1,454,000 maternity and infant cases. In the peak year of 1944, care was authorized for more than 488,000 women and infants (19). The high point in expenditures was reached in the 1945 fiscal year, covered by two appropriations by Congress totaling 45 million dollars.

EMIC was conceived and developed as a program in a nation at war. The widespread fear that it might be extended into the postwar period as a basis for a broader medical care program under governmental auspices made it a center of controversy in medical circles. Numerous irritations plagued the relationships between the practicing physicians providing the services and the Federal and state agencies administering the program. Some of the difficulties were caused by the lack of time in developing policies and procedures for the program; others were related to fundamental differences in philosophy. The end of the program was greeted with mixed feelings on the part of the medical profession. Some physicians felt that the over-all objectives of the program had been reached and that definite values had been gained, "on the grounds that lives were saved and that (servicemen's) children received a great deal of sound medical care." (20)

Specialized Health Services. Once interest in the health problems of children was aroused in the United States, developments occurred rapidly in many directions. Services for children with handicapping conditions were among the earliest to be developed. The first governmental appropriation for the rehabilitation of handicapped children was made by the Minnesota State Legislature in 1897. At first these services were purchased from an existing hospital; a new hospital was built by the state in 1911 and has been operated continuously since then (21). Following the severe poliomyelitis outbreak of 1916, New York State provided orthopedic consultation services in rural areas and other places lacking this service. This developed into a system of orthopedic consultation clinics conducted by the State Department of Health. Ohio, in 1919, was the first state to enact a law for the provision of services for handicapped children on a statewide basis (22). By 1934, services of widely varying adequacy were available in 35 states. The grants-in-aid provided under the Social Security Act facilitated further rapid expansion of services for handicapped children. At first only children with orthopedic and closely related handicapping conditions were eligible for care. The range of conditions covered has been enlarged gradually, with great interest centering in children with cerebral palsy, epilepsy, auditory and visual handicaps, and rheumatic and congenital heart disease.

The concept of rehabilitation of the handicapped has broadened since the early 1940's; children have benefited from the improved services and rehabilitative techniques provided in community rehabilitation centers and other agencies. Present-day rehabilitation centers followed varied patterns of evolution. The center in Cleveland, for example, dates back to 1889, but in different form. "It is of interest to note that its first function was the provision of recreation for children in a general hospital, later becoming interested in education and in training for jobs and employment." (23)

The pattern for a community approach to the care of premature infants was set in 1932 when the first premature center under governmental auspices was opened in Chicago. Premature infants born at home or in hospitals not equipped to give adequate care were transported to the premature center, where highly trained personnel provided the specialized care needed. Since 1945 this pattern of care has been widely followed.

Treatment of emotionally disturbed children not under private care has usually been provided through child guidance clinics under varied auspices such as voluntary or governmental general health and specialized mental health agencies, schools, hospitals, or courts. While interest in the emotionally disturbed child sprang from several sources prior to the First World War, much of what is found in current child guidance clinics was developed in the pioneer clinic for juvenile delinquents in association with the Juvenile Court of Cook County, Illinois, started in 1909. A period of rapid development of the child guidance movement followed the subsidization of demonstration clinics by the Commonwealth Fund "with the purpose of showing the juvenile courts and child-caring agencies what psychiatry, psychology and social work has to offer in the treatment of the problem child." (24)

After a slow start, dental health services for children also have undergone rapid expansion. The teaching of school children of the need for thorough toothbrushing was the earliest activity, following the widely held belief that "a clean tooth never decays." The training of dental hygienists was intended to supply an auxiliary group to spare dentists the time needed to clean children's teeth and to teach techniques of toothbrushing. The first dental hygienist was trained in Bridgeport, Conn., in 1913, mainly for work with school children; the services of dental hygienists were first legalized in Massachusetts two years later.

Private philanthropy had taken the lead in 1910 in providing dental treatment for children in indigent families with the establishment of the Forsyth Dental Infirmary in Boston. Treatment services for school children, largely for dental emergencies requiring extraction of teeth, began to develop shortly afterward. The first special unit in a state health department was organized in North Carolina in 1918. The rapid growth in public health programs was reflected in the organization of the American Association of Public Health Dentists in 1938. However, significant strides in the prophylactic aspects of the program have been made only since 1948, when the use of fluoride salts in the drinking water or by application to the teeth began to be generally appreciated as a preventive measure against dental decay.

The years since the dissolution of the American Child Health Association in 1935 have witnessed a phenomenal increase in the number, strength, and activities of voluntary health organizations concerned with particular disease problems. In many of these organizations, emphasis has been upon diseases and conditions taking their greatest toll in childhood. Here again, the appeal of the handicapped child has been justifiably used to arouse interest in health problems and to open the purse of the public for the support of programs which benefit the adult as well. National, state, and local voluntary health organizations have made increasingly valuable contributions to the health and welfare of children suffering from poliomyelitis, cerebral palsy, auditory and visual difficulties, heart disease, epilepsy, and other conditions.

Trend toward "Total Care." While organizations and programs relating to special health problems in both official and voluntary health circles have continued to grow at a rapid rate, a simultaneous trend toward bringing these various specialized services into a total health program for children has also been evident. An association of directors of maternal and child health programs was organized in 1944 mainly to cope with problems arising from EMIC. An invitation was later extended to the directors of services for physically handicapped children to join the association, and the interests of the organization were broadened in accordance with its new name, the Association of Maternal and Child Health and Crippled Children's Directors.

The appointment of the general advisory committee to the Children's Bureau in 1948 was another evidence of the return of emphasis to total child care. Smaller technical advisory committees to the Children's Bureau had been in existence for a number of years but had been concerned with rheumatic fever and other specific problems. The general advisory committee has considered such subjects as care of rural children, long-term care of children, education and training of personnel, and the encouragement of integration of existing special services for children in each area.

The Midcentury White House Conference on Children and Youth of 1950 set as its theme the total well-being of children or "how we can develop in children the mental, emotional and spiritual qualities essential to individual happiness and responsible citizenship and what physical, economic and social conditions are deemed necessary to this development." It promoted widespread citizen participation for more than two years in advance of the actual meeting. About 5,000 delegates, in addition to a large number of foreign observers, attended from all fields of activity bearing on the Conference theme.

It is probable that every professional group attending the 1950 Conference initially felt that its own contributions toward the stated objective had been slighted; most groups finally realized that their contributions could only be a small part of a much larger whole requiring skillful intermeshing of many parts. As a prominent pediatrician expressed this feeling in relation to his own medical specialty, "The medical men in attendance learned or re-learned one important fact; namely, that important as they may be in the field of improvement of child health, they are neither the sun nor the moon in the heavens, but just one of the stars." (25)

The fact-finding reports and recommendations of the Conference have found wide use as basic documents in the promotion of broad child health programs (26). The Conference sharpened the focus on the fundamental importance of personality development of children and youth to the structure of our society. In its Pledge to Children and in the recommendations in its Platform, the Conference went beyond the limits of earlier conferences. "The action taken . . . will take root in the states and their communities to mold a new understanding of the influences that affect the healthy personality development of our children and youth." (27) The National Midcentury Committee for Children and Youth functioned until the beginning of 1953 as a follow-up body to stimulate action on the recommendations of the Conference mainly by working with and through existing organizations (28). Since then, its work has been carried forward independently by two advisory councils formed originally in preparation for the Midcentury White House Conference itself.

LANDMARKS IN CHILD HEALTH SERVICES IN THE UNITED STATES

1873   Section on Obstetrics and Diseases of Women and Children formed in American Medical Association

1879   Visitation of sick infants in homes by physicians and nurses— New York City

      Section on Diseases of Children formed in American Medical Association

1888   American Pediatric Society founded

1893   Milk stations opened by Strauss Milk Charity—New York City

1894   Regular medical inspection of school children for contagious diseases—Boston

1897   Care of handicapped children aided by state of Minnesota
1902   Federal Bureau of Census authorized to issue statistics on births and deaths
       Nursing service started in schools—New York City
1906   Mortality Statistics for 1900–1904 published by Bureau of Census
1908   First municipal unit for child health—Bureau of Child Hygiene, New York City
1909   White House Conference on Care of Dependent Children
       American Association for Study and Prevention of Infant Mortality founded
       Prenatal visits started by nurses—Boston
       Clinic for juvenile delinquents—Juvenile Court of Cook County, Illinois
1910   Flexner report on medical education published
       Forsyth Dental Dispensary established—Boston
1912   Children's Bureau established in U.S. Department of Labor
       First state health department unit for child health services organized—Louisiana
1913   First dental hygienists trained—Bridgeport, Conn.
1915   Birth Registration Area established under U.S. Bureau of Census
1917   Child Health Organization formed
1918   Children's Year
       First state dental health unit—North Carolina
1919   White House Conference on Child Welfare Standards
       First law for statewide care of handicapped children—Ohio
1921–1929   Federal Maternity and Infancy (Sheppard-Towner) Act in force
1921   Maternal and Child Health Section formed in American Public Health Association
1922–1935   American Child Health Association
1927   First medical social worker in a health department—Los Angeles County, California
1930   White House Conference on Child Health and Protection—Children's Charter
1931   American Academy of Pediatrics established
1932   Premature infant care program initiated—Chicago

1933 "Maternal Mortality in New York City" published
1935 Social Security Act passed
1940 White House Conference on Children in a Democracy
1943–1949 Emergency maternity and infant care program for service-
        men's families (EMIC)
1945–1946 Nationwide study of child health services by American
        Academy of Pediatrics
1948 Committee on Child Health formed in American Public Health
        Association
        General advisory committee to Children's Bureau appointed
1950 Social Security Act amendments passed
        Midcentury White House Conference on Children and Youth
1951 American Academy of Obstetrics and Gynecology formed
1953 Federal Department of Health, Education, and Welfare estab-
        lished

CITED REFERENCES

1. VAN INGEN, PHILIP, The History of Child Welfare Work in the United States, pp. 290–322, in "A Half Century of Public Health," The American Public Health Association, New York, 1921.
2. CANNON, IDA M., "On the Social Frontier of Medicine: Pioneering in Medical Social Work," Harvard University Press, Cambridge, Mass., 1952.
3. SMITH, RICHARD M., Medicine as a Science: Pediatrics, *New England J. Med.*, Vol. 244, pp. 176–181, Feb. 1, 1951.
4. BEVAN, ARTHUR D., Chairman's Address, First Annual Congress on Medical Education, 1905, quoted by Herman G. Weiskotten, Responsibility of a Profession for the Promotion of Educational Standards, *J.A.M.A.*, Vol. 142, pp. 1119–1122, Apr. 15, 1950.
5. NORTH, CHARLES E., Milk and Its Relation to Public Health, in "A Half Century of Public Health," The American Public Health Association, New York, 1921.
6. BAKER, S. JOSEPHINE, "Fighting for Life," The Macmillan Company, New York, 1939.
7. ZIEGLER, AZELIE, "Milestones in Louisiana's Health Program for School-age Children," Quarterly Bulletin of the Louisiana State Department of Health, Vol. 15, pp. 3–33, December, 1949; courtesy of B. Freedman.
8. MUSTARD, HARRY S., "Government in Public Health," Commonwealth Fund, Harvard University Press, Cambridge, Mass., 1945.
9. GUNN, SELSKAR M., and PHILIP S. PLATT, "Voluntary Health Agencies," p. 15, The Ronald Press Company, New York, 1945.

10. "Maternal Mortality in Fifteen States," Children's Bureau Publication No. 223, Washington, D.C., 1933.
11. "Maternal Mortality in New York City: A Study of All Puerperal Deaths," Commonwealth Fund, Harvard University Press, Cambridge, Mass., 1933.
12. GORDON, CHARLES A., The Mortality Remainder, *Am. J. Obst. & Gynec.,* Vol. 62, pp. 1132–1137, November, 1951.
13. WISHIK, SAMUEL M., Program of the Committee on Child Health of the American Public Health Association, *Pediatrics,* Vol. 10, pp. 85–87, January, 1953.
14. SMILEY, DEAN F., and FRED V. HEIN, editors, "Health Appraisal of School Children," American Medical Association, Chicago, 1948.
15. BEAVEN, PAUL W., The Academy Comes of Age, *Pediatrics,* Vol. 9, pp. 1–6, January, 1952.
16. "Child Health Services and Pediatric Education, Report of the Committee for the Study of Child Health Services," The American Academy of Pediatrics, Commonwealth Fund, Harvard University Press, Cambridge, Mass., 1949.
17. Our Object: The American Committee on Maternal Welfare, *The Mother*, p. 3, Winter, 1952.
18. BEACHAM, WOODARD D., The American Academy of Obstetrics and Gynecology: First Presidential Address, A History of American Obstetric and Gynecologic Organizations and the Genesis of the American Academy, *Obst. & Gynec.,* Vol. 1, pp. 115–124, January, 1953.
19. "Annual Report of the Federal Security Agency for 1949," p. 165, Washington, D.C., 1950.
20. PEASE, MARSHALL C., "A History of the American Academy of Pediatrics," p. 181, The Academy, Evanston, Ill., 1952.
21. BEER, JOHN J., Personal communication, 1952.
22. STERN, BERNHARD J., "Medical Services by Government—Local, State and Federal," p. 136, Commonwealth Fund, Harvard University Press, Cambridge, Mass., 1946.
23. GREVE, BELL, The Cleveland Rehabilitation Center, in "Rehabilitation of the Handicapped: A Survey of Means and Methods," William H. Soden, editor, The Ronald Press, New York, 1949.
24. RAYMERT, MARTIN L., The Organization and Administration of a Child Guidance Clinic, in "Handbook of Child Guidance," edited by Ernest Harms, Child Care Publications, New York, 1947.
25. SISSON, WARREN R., "The Midcentury White House Conference on Children and Youth," American Academy of Pediatrics News-Letter, February, 1951.
26. "The Official Conference Proceedings," Health Publications Institute, Raleigh, N. C., 1951.
27. Midcentury White House Conference on Children and Youth, editorial, *J.A.M.A.,* Vol. 144, pp. 467–468, Dec. 23, 1950.

28. "National Midcentury Committee for Children and Youth, Report on Children and Youth, 1950–1952," Health Publications Institute, Raleigh, N.C., 1953.

ADDITIONAL REFERENCES

1. This First Half Century, Symposium, *J. Am. Dent. A.,* Vol. 40, pp. 644–768, June, 1950.
2. SINAI, NATHAN, and ODIN W. ANDERSON, "EMIC (Emergency Maternity and Infant Care): A Study of Administrative Experience," University of Michigan School of Public Health, Ann Arbor, Mich., 1948.
3. QUIGLEY, JAMES K., Then and Now. Obstetrics in 1900 and in 1950, *Am. J. Obst. & Gynec.,* Vol. 63, pp. 241–250, February, 1952.

5 ADMINISTRATIVE RELATIONSHIPS

Many of the landmarks in child health services were, as we have seen, not only pioneer efforts for children, but they were the first community efforts in meeting different health problems in any age group. Regular supervision of the health of presumably normal individuals found its first application in the child health field. Among the first Federal grants-in-aid for any type of health services to states were those made for the promotion of maternity and infant care under the Sheppard-Towner Act. The earliest community health services for handicapped persons were developed for children. Rheumatic fever and rheumatic heart disease programs in childhood preceded by a decade the organized attack on heart disease in adult life. These few examples have been cited to indicate that community health services for children have often preceded and spearheaded similar approaches to health problems in the adult.

OFFICIAL HEALTH AGENCIES

Many of the specialized services now provided by governmental health agencies originated as functions of the division or bureau administering the maternal and child health program. Nutrition services in a number of state and local health departments have begun with the employment of a nutritionist in the maternal and child health unit. Starting perhaps with the education of pregnant women and mothers of infants in the fundamentals of good nutrition, her activities gradually broadened. With the addition of other nutritionists, all age groups and the various health programs having nutrition components were served; this culminated in the formation of a separate unit for nutrition services. Yet, even in 1950, 34 of the 45 state nutrition units were still to be found within the divisions or bureaus of maternal and child health (1).

This is true to a lesser extent of dental health services, of medical social work in health departments, and of various types of specialized services for handicapped persons in both health departments and other governmental agencies. The availability of Federal grants-in-aid for child health services was an important factor in these developments.

Several other reasons have been advanced for the pioneer role of child health services. Preventive services during the prenatal period and the early years of life are often more effective than similar measures at later ages. Many specific problems of health and disease in childhood are more susceptible to attack through an organized program than comparable problems in adult life. Moreover, health benefits to children carry over for a longer proportion of the life span than those to individuals in the middle or later years of life. These three reasons are often only theoretical considerations; in practice they may be of less importance than the child's emotional appeal to the public and to legislative bodies.

The compelling factor of national defense has also strengthened the case for more adequate health services for children, based on the findings of the selective service examinations in two world wars. The conclusion has been drawn that some, at least, of the rejections for military service could have been avoided if more attention had been paid to the health problems of the selectees when they were children. Studies have also shown that a large proportion of youths rejected for military duty for health reasons showed evidence of the same conditions in their school medical examinations fifteen years earlier (2).

Health services for children have therefore been developed for a variety of reasons. Some are based on sound principles of public health planning. Often, on the other hand, new services are initiated as a result of popular pressure, even though more urgent and readily solvable problems remain untouched. The practicing physician should realize that health officers bear the responsibility of carrying out the mandates even of laws whose passage they may have opposed (3). Under such circumstances, health officers must administer the required services for the maximum benefit of the community and with the least disturbance of possibly more essential activities.

Patterns of Administration of Child Health Services. The provision of health services for mothers and children has been set forth as one of the six essential functions of a local health department (4). The platform of the American Medical Association devotes 2 of its 10 points to prenatal care and childbirth and infant and child care (5). Singling out the problems of mothers and children among the essentials of public health services by leading medical and public health groups points to the need of maintaining the integrity of these services.

The field of child health has sometimes been called public health with age limits. This statement neglects the different approach needed in child health services, since the child is a growing organism with special physical and emotional needs. Nevertheless, it does bring out the fact that the diversified services of health agencies must somehow be brought together to serve the best interests of children as individuals, that is, they should be child-centered as well as service-centered.

Two patterns of organization have grown up in the administration of child health services. Under the first, the various types of health services for children are brought together in a single major unit within the health department. Under the second, specialized services may be set up under separate units to serve all age groups including children. The former is better suited to meeting the needs of the children as individuals, but it is more difficult to use the services of medical and other specialists efficiently under this administrative pattern. The latter arrangement has the advantage of using specialists on the staff to serve both children and adults, but carries with it the danger that the total needs of the child will be lost from sight in focusing on the specific disease or disability.

In practice, historical developments and personal interests may decide the type of administrative pattern, although sound arguments have been advanced for both arrangements. Whatever the arrangement, one person within each department should have specific responsibility to examine proposed or existing programs to advise on their place in promoting the total health of children. It is immaterial whether this person is given an official title such as coordinator of child health services or if he is simply the director of maternal and child health services with a dual responsibility.

Interrelationships of Official Health Agencies. Health agencies in local, state, and Federal governments are doing a single job with the same objective in mind. If adequate local health departments existed throughout the nation, it would be possible to approach the ideal of having all official health functions funneled through them, whatever the ultimate source of supporting funds. Unfortunately only about two-thirds of the population of the United States live in communities with full-time local health departments, and many of these departments are very poorly developed. State health agencies have therefore had to provide direct services for children in wide areas of the country, when they have been provided at all. In the smaller and more sparsely populated states, direct services to children by states agencies have been and probably will continue to be extensive. Even Federal health agencies deal directly with individuals in the distribution of booklets on health education, and some even provide health services to individuals and organizations in local communities.

Local Health Agencies. All services of local health departments bear directly or indirectly upon the health of children. A brief review of the five essential health services other than maternal and child health, as outlined by leaders in the public health field, brings this out more clearly (4):

1. Recording of births, sickness, and deaths; their verification for completeness and accuracy; their tabulation, interpretation, analysis, and publication. Without these data it is impossible to determine where problems exist, to plan services adequately, and to evaluate the results of services.

2. Control of all communicable diseases affecting or threatening the people in the area. The child health program is specifically concerned with the prevention and control of the major communicable diseases of childhood, but even these cannot be adequately controlled unless the whole population is considered. Furthermore, in some areas, communicable diseases not falling into the group of childhood diseases may be a more serious threat to the child than, say, diphtheria or scarlet fever. Hookworm, malaria, and other parasitic diseases, although affecting the population as a whole, may take the greatest toll in childhood. Typhoid fever, although less severe in children than in adults, can be controlled only by community measures.

3. Making the environment of man one of sanitary safety. The provision of safe water and milk supplies has been a major factor in the reduction of infant mortality and morbidity in the past half century. Environmental sanitation must also be given major credit for control of the parasitic diseases previously mentioned and for the control of dysentery of bacillary origin, which was the major causative factor of much of the diarrheal diseases of infancy of past years. Environmental

sanitation has recently been called upon to provide new types of services. This profession supervises the introduction of fluoride into drinking-water supplies to reduce the incidence of dental caries, which is being widely adopted as a routine public health procedure. Environmental sanitarians may license and supervise commercial infant-formula services where these exist.

4. Provision of diagnostic laboratory procedures essential for early and accurate diagnosis of at least the locally important communicable diseases and to give scientific basis for control of environment. To this may be added the purchase, distribution, and even the preparation of biologicals for the prevention and treatment of communicable diseases. Health departments also distribute capsules of silver nitrate solution for the prevention of ophthalmia neonatorum.

5. Health education. Although health education is inherent in every phase of maternal and child health activities, as will be discussed later, all health education which affects family living and the assumption of community responsibilities for health will influence the health of children as well.

Patterns of Local Health Services. Local health jurisdictions range in size from that of New York City, with a population of nearly 8 million, to small county health departments covering less than 10,000 persons in sparsely settled areas. The diversity of administrative patterns between these two extremes is naturally enormous. The larger the health unit, the greater is the degree of specialization possible. In New York City, for example, the child health unit is headed by an assistant commissioner and has major subdivisions responsible for the supervision of maternity and newborn services, for school health services, for the care of physically handicapped children, and for the supervision of day care and institutional care of children. It even has a smaller unit responsible solely for the administration and supervision of child health conferences. Full-time and part-time specialized medical, nursing, and other professional personnel are employed in each unit. In the small full-time health departments, the entire professional staff often consists of only the health officer, a public health nurse, and a sanitary inspector. In many of the smaller county health departments, the health officer conducts child health conferences and immunization clinics himself, further reducing the time available to him for planning and coordination of health services in the area.

No one health department provides all or nearly all the services described in this book, nor are all the services needed universally. In like manner, there is no typical pattern of administration of child health services in the county and city health departments of the nation. In practice, child health services may be administered by several units of a local health department, even when the unit has a full-time director of maternal and child health. Conversely, the child health unit may be responsible for certain programs serving adults as well, such as nutrition, medical social work, mental health, and home accident control programs. Local health units even supervise and license day-care centers for children.

State Health Services. State health departments are in a strategic position in relation to Federal and local health agencies. They are usually in a stronger financial position than local health departments. In addition, state health agencies are the receiving and disbursing agents for Federal grants-in-aid. The state agencies exert a strong influence on the direction and character of local health services through financial aid from both state and Federal sources, through the development and maintenance of standards, and through their supervisory and consultative functions.

In most states, the primary responsibility for safeguarding the health of the population rests with the state government and is delegated by law, with specified limitations, to the counties and other local jurisdictions; some of the largest cities may operate independently to a greater degree. It has been common for child health services to develop first in large metropolitan centers. When this has occurred, it has served as a stimulus for similar developments in the state health department. The first concern of the newly established unit in the state health department has generally been the promotion of new services in areas of the state outside the large cities. This development was stimulated also by funds available under the Social Security Act, which requires that special attention be paid to rural areas and areas in special need in the use of these funds. In recent years, more state aid has been made available to large cities as well as to rural counties. Instances may also be cited of close cooperation in special studies and in-service training programs for child health personnel on the part of state and large city departments of health.

Administrative Variations in State Health Departments. Under the Federal Constitution the responsibility for safeguarding the health and welfare of its citizens is reserved to the states. This fact of local jurisdiction is the major reason for the wide variation in child health programs in the various states. A single urgent problem or dramatic incident often precipitated the start of programs and determined their nature and content thereafter.

Many official health services for children are administered by agencies other than health departments in numerous states. Services for physically handicapped children are administered by welfare departments in nine states or territories, by state universities in four, by special commissions in six, and by departments of education in three. In only 31 states or territories are these services administered by health departments, in 14 as separate units and in 17 combined with the maternal and child health unit (6). Administration of school health services is divided between state departments of education and health. Supervision of hospital services for mothers, newborn infants, and older children, with or without licensing powers, may be a function of the state maternal and child health unit, or it may reside in a special commission, in a welfare department, or in another unit of the health department. The tendency is toward increased complexity in the administrative structure of health services. In 1940 there was a range of 6 to 18 agencies of state government participating in health services of all types, as compared with a spread of 7 to 32 in 1950, when 16 states exceeded the maximum of 18 a decade earlier (7).

Financial Support. The costs of health services for children are met from a diversity of sources. Tax funds and public contributions to voluntary agencies, even when expenditures for medical care by welfare agencies are included, constitute only a small fraction of the total expenditures. The greater part of the costs is met by families from their own resources. It is probably true that the relative proportion has not changed significantly in the past several decades, despite the great increase in governmental appropriations and in an even greater proportional increase in the amount of funds donated by the public to the voluntary health organizations.

Where a county or city health department is functioning, the costs of maternal and child health services are usually included in the total health budget of the department. In many states, a varying proportion of these costs are met by the state in the form of state aid. In addition, direct grants for specific services may be provided by the state, using either state tax funds or Federal grants-in-aid. In some of the smaller states, all local governmental health services are provided directly by the state department of health, or the full costs of the local health services, though administered locally, are met in full by the state. In some of the larger states not well served by county health departments, the states may provide local health services directly through districts covering several counties. The costs of services for handicapped children are still met largely from state and Federal funds although, in the wealthier states, localities are bearing an increasing share. The costs of medical care of handicapped children in state-university hospitals and in related services are usually covered in the budget of the medical centers from state appropriations.

Federal Health Agencies. Health services for children in the Federal government are to be found in a number of agencies, mainly located in the Department of Health, Education, and Welfare. The reorganization plan which created the department from the former Federal Security Agency in 1953 permitted the department head, a secretary with cabinet status, to establish new central services within the department. It did not alter the previously existing responsibilities of individual units of the Federal Security Agency.

The major portion of health services for children in the Department of Health, Education, and Welfare are concentrated in the Children's Bureau. The Bureau has consistently fought over the years for improved standards of child care. It was a pioneer in promoting the adoption of adequate merit systems for personnel employed in state and local child health programs. The major responsibility of the Children's Bureau in relation to the states and localities is its administration of the grants-in-aid program for the extension and improvement of maternal and child health and crippled children's services.

The regulations of the Children's Bureau set forth the manner in which the states must meet the general requirements of the Social Security Act in the use of Federal funds. Each state must submit a plan covering services financed either directly by Federal funds or by state matching funds, that is, through funds appropriated by the state or local governments, for child health services. The grants-in-aid must be allocated only to state health departments and special crippled children's agencies for use in the manner set forth in the state plans. The grants-in-aid are divided into two parts. One portion, Fund A, is made available to each state according to a formula based on the birth rate, the extent of the rural area, and the per capita income of the state; this portion must be matched by an appropriation of state and local funds. The other part, Fund B, does not have to be matched by the states. A portion of Fund B is allocated on the basis of the health needs of each state. Another portion of Fund B is reserved for the development of new types of services and model programs or for special training programs which serve the needs of several or all the states. As was the intention at the time of passage of the Social Security Act, the grants-in-aid have stimulated increasing state and local appropriations for child health services.

Through its Division of Research in Child Development the Children's Bureau continues to serve its original function of investigating and reporting upon all aspects of child life. This division cooperated closely with the American Academy of Pediatrics in its study of child health services. The Clearinghouse for Research in Child Life was organized as a function of the Children's Bureau in 1948. The Clearinghouse gathers information on all studies being carried out throughout the nation that bear on the health of children; it makes this information available to research workers in order to prevent duplication and to disclose areas of research which are apparently receiving insufficient attention. The Children's Bureau has also contributed a noteworthy public service in its series of "Bulletins for Parents." The most famous of these, "Infant Care," has been distributed in millions of copies and has been translated into a number of foreign languages.

The Children's Bureau has decentralized many of its functions through the regional offices, bringing it into a closer working relationship with the states. Grants-in-aid are administered through these offices. Equally important, however, are the consultative services offered through the regional offices to the states. The regional staffs of the Children's Bureau are in reality teams of specialists covering the medical, nursing, medical social work, and nutrition aspects of child health programs. Additional specialized consultants in dental health, mental health, and other fields are available from the Washington office of the

Bureau. These consultative services have been of particular value in fostering continuity of services in states in which frequent changes in administrative personnel have occurred.

The Public Health Service carries out many functions which bear directly and indirectly upon the health of the nation's children. It promotes more adequate state and local generalized public health services, and it administers grants-in-aid for general public health services and for specialized programs for the control of tuberculosis, venereal diseases, and cancer, and several other types of health problems. Its grants-in-aid for mental health services are used extensively for child guidance clinics and for the training of personnel needed for the treatment of emotionally disturbed children. Through special appropriations for the purpose, it has sent out demonstration teams to the states for the application of sodium fluoride to the teeth to reduce the incidence of dental caries. These demonstration teams have been a major factor in the rapid extension in the use of this prophylactic procedure by public health agencies and by dentists in their private practices. Grants to the states for community programs for the control of heart disease have included services for children with rheumatic and congenital heart disease. The Public Health Service may make a portion of its funds available directly to local communities and institutions (8).

The National Institutes of Health administered by the Public Health Service conduct basic and clinical research in many problems of disease in childhood, such as dental caries, communicable diseases, and heart disease. One large grant supports a long-range study by the Child Research Council of Denver. This study seeks to develop more reliable methods for determining patterns of normal growth and development by correlating the physical, mental, and emotional factors involved.

The National Office of Vital Statistics, transferred to the Public Health Service from the Bureau of the Census in 1946, is responsible for gathering and studying statistics relating to birth, mortality, and morbidity. It has promoted more complete and more accurate reporting of births and deaths.

The Office of Vocational Rehabilitation is responsible for administering grants to the states for services to handicapped persons over fourteen years of age who can be rehabilitated for part- or full-time employment. Needed medical treatment is provided as part of the rehabilitation process, along with vocational training and guidance.

VOLUNTARY HEALTH AGENCIES

A voluntary health agency has been defined as

an organization that is administered by an autonomous board which holds meetings, collects funds for its support chiefly from private sources, and expends money, whether with or without paid workers, in conducting a program directed primarily to furthering the public health by providing health services or health education, or by advancing research or legislation related to health, or by a combination of these activities. (9)

There are probably over 20,000 national, state, and local voluntary health agencies in the United States. The extraordinary development of the voluntary health agency has been typically a phenomenon of the democratic scene in the United States. It is based on the desire of persons, individually and in groups, to solve health problems, as they see them, by their own voluntary activities. The financial support of the voluntary agencies has come mainly from a multitude of small contributions, in contrast to the few large endowments which established the great philanthropic foundations.

Since the dissolution of the American Child Health Association, no one organization has concerned itself on a national scale with the health of the child as a whole. Nevertheless, children have benefited greatly from the services rendered by many specialized voluntary health agencies. A number of organizations have based their appeal on the needs of children and have devoted the major portion of their funds to health services for children. These funds are now a highly significant portion of the total health budget of the nation. Most of the funds collected by voluntary health organizations would otherwise go into socially less productive channels. In 1949 a total of 300 million dollars was recorded in philanthropic contributions for health services by the American people. There is no way of estimating what proportion of this sum was devoted to health services for children.

Functions of Voluntary Health Agencies. Voluntary agencies differ widely in the types of services they render. Formed in most instances because of the existence of some unmet health need, the new agency has usually concentrated on a campaign to bring the problem to the attention of the general public. Health education has thus been a basic function of most voluntary health agencies. Some agencies have restricted themselves to this function and to working with other groups in the community to promote the needed services. Most voluntary health agencies have gone beyond this, to finance programs for the discovery and treatment of individuals suffering from conditions with which the agencies are concerned, even to the extent of financing prolonged hospitalization and aftercare.

Voluntary health agencies make their greatest contribution by invading new fields of health activity and by developing new techniques which have not been well enough established to be included as routine public health activities. Conversely, some voluntary agencies have called attention to outmoded public health activities while demonstrating new methods.

Demonstration of the value of these new activities, at least as far as a particular community is concerned, draws public attention and develops public and professional support for the projects. Local voluntary health agencies may tip the balance in favor of a major expansion of needed services by supplementing available funds for items which are not readily budgeted at first from other sources. The actual monetary contribution may be small, possibly only enough to cover the salary of a medical social worker, or the purchase of material needed to maintain a roster of handicapped children, but it may make the difference between success and failure of a proposed program. When direct medical and hospital care has been financed on a broad scale by voluntary health agencies, organizations as wealthy as the National Foundation for Infantile Paralysis have found themselves in financial straits and have had to issue emergency appeals for funds. The steadily rising costs of hospitalization, the complexity of the services required, and the increased case load resulting from education of the public in the value of the health services provided have been some of the factors responsible for this dilemma.

Nongovernmental health agencies on the local scene are legion, particularly in relation to orthopedically handicapping conditions in childhood. Many of these are concerned with the development and maintenance of a single institution for treatment or rehabilitation. Quarters and other physical facilities for special rehabilitative units for handicapped children may also be provided from voluntary funds, often with the idea in mind that the costs of services provided in these centers will be gradually assumed by official agencies.

Other types of organizations with primary interests outside the health field assist with the provision of health services for children as well. Local service clubs often make contributions that cannot be obtained readily through other sources. They may provide funds for eyeglasses, braces, and hearing aids. This is frequently done on a highly personal basis. A club may "adopt" or sponsor a particular physically handicapped child and arrange for his complete medical care and even education. Some major service organizations have built and maintained large hospitals and clinics for handicapped children, especially those with orthopedic problems. Service clubs and similar organizations are generally not interested in ferreting out and studying health problems. They are more likely to lend their support to health projects already prepared in package form, so that they may have a clear idea of what needs to be done and what the cost will be.

A change in attitude toward all philanthropic endeavor has permeated the health field as well. The slogan, "not so much in helping people in trouble as in helping people out of trouble," was coined about 1930. Since then this has been "broadened into also helping people to avoid trouble, and helping them to realize their own full capacities for work and play and growth." (10) In the health field this tendency has expressed itself in increasing attention to basic research relating to each condition. Some of the major agencies have contributed large sums of money for research into the prevention, causes, and treatment of disease. Several of these agencies have expressed the desire to spend even greater amounts for this type of work. They have been unable to do so because the rapidly increasing costs of medical and hospital services have drained their financial reserves.

Fear has been expressed that the multiplicity of new specialized voluntary health agencies would result in decreased public support for all. Though this may be the ultimate outcome, there is still no evidence that it is actually happening. More agencies than ever, operating in different fields and sometimes even competing for funds to meet the same problem, have been the beneficiaries of generous public support.

The danger of throwing the community child health program out of balance by the newly developed, specialized services has also been pointed out. Granting this danger, practical advantages may well outweigh it in the long run. For example, some of the agencies interested in specific disease problems have been confronted with the perennial scarcity of specialized professional and technical personnel, as in physical and speech therapy. Having created a demand for such personnel, the agencies concerned were in a position to provide fellowships and to encourage young people in other ways to enter these fields. Thus, therapists became available for treatment of children with certain handicapping conditions other than those for which they were originally trained. Gross imbalance of services for different conditions becomes obvious to a community in the long run. The very imbalance provides an increasingly powerful argument for the development of other badly needed services.

Services of Volunteers. Apart from a core of paid full-time workers, the organizational activities of voluntary health agencies are usually conducted by persons who donate their time and energies without remuneration other than the satisfaction and prestige inherent in the activity. In addition, some voluntary agencies assist through the provision of volunteer service in more direct health activities. The volunteer may participate in a health survey, help in hospitals or clinics, or transport children and their parents who cannot reach hospitals and clinics without help. Local organizations of an essentially social nature may require a specified amount of volunteer work each year for persons to gain or maintain membership in the group.

When volunteer assistance is provided, it is most effective when done on an organized basis with definite assignments and alternates for each assignment. Volunteers must be selected and trained carefully for their duties. Volunteer service is a very useful function and one that may be more productive than contribution of funds. Volunteers should be given full recognition for their services if they are to be expected to continue to provide services over a long period.

Foundations. The foundation differs from the voluntary health agency in that its income is generally derived from endowments by single individuals or families, rather than from drives for public funds. The trustees of the foundation are selected and serve under the terms of the endowment, in contrast to the autonomous board of the voluntary agency. Some of the voluntary health agencies which have the word *foundation* in their names are not foundations in the sense of this definition.

Foundations for health purposes rank third in number, after those devoting attention to education and social welfare (10). Some of the largest and wealthiest foundations, however, have concentrated entirely or largely upon health problems. Several of the foundations which have made the greatest contributions to public health and especially to the well-being of children have been self-liquidating over a specified period. Under the terms of their endowment, a set portion of the capital must be spent each year in addition to the income. The best example of this was the Couzens Children's Fund of Michigan which went out of existence in 1949 after twenty years of noteworthy service. The Commonwealth Fund supported basic demonstrations in the child health field in the 1920's (11). At the present time foundations are active in breaking new ground in the areas of nutrition, mental health, and regionalization of hospital and medical services. A recent development has been the establishment of foundations by large industrial corporations for the support of research in pediatrics and other health fields.

PROFESSIONAL ORGANIZATIONS

Organizations of professional personnel resemble the voluntary health agencies in some respects. Professional organizations and voluntary health agencies have a common goal of improvement of health and related services. Both have made major contributions in promoting and extending health services for children. The differences in approach to health problems have been determined largely by the nature of the membership of the two types of organizations.

As representatives of groups of individuals with common professional and personal interests, professional organizations must and should be concerned with safeguarding and promoting the prerogatives and interests of their membership. In almost all instances this has been done in such a way as to raise the standards of care rendered the public. Many professional organizations have developed minimum qualifications for membership which have been adopted widely by official and voluntary agencies as guides in their own personnel policies. Others have suggested sets of qualifications for the express purpose of providing guides to other groups (10).

Educational Functions. Beyond their original functions, professional organizations have participated in broad programs for the improvement of child health in cooperation with other agencies. Education of their own membership is, however, the function they can best carry out and which can be performed to only a limited extent through other means.

Because they are representatives of their own professional groups, they find their membership receptive to their guidance and advice. They are an excellent medium for graduate professional education through technical programs at meetings, regular or special publications, radio programs, and more recently, through television. Some provide technical consultation services by distribution of reference material on request.

Types of Organizations. Professional organizations range in membership from those consisting of persons in a single specialty or even subspecialty to those embracing all types of professional personnel in a broad field. The former is typified by the American Academy of Pediatrics. At the other extreme is the American Public Health Association, which admits to membership not only professional personnel but also nonprofessional persons who are interested in public health in general or in any special field within public health. There are also variant patterns of administrative structure. The American Heart Association, for example, originally consisted only of professional persons, almost exclusively physicians with primary interest and training in heart disease. In 1948 the Association broadened its activities to become one of the leading voluntary health agencies, soliciting and obtaining large contributions by mass drives for funds. At the present time there are organizations in existence representing personnel in the broad fields of medicine, dentistry, nursing, medical social work, and nutrition, and in physical, speech, occupational, and other specialized types of therapy as well as in specialties in these and other fields. The contributions of some of the broader organizations have been presented in Chapter 4.

CITED REFERENCES

1. Nutrition Programs in State Health Departments, Prepared by a Subcommittee of the Commitee on Diagnosis and Pathology of Nutritional Deficiencies of the National Research Council, *Pub. Health Rep.,* Vol. 65, pp. 411–445, Mar. 31, 1950.
2. CIOCCO, ANTONIO, HENRY KLEIN, and CARROLL E. PALMER, Child Health and the Selective Service Physical Standards, *Pub. Health Rep.,* Vol. 56, pp. 2365–2375, Dec. 12, 1941.
3. ANDERSON, GAYLORD W., Public Health—A Mandate from the People, *Am. J. Pub. Health,* Vol. 42, pp. 1367–1373, November, 1952.
4. EMERSON, HAVEN, Public Health and Medical Care for the Community and the Individual, *J.A.M.A.,* Vol. 148, pp. 41–44, Jan. 5, 1952.
5. The Ten Point National Health Program of the American Medical Association, *J.A.M.A.,* Vol. 136, pp. 261–266, Jan. 24, 1948.

6. "Services for Crippled Children in the States," Folder No. 38, Children's Bureau, Washington, D.C., 1952.
7. MOUNTIN, JOSEPH W., EVELYN FLOOK, and EDWARD E. MINTY, "Distribution of Health Services in the Structure of State Government, 1950—Part 1: Administrative Provisions for State Health Services," Public Health Service Publication No. 184, Washington, D.C., 1952.
8. WARNER, ESTELLA F., and EVELYN FLOOK, Resumé of Public Health Service Grant-in-aid Programs Providing Medical Services, *Pub. Health Rep.,* Vol. 66, pp. 167–182, Feb. 9, 1951.
9. GUNN, SELSKAR M., and PHILIP S. PLATT, "Voluntary Health Agencies," The Ronald Press Company, New York, 1945.
10. ANDREWS, F. EMERSON, "Philanthropic Giving," Russell Sage Foundation, New York, 1950.
11. DINWIDDIE, COURTENAY, "Child Health and the Community: An Interpretation of Cooperative Effort in Public Health," Commonwealth Fund, Harvard University Press, Cambridge, Mass., 1931.

ADDITIONAL REFERENCES

1. MOUNTIN, JOSEPH W., and JACK C. HALDEMAN, State Health Organization Today and a Decade Ago, *J.A.M.A.,* Vol. 151, pp. 35–37, Jan. 3, 1953.
2. ANDREWS, F. EMERSON, "Corporation Giving," Russell Sage Foundation, New York, 1952.

6 IMPLEMENTING THE CHILD HEALTH PROGRAM

Knowledge that a health problem exists and planning a program designed to overcome the problem are only preliminary steps in bringing the program into being. Many factors, tangible and intangible, may obstruct full application of a program considered desirable by leaders in civic and professional circles in a community. Lack of general community understanding of the value of the proposed services may be a major stumbling block. Outmoded laws may require health activities inconsistent with the real needs of the community; even the absence of enabling legislation may prevent the development of needed services. Poorly developed standards of care may result in services of lower quality than the resources of the community warrant.

Several techniques are in general use in promoting and maintaining community child health services. These techniques are basic functions of the program itself. Public acceptance of the program may be sought through special demonstrations or as one of the aspects of public health education. Adequate standards for community health services must be developed as an aid to services of the best possible quality. The physician in private practice should have a deep interest in these activities because they affect not only his professional relationships with the public, but also relationships with patients in his own practice. General information in booklets on child care, for example, suggest questions which parents may raise with their physicians. Most health agencies are eager to have the comments or criticisms of practicing physicians on any aspect of their work; the physician who feels that the content of any educational material is unsound should not hesitate in making his feelings known to the agency concerned, especially if he has constructive suggestions to offer.

Similarly, the practicing physician has an opportunity to influence the quality of community health services by contributing the fruits of his experience when his advice is sought as an individual or as a member of a medical organization in the formulation of standards for various health services.

STANDARDS, LAWS, AND REGULATIONS

Improvement of health services for children requires the development and maintenance of standards in all aspects of the program. Standards are potent guides to the achievement of better health for children, never ends in themselves. Unless they are carefully conceived, diligently promoted, and revised periodically in the light of changed conditions and newer knowledge, standards are apt to become dead letters or even drags on progress. Continued use of antiquated or ill-conceived standards diverts attention from more productive activities. Of even greater importance, the agency responsible for the promulgation of unrealistic standards suffers the loss of respect of the individuals and groups expected to meet the standards.

Standards in health work are guides for measuring the adequacy, quantitatively and qualitatively, of health services and facilities. They may be set up as minimum standards, usually in the form of regulations or laws; or they may be developed as optimum standards or desirable goals. Each type of standard has its own essential role, whether used by governmental or voluntary agencies. Minimum standards should not be put into effect unless there is a strong likelihood of obtaining broad compliance with them at the time they become effective; if certain of the regulations require a period of time for compliance, the effective date for these should be set at a later date. Standards of more than a minimum nature, as goals for achievement, are not set up with an effective date in mind, but even these should not be set so high as to be impossible of attainment with reasonable effort and expenditure of funds.

Uses of Standards. Standards in the sense of desirable goals have been developed extensively by both official and voluntary agencies. Good examples of these are the recommendations on hospital care of full-term and premature infants issued by the Children's Bureau and the American Academy of Pediatrics (1). These standards are extremely useful guideposts in evaluating existing hospital facilities and services and in planning new hospital nurseries. They are entirely of an educational nature, unless they are adopted in unchanged or modified form by some agency which has the power to promulgate and enforce minimum standards. Evaluation schedules, described earlier, are really goal-setting standards.

Minimum standards are used by voluntary agencies in two chief ways. Voluntary agencies may set standards which facilities and services operating in a given field must meet to be approved or accredited by the agency. The American Heart Association, for example, has developed minimum standards for cardiovascular clinics which are used by the Association in its approval of clinics (2). The request for such approval on the part of the clinic administrator is entirely voluntary; approval is desirable for the prestige it brings to the clinic in the community. Standards of hospital care have been raised over the years by the activities of the American College of Surgeons and other organizations. The other use of minimum standards is in relation to direct health services which voluntary health agencies administer or finance. By insisting that personnel or facilities in these services meet the standards set, the voluntary health agencies can do much to maintain the quality of these services.

While governmental health agencies make frequent use of minimum standards for the services they administer, they also develop and enforce minimum standards for services affecting the community at large when the welfare of the community is shown to be involved. Laws granting these powers must be within limitations of the state constitution or the local charter, or in the case of regulations, they must be within the scope of the law on which they are based. An objective may be gained by different approaches without necessarily introducing new legislation. For example, the physical arrangements and nursing techniques in nurseries for newborn infants may be covered in a regulation aimed at control of diarrhea of the newborn, which in turn may derive from the general responsibility of the health department to prevent the spread of communicable diseases wherever the danger of outbreaks exists. An existing law may require the licensing and supervision of the entire hospital; in that event, standards for maternity and newborn services could be approached directly as part of the total hospital supervision program. When the licensing function is placed in some unit of government other than the health agency, the latter may be called upon to assist in the development of standards and in the associated educational campaign to bring services above the standards.

Laws and regulations are minimum standards which should never be put into force unless there is full intention and possibility of carrying them out completely and fairly promptly. That this is often not the case in practice is not necessarily the fault of the agency given the responsibility for enforcement. Laws should be stated in general terms, with the objectives clearly set forth and the limits of power of the enforcing agency defined. Detail in the law is undesirable, since it fixes practice which cannot be changed unless the law is amended. This is possible in some states only after a lapse of two years since many state legislatures meet biennially and they may be disinterested even then in apparently minor administrative changes. The law should also state specifically what type of regulations is needed to implement its provisions. The power of drawing up regulations for enforcing a law may be vested in a commissioner of health, in a general board of health, or in a special board or commission.

State laws and regulations usually take precedence over local laws and regulations, unless localities are specifically exempted from their provisions. On the other hand, Federal laws relating to child health services officially have no bearing on local and state practices. Actually, the Social Security Act and the regulations of the Children's Bureau based on the Act have profoundly affected the standards of health services for children in their own communities almost as if they were local ordinances. The reason for this has been presented before: the various states cannot obtain Federal funds for child health services unless they meet the requirements of Federal regulations not only in services financed by the Federal funds, but also in services financed by state and local funds budgeted by the states to match the Federal funds.

Development and Maintenance of Standards. It is a rare exception when standards must be developed without some precedent as a guide. Recommended standards for many types of services are available from the Children's Bureau or Public Health Service, or from the American Medical Association, the Academy of Pediatrics, the American College of Surgeons, and other professional organizations and voluntary health agencies listed in the Appendix. These should be studied along with standards developed by state and local health departments or crippled children's agencies, which can be obtained by communicating with the agencies mentioned. When parts of the proposed standards can be tested experimentally, this either may be done locally or the services of an outside agency may be obtained for the purpose. The advice of technical experts in the field should be sought at the start of the process, and they should be consulted regularly until the final draft is completed.

The approach to achieving and maintaining standards should be thought of as an educational process to the greatest possible extent. In the case of more than minimum standards, implementation must be entirely through educational means, since there are no legal teeth in the standard. Even in the enforcement of health laws and regulations, use is rarely made of implied or actual police powers except as a last resort for a few serious offenders. Efforts are generally exerted by health agencies to raise standards as near to the optimum as possible, rather than aiming only at compliance with minimum requirements.

In the educational process, all the techniques of consultation and advisory services may be used. Special institutes, in which full participation by professional groups is encouraged, may be held in different localities. Articles may be prepared for publication in professional periodicals. A valuable device is the use of questionnaires for the persons and agencies affected by proposed requirements, so that they may have an opportunity to review their own situation. All these activities should be carried out before the new minimum standards go into effect, whenever this is possible.

It is often the first thought of legislators to impose a system of licensure as a means of raising standards of health services. Licensing by itself cannot improve standards; it must be accompanied by an educational campaign with consultative services to the institutions or facilities being licensed. Under some circumstances, licensing may defeat its own purpose. In some states having hospital licensure systems, the limited number of available hospital beds in certain areas has forced the licensing agency to issue licenses to hospitals with obviously poor standards. Continued licensing of these inadequate institutions tends to sour the better hospitals to any recommendations of the licensing agency for improvement of their services above minimum requirements for licensure.

Supervision of midwives provides another example of the limitations of licensing procedures. In many rural areas with large Negro or Spanish-speaking populations, the only care available during pregnancy and delivery is that provided by poorly educated and untrained midwives. It would be highly undesirable to have licensing standards low enough to approve the type of maternity care given by the local midwives. It is more reasonable to require registration of the midwives to bring them to light first. After this has been done, a gradual but rudimentary training of the midwives can be instituted until more stringent control is feasible. In many states in which obstetrical care by physicians is generally available, strict licensing laws are in force which make it almost impossible for a new midwife to obtain a license.

The full process of developing and maintaining standards is exemplified in the New York State program for the control of diarrhea of the newborn in hospital nurseries (3). In the development of a new regulation of the state sanitary code to cover minimum standards for newborn nurseries, including space requirements, nursing personnel, unit care of infants, "suspect" nurseries, and terminal heating of formulas, a number of steps were taken. The records of the investigations of outbreaks of diarrhea of the newborn in the state and elsewhere were reviewed to disclose the causative factors, so that measures to eliminate these danger spots could be required in the proposed regulation. Recommendations of the American Academy of Pediatrics and the Children's Bureau were reviewed carefully, along with the findings of the research program of the Michigan Department of Health. Laboratory studies were carried out on the efficacy of several methods of terminal heating of infant formulas to destroy test organisms. Technical experts from various fields were consulted. As the basic requirements took shape, they were reviewed in detail with representatives of the Medical Society of the State of New York and of the hospital association. The regulation as enacted by the state's Public Health Council permitted deferment for a period of two years of the requirements on size of nurseries and maximum number of infants per nurse.

Prior to enactment of the regulation, a series of institutes were held throughout the state, at which obstetricians and pediatricians in charge of hospital services, hospital administrators, and nurses had opportunity to discuss the proposals at length. Detailed questionnaires were prepared to help responsible persons in each hospital review their own situation prior to taking necessary action. The questions concerning minimum requirements were underlined, but a series of additional questions were asked to encourage hospitals to raise their standards as far above the minimum as possible. In a number of instances, the physicians in charge of the newborn nurseries and the hospital administrators privately welcomed the new requirements in giving them the ammunition they had needed for a long time to obtain approval from their hospital boards for badly needed changes in the newborn nurseries. Consultant medical and nursing personnel from the State Department of Health reviewed the problems in various hospitals on the spot with representatives of the hospitals. Intensive institutes of one and two weeks duration in the care of newborn infants were held for supervising public health nurses and hospital nurses. Responsibility for periodic inspection and review of hospital newborn nurseries rested with the local health department or state district health office in whose area the hospital was located. Through this educational process alone, nearly all the hospitals vastly improved their newborn nurseries, often into model nurseries far beyond the requirements of the sanitary code. As it turned out, the program attained far more than its stated objectives.

This description of the process of developing, implementing, and maintaining standards is not intended to imply that sole or even major credit for the success attained rested with the program as presented. The standards were developed at a time when problems in newborn nurseries were receiving nationwide attention on the part of hospital, medical, and nursing groups. Hospital construction or renovation was taking place on a grand scale, so that entirely modern newborn nurseries could be provided in many hospitals with a minimum of effort and expense. The program centering about the sanitary code standards served to crystallize the widespread interest and provided the consultative and training facilities needed particularly by the smaller hospitals to help effect the subsequent improvements.

Technical Advisory Services. The subject of technical consultants and advisory committees and groups is considered here because one of their chief functions is assistance in the development of standards. Advisers, individually or in groups, should not have administrative functions, nor should they be expected or permitted to make final decisions of any kind. The responsibility for such decisions must rest with the head of the agency with which the advisers are working. If this is not made clear to the physicians being asked to serve in an advisory capacity, they should request an unequivocal statement of their functions and responsibilities. The advisers should be chosen on the basis of their outstanding technical knowledge and judgment and their accepted preeminence in their chosen fields. The prestige of an advisory group is often of great value in gaining acceptance for new standards.

Consultants should not be appointed simply because they represent particular organizations, nor should appointment in an advisory capacity be used as a means of conferring recognition upon them. The advisers, in other words, should be individuals in whom the program director and his staff can place utmost confidence. When liaison functions between organizations are to be served, these can best be carried out through coordinating groups representing the organizations concerned. Technical consultants and advisory groups should be appointed for a specified period. This will prevent misunderstanding if an advisory group should be dissolved after the function for which it was appointed has been discharged, and it will allow changes in these groups when points of emphasis in the program are modified.

DEMONSTRATIONS

It is rare, indeed, for a community-wide child health program to spring into being all at once. The usual course is one of spasmodic evolution, at a slow pace at first, but with more rapid progress when community acceptance and support have been won. For acceptance to be gained, the values of the services must be demonstrated. Demonstrations may take several forms in local health programs. Services may be concentrated within a limited geographic area, with the hope of expansion as soon as additional funds and facilities can be obtained; or they may be provided for a limited time with the understanding that continuing support will be forthcoming if the merits of the services are shown. In either case, care must be taken to provide a service of satisfactory quality and quantity under adequate supervision to ensure the results desired. A service of poor quality or one with insufficient personnel to make its influence felt in the demonstration area may well "demonstrate" an undesirable service, which may be used as an argument against such services for years to come. A third type of local demonstration is the provision of a single service of superior quality. A child health conference staffed by highly qualified physicians and nurses may be used to promote child health supervision in the entire community through private resources. A child health conference of this quality may also serve as a training facility. There may be no need under local conditions to extend this type of service. Finally, specific services rendered by nutritionists, dental hygienists, and other types of personnel may be demonstrated by their loan to communities for a predetermined period of time.

Demonstrations under State and Federal Auspices. State and Federal health agencies promote the development of local child health services through the use of demonstrations. These are similar in principle to demonstrations within local programs, but they generally cover a broader geographic area or offer a more complete service. An entire county or state may be selected as a demonstration area. Administrative responsibility for the demonstration may reside in the local health department, or rest with the state or Federal agency providing the funds.

The Children's Bureau does not have direct responsibility for demonstration programs, even when these are financed from Federal grants-in-aid. In practice, the Bureau has broad powers in determining the policies governing such programs since it must approve the plans submitted by the state agency. For example, special rheumatic fever programs planned by states were supported for about a decade after 1939 from a special grant of Federal crippled children's funds. The Children's Bureau required that such programs be "complete," that is, that they provide well-rounded services for children with rheumatic fever, including facilities for diagnosis, hospitalization, and convalescent care and adequate follow-up services, with attention to medical-social and nutritional aspects of care as well. The amount of funds made available to any one state was generally enough to support a program covering only one or two counties of a state, unless additional state and local funds were available. Interpretation of the nature of "completeness" of demonstration programs caused friction between state health agencies and the Children's Bureau. Experience has, however, confirmed the wisdom of the general requirement in that patterns of adequate care have been established by concentrated programs, whereas more diffuse use of the funds would have dissipated them without pointing up the public health problem and its possible solution.

The Children's Bureau has defined demonstrations in its regulations in two specific ways: (*a*) the provision in a county, district, or community of more and better services than are available in any comparable area in the state, to establish standards of care and service that are practical, effective, and adequate to improve the health of mothers and children; (*b*) the provision of a special type of service to prove its value and to obtain information on cost, methods of development, techniques of provision, and administration of a given type of health service not generally available to mothers and children (4). It is difficult to draw a line between the second type of demonstration and a frankly experimental or research program. Perhaps attempting to draw too fine a distinction would only hamper progress, but, in general, in a demonstration program the clinical techniques used must meet with professional acceptance and only their public health or mass application is in question.

The Public Health Service may work through the states or directly with local agencies in some of their demonstration programs. In its dental health program the Public Health Service has been required by Act of Congress to provide teams of dentists and dental hygienists to localities within the states to demonstrate the application of sodium fluoride solution to the teeth in the prevention of dental caries; the Service has not been allowed to provide funds to the states or localities for this purpose. The Public Health Service also loans personnel for extended periods of time to states and communities for specific purposes.

HEALTH EDUCATION

The individual approach to health education is implicit in every phase of the health program for mothers and children. Health educators now realize that motivation to achieve better health for self and family must come from within the individual as part of a drive for the attainment of desirable ends more tangible than health in the abstract (5). Immediate desirable goals might be success in business or marriage, a more satisfying social life, or better opportunities for the development of children in the family.

At certain stages in life, which are highly charged emotionally, the individual may be more readily influenced by properly directed health education. Some of the major events in human development occur at times when parents and children are recipients of health services—in preparing for marriage, during pregnancy, in caring for the new baby, in getting the child ready for school, or during illness. The physician stands in a key position at all these strategic points; in his private practice or as a participant in clinic activities, he is expected to provide health guidance. He has the opportunity and responsibility to seize these favorable moments to motivate behavior in the hope that it will carry over to less receptive periods of life.

Functions of Health Education. Health education of the public seeks first to motivate the public, individually and collectively, through change in attitude and behavior, to act in the promotion of their health, and to obtain early and adequate care in the event of ill health from any cause.   .

The aim of health teaching should be the same as for all good teaching— to help the learner discover material which he can adapt to his own needs, not the mere giving of ready-made answers. . . . Ours is the job of emancipating people from a slavish reliance upon what the expert says and of helping them make intelligent decisions, each in keeping with his ability, yet each within the permissive atmosphere of a free society. (6)

Mass mediums of communication—the daily press, the radio, television, the screen, distribution of booklets—are all used to achieve these objectives. Talks, demonstrations, and panel discussions on health topics may be included on the programs of community organizations. Special meetings may be convened for the same purpose, but the topic must have a dramatic appeal or be keyed to matters of immediate concern if the time and energy entailed in such efforts are to be productive. The group approach to public health education is necessary because of the sheer size of the problems being attacked, but it should supplement rather than replace the approach to the individuals composing the group.

The second major function of public health education is to make the public aware of the nature and size of health problems in the community and to guide it in the support of measures to solve these problems. The availability of community facilities must be publicized to promote their use. Promotion of community participation and support in meeting these needs through a rounded program may be obtained through showing how these problems affect each individual. This aspect of public health education is closely related to community organization. Mass mediums of communication find even wider use in this aspect of public health education.

Publicity and fund raising for specific activities by official and voluntary health organizations as ends in themselves are not infrequently confused with health education. Good public relations are necessary in implementing the child health program. "In the field of public health, public relations refers to winning good will for an organization or for one of its programs; health education aims to facilitate learning about health and health problems and motivating good individual and group health practices." (7)

Fear as a Motivating Force. Scare psychology has no place in health education, although frequent examples are found in publications of reputable health organizations as well as in the commercial press. Articles in popular women's magazines have created needless anxiety by presenting the dangers of rheumatic fever and erythroblastosis fetalis in a lurid manner; this has had a particularly bad effect on readers living in areas in which facilities for care are lacking. The popular magazine has even been used as a means of discouraging the use of silver nitrate solution as a preventive of ophthalmia neonatorum when the supposed superiority of antibiotics had not been established.

There are times when it is necessary to point out actual and potential dangers to prevent serious accidents. This must be done carefully, preferably in the general context of health education of parents and children. Indiscriminate resort to fear may be temporarily effective, but it soon loses its force; in any event, its total effect is destructive. Equally harmful is the use of techniques which arouse feelings of guilt as a key to action. The resulting resistance on the part of the public may carry over to other aspects of the health program as well or, in parent education particularly, it may create new problems in parent-child relationships as serious as the ones supposedly corrected.

RESEARCH

Research in child health may be thought of as any activity which seeks to obtain new knowledge, or to develop or improve techniques for the application of available knowledge through the medium of the child health program. At one extreme, research as a means of implementing the public health program merges into clinical research. At the other, it cannot be distinguished from administrative planning and practice which requires periodic testing and review of techniques. Without research activities of some sort, a program tends to become routinized and sterile. Even when members of the staff of the health agency participate in studies to only a limited degree, it may give them a feeling of accomplishment beyond that obtained from their usual activities.

Research studies should not be attempted by agencies whose primary responsibility is the provision of health services before these services are well launched in the community. They should be designed to make the services more effective, rather than as ends in themselves, apart from the program. In smaller areas, there is a fruitful field for experimentation in adapting relatively complicated techniques to simpler situations. Participation in broader studies covering a number of communities is also possible. This is especially desirable when variation in social and economic conditions and in community resources and attitudes are among the factors under investigation. The follow-up services of health agencies are also invaluable in clinical studies in fields related to public health services. Facilities of health agencies may also be made available for graduate students and other investigators.

In larger local agencies and in state health agencies many fields are open for study, some of which can be made by no other agencies. Studies of the prevalence of many conditions of infancy and childhood can best be done on a community-wide or statewide basis to prevent the distortion when data from only a limited number of hospitals are used. Studies primarily of an evaluative nature and the roles of Federal agencies in research have already been discussed.

CITED REFERENCES

1. (*a*) "Standards and Recommendations for Hospital Care of Newborn Infants: Full-term and Premature," Children's Bureau Publication 292, Washington, D.C., 1943; (*b*) "Standards and Recommendations for Hospital Care of Newborn Infants—Full-term and Premature," Committee on Fetus and Newborn, American Academy of Pediatrics, Evanston, Ill., November, 1948.
2. "Recommended Standards and Minimum Requirements for a Cardiovascular Clinic," Committee on Cardiac Clinics, American Heart Association, New York, December, 1949.
3. Program developed under immediate direction of Dr. Ray E. Trussell, described in detail in (*a*) TRUSSELL, RAY E., Diarrhea of the Newborn: An Approach to Control through Minimum Standards of Nursery Care, *New York State J. Med.*, Vol. 49, pp. 2789–2791, Dec. 1, 1949; (*b*) KORNS, ROBERT F., EDWARD R. SCHLESINGER, and MADELEINE Y. PHANEUF, The Control of Communicable Disease in Hospital Nurseries for the Newborn: Progress Report, New York State Plan, *New York State J. Med.*, Vol. 52, pp. 39–42, Jan. 1, 1952.
4. "Regulations for Maternal and Child Health and Crippled Children's Programs," Children's Bureau, abstracted from the *Federal Register*, Washington, June 28, 1949.

5. GALDSTON, IAGO, Motivation in Health Education, *Am. J. Pub. Health,* Vol. 39, pp. 1276–1283, October, 1949.
6. ANDERSON, ELMER, J., Ideological Barriers to Effective Teaching by Health Workers, *Pub. Health Rep.,* Vol. 65, pp. 661–669, May 19, 1950.
7. DERRYBERRY, MAYHEW, in Health Education and Public Relations: A Symposium, *Am. J. Pub. Health,* Vol. 40, pp. 251–259, March, 1950.

7 SERVICES OF PROFESSIONAL PERSONNEL

A community child health program requires the services of personnel from a variety of professional and semiprofessional disciplines. Physicians and dentists, in administrative capacities and in all phases of clinical services from diagnosis through treatment and rehabilitation, are at the hub of the program. Nurses, social workers, nutritionists, dental hygienists, and various types of technical personnel and therapists have valuable contributions to make, based on their specific training and experience. An understanding of their functions is of direct concern to the physician in private practice since their services are often available for patients under his care, as well as in the health services subsidized by community agencies.

Each member of the staff of a health agency, whether employed full-time or part-time, has an important function to perform, and each person should be used to take maximum advantage of his training. The longer and more expensive the training, the greater should be the effort to employ their professional skills at top grade, using other staff members with less training for functions which require a smaller amount of training and experience. A dentist should not be expected to spend his time in routine prophylactic services; dental hygienists are available to clean teeth, for topical application of sodium fluoride, and to carry out certain educational functions. When existing laws or regulations do not permit dental hygienists to apply sodium fluoride to the teeth, every effort should be made to remove this barrier to efficient service. Orthopedic surgeons should not have to do routine muscle testing, when physical therapists are available for the job. Functions which can be routinized without damage to the services may often be assigned to clerks and stenographers, to allow specially trained personnel to devote full time to their professional or semiprofessional duties.

Employment on personal merit, and security through safeguards on the job and by an adequate retirement system, form the basis for sound personnel relationships. More important than this, each staff member in the various community health agencies should have a sense of participation in a worthwhile undertaking. At an institute on interpersonal relations, the conclusion was reached that

"organization charts ought not be used as indicating status or authority." The members of the institute considered that such charts represent primarily maps of channels of communication. Once such channels are established, everyone in the organization should be regarded on the same human level. Each one is respected as the person who is the recognized expert on his own job, whether that job be that of the health officer who plans the total program or that of the janitor who cleans the floors. (1)

In this chapter, special attention will be devoted to the general functions of physicians, nurses, and medical social workers in the total child health program. The functions of the other types of professional personnel will be considered in relation to dental health, nutrition, and other specialized programs in which they work.

PHYSICIANS

The administrative functions of physicians as health officers or directors of child health programs have been implied in the discussion of planning and implementing the child health program. How physicians participate, directly or indirectly, in the clinical aspects of the child health program deserves further consideration. These services may be provided in the immediate care of children in clinics, hospitals, or convalescent institutions, or the care may be given in the physician's own office or in the child's home. The physician may provide indirect services by the supervision and direction of other professional and semiprofessional personnel.

The method of obtaining the clinical services of physicians varies widely in different programs and areas (2). Physicians may devote all or only part of their time to community health work. Others are employed full-time or part-time for medical services in a hospital or convalescent institution from which services are purchased for individual children under the program. Physicians may be reimbursed at a stated fee per day or per clinic, and special arrangements may be made to cover time involved in travel. In the treatment of handicapped children, unless the care is given by physicians working full-time in state medical centers and similar institutions, physicians usually receive a set fee for every service performed. In certain programs involving large numbers of persons receiving similar types of services, as under EMIC, a flat fee may be paid per case, regardless of the amount of care rendered; the theory behind this method of payment is that the amount of service rendered tends to average out in a long enough series of cases.

Each method of obtaining the services of physicians has its advantages and disadvantages. The acceptability of a given method to the medical profession and the government fiscal authorities often determines its selection. In clinic services requiring medical specialists, it may be simpler to have full-time physicians conduct the clinics in a given area. Indeed, there may be no alternative to this arrangement when there are no specialists available in the immediate area, and when none can be induced to travel to staff the clinics. The disadvantage of this method is that, should the full-time specialist leave for any reason, the service must automatically be discontinued until another full-time physician can be found. If local specialists are employed on a part-time or session basis, the service is not interrupted if one of the physicians discontinues his service.

When the services of specialists are not required, there is an additional cogent reason why local physicians should be induced to participate in clinic services. Physicians in private practice who conduct a child health conference or other service can be reached in in-service graduate refresher programs. There is a good possibility that they will then carry over their interest and knowledge in improved care of children in their own practices. This is admittedly a long-term program if real gains are to be registered. On the other hand, these gains are likely to be more permanent than when a full-time person is employed and brought into the community only for the clinics.

Rosters of Specialists. It is desirable for the official health agency, usually the state health department or state crippled children's agency, to have a roster of specialists available. For certain types of services, only specialists are acceptable under the program. For example, the surgical correction of various handicapping conditions or consultations in complicated cases require the services of medical specialists. When specialists and general practitioners provide the same type of service, as in child health conferences, a differential fee may be allowed the specialists in some areas.

There is general agreement that a listing of specialists is desirable and necessary, but there is much controversy as to the best method of attaining this objective. Licentiates and diplomates of the various specialty boards are usually included, along with those physicians whose training and experience make them eligible for examination by such boards. In questionable cases, the advice of a medical board of review, preferably designated by the medical society, is often sought, even though the final responsibility for inclusion of a physician on the roster must remain with the health agency using the roster in its services. When an understanding is reached between the medical society and the health agency on the purpose and use of the roster, the advice of the former, based on careful review of the professional qualifications of each physician, will almost always be followed.

Consultation Services. Pediatrics has developed rapidly as a specialty since 1930. Unlike most other specialties within medicine, pediatrics has a dual role. It is often general practice with an age ceiling, at whatever age ceiling may be set in different areas. The consultative function, while relatively less frequently called upon than in former years, is as important as ever.

Although pediatrics has grown rapidly as a specialty, pediatricians are concentrated in a relatively few areas, and especially in urban centers around medical schools. One or more practicing pediatricians, only half of whom are certified as specialists by the American Board of Pediatrics, were to be found in only one out of every six counties of the United States in 1946 (3). At that time 75 per cent of all medical care for children was provided by general practitioners.

Pediatric consultation services provided to the general practitioner in an area otherwise lacking such services brings him definite values. It improves his relationships with his patients by assuring them that they are obtaining specialized attention within their own communities. The professional stimulation from the opportunity of discussing more difficult medical problems with a specialist carries over to other children under the general practitioner's care. Adequate consultation services permit earlier diagnosis when the child's medical condition may not require complicated care.

The following statement of the principles involved in pediatric consultation services is of interest in this connection (4):

The Medical Society of the State of New York and the New York State Department of Health agree on the principle that adequate pediatric consultation services should be available to general practitioners. Such pediatric consultation services are primarily a technic of graduate education which will in the long run improve the quality of medical care to all the children of the State. As such it is of concern to the two organizations issuing this statement.

Private practitioners should be encouraged to make greater use of pediatric consultation services. For patients who cannot obtain the needed consultation services, including indicated laboratory and x-ray examinations, such services should be made available to general practitioners through the instrumentality of the public health program on a regional basis radiating from a pediatric center. . . .

In the development of pediatric consultation services, major emphasis should be placed upon consultations for groups of patients in such locations that the needed laboratory and x-ray examinations may be readily provided. The referring physician is required and other physicians are encouraged to attend the group consultation. In connection with such group consultations, teaching conferences and other educational devices should be arranged for the pediatric consultant. In view of the varying circumstances in each case, the referring physician must be the individual to determine if pediatric consultation service including indicated laboratory and x-ray examinations, is otherwise available to his patient.

Promotion of Consultation Services. The prerogatives of the physician in private practice must be carefully observed, and the quality of consultant service rendered must be sufficiently high to be of practical help to the physician. No amount of promotion will be effective in selling the service, if the referring physician is not convinced by experience that the service is useful to him. Consultations for cases of suspected communicable disease may be offered as the initial consultation service or as part of the continuing program.

It has been a common experience in the early development of pediatric consultation services that the only problems referred are those about which little of a remedial nature can be done. This is by no means waste effort. By providing a second opinion, which bolsters the referring physician's opinion in these cases, the consultant builds confidence in the consultation service. In addition, through discovery of these children with irremediable conditions, steps can be taken for their proper disposition and the families can be helped with the social and emotional problems involved.

Group Consultations or Clinics. A group consultation or clinic is the method of choice in providing pediatric consultation services in many areas. It is more efficient in that a pediatrician, who may be brought from a distance, can see a group of children at a single session in a properly prepared medical setting. Arrangements for diagnostic laboratory and x-ray studies can be made more readily. Patients are aware of the services to be offered and the nature of the consultation, permitting the consultant to work more efficiently.

An effort is generally made to have the referring physician present at the consultation clinic for a personal discussion with the consultant. If this is not possible a written report is sent to the family physician; the child is usually returned to the referring physician for information and further care, unless the family physician specifies that such information should be given directly to the family at the clinic. Physicians who have referred children to the clinic may remain during the entire session for a discussion of the other medical problems reviewed.

Individual Consultations. Consultations for individual children may be provided by a full-time pediatrician on the staff of the health agency or by pediatricians in private practice under a variety of arrangements. These consultations may be given in the general practitioner's own office or in a local hospital. In some areas, the children are taken to the office of the pediatrician some distance away from the child's home. This saves the time of the pediatrician, but it nullifies one of the major premises of the consultation services, that the child be cared for in his own locality in so far as possible. It also means that the referring physician will not be present during the consultation so that important benefits inherent in the service are lost.

Consultations for individual children are expensive and an inefficient use of the consultant's time. Their use is usually restricted to children who cannot be seen at a regularly scheduled clinic either because delay would be inadvisable in view of the acuteness of their condition, or because they cannot be transported for medical reasons. The provision of individual consultation services in some states by a full-time or part-time physician on the staff of a health department is justified on the ground that the favorable relationships developed with the medical profession carry over into other phases of the child health program.

PUBLIC HEALTH NURSES

The public health nurse, as is the case with the entire nursing profession, has often been referred to as an agent of the physician in many of her functions. She spares the physician in his office and in the clinic by interpreting his recommendations to the family and by assisting in locating community services in accordance with these recommendations. She encourages the family to seek medical care for any member of the household suspected of any deviations from normal health. She advises the family to return for care as needed, as part of her follow-up services. Yet the public health nurse has her own special contributions to make as a professional person with training and experience different from all other groups (5). Her relationship with the physician is one between two professional persons, each having particular functions to perform.

In essence, public health nursing is a family service (6). A public health nurse assesses the total health needs of the family, whatever the immediate reason for a home visit. By serving the family in its home setting, she is in an advantageous position to gauge the relationships among members of the household. From her knowledge of the total family situation obtained through direct observation, she can draw upon strengths within the family itself for solving its own problems. To do this, instruction or demonstration of simple techniques of bedside care or assistance in better use of available foods to improve family nutrition may be all that is necessary. When some form of outside help is needed to tide over an acute situation or to help with a chronic problem, the public health nurse calls upon her knowledge of community resources. This is more than a mechanical referral. If she has established a sound relationship with the family, she provides an invaluable function in aiding in transferring this relationship to the new agency, as well as in interpreting the needs and attitudes of the family to the agency.

In a number of respects the services of a public health nurse are unique. She visits socially isolated families which do not participate in local organizations and which are not reached by the usual mass mediums of public health education. Through her contacts in the community she hears of pregnant women, for example, who have not sought medical care. More than any other person, the public health nurse can promote positive health in situations in which it is not otherwise possible to do so.

The generalized public health nurse provides services to women during the maternity cycle and to children from birth through adolescence as part of her services to the family unit. As in so many other phases of the child health program, it is not possible nor is it desirable to separate out these child health functions with any degree of precision. Focusing of attention on the child's problem exclusively may be detrimental to the child. For example, a nurse may visit the home of an orthopedically handicapped child to be sure that certain exercises demonstrated in a clinic are being carried out; if the nurse is not aware that the mother is concerned at the moment about her husband's illness, and unless she takes steps to help with this problem first, she is not likely to be successful in her follow-up service with the child.

Administration of Services. Under the general heading of public health nurses are included nurses employed by health departments, visiting nurse associations, educational systems, life insurance companies, and a variety of voluntary health agencies. Visiting nurse associations are found mainly in metropolitan centers; their primary service is the provision of bedside care in the home, with accompanying emphasis upon instruction of the family in the techniques of care (7). The practicing physician is more apt to be in closer contact with public health nurses employed by visiting nurse associations, where they exist, than with other types of public health nurses. Public health nurses employed by official health agencies spend a greater proportion of their time in health promotion, rather than in nursing care during illness. In rural areas, when a sufficient number of public health nurses employed by health departments are available, the public health nurses often provide bedside nursing services as well.

The trend throughout the country, with some notable exceptions, is toward generalized public health nursing. The specialized staff maternal and child health nurse is rapidly disappearing. In spite of many difficulties, the services of voluntary visiting nurse associations are slowly being merged with official health departments, and the nurses in each formerly distinct agency are taking on combined functions. The home nursing services provided by life insurance companies and by such agencies as the American Red Cross are rapidly being disbanded as public health nursing services by official health departments and visiting nurse services have expanded. Specialized school nursing is slower in fitting into this general trend, especially in those areas of the country in which this specialized type of service preceded the formation of local health departments or, in fact, where such departments still do not exist.

Supervision and Consultation. Since the generalized public health nurse has such broad responsibilities and since new technical developments in child health and other fields crowd closely upon each other, it is essential that she have adequate supervision by more experienced public health nurses. It is manifestly impossible for a supervising nurse to have the latest information in all public health fields constantly at her finger tips and to have a thorough knowledge of the techniques for imparting this to her staff. For this reason the larger local health agencies and the state health agencies employ specialized consultant nurses in various fields. Some of these consultants cover the entire maternal and child health field. Other consultants devote themselves to either maternal health or child health exclusively, or to one or more types of special health problems; still others provide consultation in hospital maternity and newborn services (8). Additional consultants in mental health and other fields may further round out the consultant program. Consultants work primarily with supervising nurses, but they also take part in institutes, staff meetings, and individual visits and conferences with staff nurses depending on the size of area and number of professional personnel served. Consultants also concentrate their work in programs in which new techniques are being tried out or where a model program is being developed.

MEDICAL SOCIAL WORKERS

Medical social workers are equipped by their training and experience to deal with the social and emotional aspects of illness. The medical social worker studies personal or environmental factors which prevent the patient from obtaining full benefit from his medical program and which interfere with his return to normal activity. At times this may even lead to the study of factors present before the illness which may have resulted in a poor social adjustment and which may have become aggravated by the illness. The medical social worker does not function independently. She uses her special equipment as a member of a team, interpreting the emotional and social needs of patients to physicians, nurses, and others, and assisting the patient and his family in adjusting to illness. She arranges with other social agencies and individuals to meet the social needs of patients.

Originally, the services of medical social workers were developed in connection with hospitals and clinics. With their background in a hospital setting, the transition to work in a community health agency would seem to be a natural one, but a lapse of twenty-two years occurred between the time of their first employment in a hospital and their inclusion in a health department program. Health departments and voluntary health organizations must deal with other community social agencies in the course of their work. It is generally accepted that every large health department should have at least one medical social worker on its staff. Nearly all states have medical social work positions, and most of the handicapped children's agencies not in health departments also have the benefit of such services. Voluntary health agencies also employ medical social workers, usually in specialized programs.

A medical social worker in an official health agency makes her greatest contribution by functioning in a consultant capacity within the organization and in a liaison capacity with other agencies in the community (9). She works with the health officer and with the directors of the various programs to promote inclusion of the social aspects of care in health services. Her experience and training are useful in helping public health nurses cope with social problems which interfere with acceptance or fullest use of health services. She may do this on a regular basis at staff conferences; or she may work directly with patients in clinics and interpret the results of these interviews to the public health nurses providing follow-up care in the home. As a liaison agent for the health department, she interprets the work of the department to other community social agencies. At the same time, she keeps health department personnel informed of the services available through these other agencies and of the most efficient channels for using them.

Medical social workers may be employed full-time on specialized programs for direct service to patients. This is particularly true of programs for physically handicapped children under the administration of welfare departments or other agencies conducting special programs. Under such circumstances, the medical social worker functions essentially as her colleague does in a hospital outpatient department when home visiting and work with other social agencies are included in the latter's duties.

In areas where other social work services are extremely limited or absent, the medical social worker on the staff of a health agency may have to provide services not specifically of a medical social character. She may have to find and supervise a suitable foster placement for a handicapped child to enable him to secure needed care not available near his own home. These types of services are usually considered of a temporary nature only, until such time as the community employs a child welfare worker. In such poorly staffed areas, the consultant functions of the medical social worker in relation to public health nurses are all the more important, since the public health nurse must assume greater responsibilities and needs more help with the social problems of families under their care.

PROFESSIONAL TRAINING

Each type of professional personnel in the community child health program is really working within a specialty in his own field. Specialty status has been recognized clearly in the case of health officers and other full-time physicians who may become diplomates of the American Board of Preventive Medicine and Public Health after examination in their medical specialty; they are eligible to take the examination after graduate study at a school of public health and after a specified period of experience under supervision in approved areas. The Committee on Professional Education of the American Public Health Association has developed suggested standards of experience and training for various types of personnel employed in health agencies.

In-service Training. Most health agencies conduct continuing training programs on the job for professional personnel employed either on a full-time or a part-time basis. In a sense, every contact between supervisor and staff, between consultant and supervisor, or consultant and staff is a part of this process. In-service training is a two-directional affair; the supervisor or consultant replenishes his experience by contacts with staff members, and he passes on the fruits of this experience to others as the occasion arises.

When professional training is mentioned, a more formal approach is usually intended. Periodic staff conferences are a useful technique, provided they are planned carefully to use the time of the staff members to best advantage. Too frequent staff conferences may defeat their own purpose by becoming routine or by producing an adverse effect on the public or appropriating body, which may not understand that the conferences are intended to raise the quality of the service rendered.

Institutes of one or two days duration are generally reserved for the introduction of a new type of program or to bring about a major change in approach in an established program. They are also used to bring together personnel of a number of agencies in a community or region to present a rounded picture of a given problem. A larger group can be attracted by outstanding figures in the field under discussion; the presence of the larger group makes it worth while to bring the panel together. For example, institutes for hospital administrators, obstetricians, pediatricians, and supervising hospital nurses may be held at the start of a premature infant care program for discussion of different aspects of the care of the obstetrical patient and the premature infant of interest to these groups.

Academic Training. For supervisory and consultant health personnel, more extended and formal training is frequently subsidized by the employing agency, so that the agency may have the benefit of a person on its staff with the latest knowledge and techniques at his command. In certain fields, the shortage of trained personnel is so acute that specialists may be granted a stipend and tuition for a more extended period of training to qualify them for highly specialized types of care. This type of training is even extended to part-time professional personnel. A stipend may be granted to an orthopedist in the community to spend some time in learning details of the care of children with cerebral palsy; or an internist or pediatrician may be given an opportunity to obtain added experience in the care of children with rheumatic fever or epilepsy so that he may participate more effectively in the local rheumatic fever or epilepsy program.

The shortage of skilled personnel has been so acute that a health agency will occasionally subsidize the basic formal training of such specialized technical personnel as physical, occupational, or speech therapists. This cannot be considered in-service training, however, since the person so trained was either not previously on the staff of the agency or, if on the staff, he was not in the field in which he is being trained. A fair proportion of the Federal funds available for maternal and child health and crippled children's services is used for both basic and in-service training of personnel participating in child health programs. Voluntary agencies such as the National Foundation for Infantile Paralysis have also generously provided fellowships for the training of generalized public health personnel.

Regional Programs. The discrepancies in consultation and postgraduate medical education services between metropolitan centers and rural and semirural areas have been attacked in several areas on a regional basis, centering about a teaching center. Various types of programs have been developed, embodying different combinations of services (10). Formal courses may be offered at the medical center for physicians from outlying areas. Pediatric residents from the teaching center may spend a few months in outlying hospitals, giving them experience outside a highly developed medical setting and providing stimulation to the staff of the hospitals they serve. Consultants from the center may visit different parts of the region periodically, to review difficult medical problems and to conduct ward rounds and special conferences. These programs are most effective when they are adapted to existing facilities.

CITED REFERENCES

1. A Suggested Attitude toward Posts and People, editorial, *Am. J. Pub. Health,* Vol. 41, p. 94, January, 1951.
2. GOLDMANN, FRANZ, (*a*) Methods of Payment for Physicians' Services in Medical Care Programs, *Am. J. Pub. Health,* Vol. 42, pp. 134–141, February, 1952; (*b*) Payment for Physicians' Services under Crippled Children's Programs, *Pediatrics,* Vol. 6, pp. 660–669, October, 1950.
3. "Child Health Services and Pediatric Education, Report of the Committee for the Study of Child Health Services, The American Academy of Pediatrics," Commonwealth Fund, Harvard University Press, Cambridge, Mass., 1949.
4. Council Committee on Public Health and Education of the Medical Society of the State of New York, announcement, *New York State J. Med.,* Vol. 48, p. 623, Mar. 15, 1948. Reprinted by permission of the *New York State Journal of Medicine.*
5. KAISER, ALBERT D., The Role of the Public Health Nurse, *Pediatrics,* Vol. 6, pp. 485–487, September, 1950.
6. FREEMAN, RUTH B., The Public Health Nurse as a Family Counselor, *Am. J. Pub. Health,* Vol. 42, pp. 1379–1387, November, 1952.
7. SHEPARD, WILLIAM P., and GEORGE M. WHEATLEY, Visiting Nurse Service: Community Asset for Every Physician, *J.A.M.A.,* Vol. 149, pp. 554–557, June 7, 1952.
8. PORTER, WINIFRED H., The Specialized Public Health Nursing Consultant in State Health Departments, *Am. J. Pub. Health,* Vol. 41, pp. 13–19, January, 1951.

9. HALL, BEATRICE, The Role of Medical-social Service in the Public-health Program, *Child,* Vol. 9, pp. 127–130, February, 1945.
10. Regional Planning for Pediatric Education and Services, Chap. V, Report on Better Medical Care for Children, Committee for the Improvement of Child Health, American Academy of Pediatrics, *Pediatrics,* Vol. 6, pp. 532–544, September, 1950.

ADDITIONAL REFERENCES

1. PEROZZI, LUCILE A., Public Health Nursing in Relation to Child Health Services, *Am. J. Pub. Health,* Vol. 40, pp. 395–399, April, 1950.
2. LIT, HELENE S., For the Child as an Individual: Case Workers in Health Programs Help to Meet Children's Social and Emotional Needs, *Child,* Vol. 16, pp. 90–93, February, 1952.

8 HOSPITALIZATION AND RELATED SERVICES

The public looks to the hospital as a place for maintaining or regaining health; this contrasts with the attitude, prevailing not so far in the past, that admission to a hospital was tantamount to a sentence of death (1). Public acceptance and support of hospitals and related institutions for medical care have encouraged the integration of obstetrical and pediatric services in hospitals into the community maternal and child health program. The wall that still separates the hospital from other community health services is gradually being leveled in many places, making possible better care through more efficient use of all health services. Practicing physicians, both as members of hospital staffs and as participants in other community health services, can hasten this development.

Few communities have hospital and related facilities in sufficient variety and quantity to permit a full range of selection of the type of care needed by all children. A child in one community may be given care at home, whereas a child with a similar clinical condition elsewhere may be admitted to a general hospital, to an institution for convalescent care, or to a foster home, depending on the availability of the different types of facilities, on conditions in the child's home, and on the decision of the child's family and physician. With an adequate range of institutional facilities, it is possible to use each to best advantage in providing the type of services for which they were designed, calling upon other facilities as the child's condition changes.

Whatever the degree of adequacy of the different types of institutional facilities, coordination of these facilities with health services reaching more directly into the homes of children will increase the value of both. Systems of referral are in use which facilitate rapid exchange of information about patients to ensure continuity of care. Prior to discharge of a premature infant, for example, a public health nurse may be requested, through such an interagency referral system, to assist the parents in preparation of the home for proper care of the infant and to notify the hospital when home conditions are safe for the infant's reception; or a child being discharged from a hospital with residual paralysis following poliomyelitis may be referred to a rehabilitation center or to an agency providing physical therapy in the home. By this type of referral system, hospital medical staffs benefit directly from the resulting close working relationship with health agencies in the community; they obtain help in follow-up of patients from the viewpoint of providing better care and of securing information needed to evaluate the results of hospital care.

Acute Care in Hospitals. Obstetric and pediatric care in hospitals have developed in divergent directions. Hospital care during delivery and for at least a few days of the postpartum period has become the accepted practice in most parts of the country. The amount of pediatric care in hospitals, on the other hand, has tended to decrease in proportion to the size of the child population. At the same time, the patterns of hospitalized illness are changing constantly. Most children with communicable diseases, with the major exception of poliomyelitis, are cared for at home; even secondary infections are usually prevented or managed without hospital care. Many special communicable disease hospitals are being closed or converted to other uses such as rehabilitation or chronic disease services; instead, children with communicable diseases requiring hospitalization are being admitted to general hospitals under proper precautions (2). It is urged in authoritative circles that patients with communicable disease who require hospitalization should be admitted to general hospitals because of immediate availability of adequate diagnostic and therapeutic facilities and consultation services and to provide training for more professional personnel in the field of communicable diseases (3).

Other factors have been operating to change the pattern of pediatric care in hospitals. Outpatient facilities of hospitals and special diagnostic clinic services of other agencies have reduced the need for hospitalization for diagnostic purposes in some communities. Periods of hospitalization for conditions such as osteomyelitis and appendicitis have been greatly reduced, largely as a result of the availability of chemotherapy and antibiotics. The increased daily cost of hospitalization to the family has also made for lesser use of pediatric beds. Partially offsetting these factors have been recent medical and surgical advances which have brought many conditions, such as certain types of congenital cardiovascular disease, within the realm of remedial care, demanding new types of diagnostic and therapeutic facilities in the hospital.

Under ideal circumstances, acute care in hospitals, because of certain dangers to the child, would be reserved for children with conditions requiring either intensive medical and nursing attention or complicated diagnostic services which cannot be provided in a physician's office or on an outpatient basis. Hospital care presents a particular hazard to children with rheumatic fever, for example, since exposure to a new strain of Group A hemolytic streptococci may produce a flare-up in the disease process. More important is the possible emotional trauma to all children in the hospital experience itself, inherent in a situation in which the attention of the staff is frequently riveted upon a succession of serious emergencies. The hospital experience is often the first physical separation of the child from his family; the feeling the child may have that the separation is in itself a form of punishment is exaggerated by the strange and, at times, painful procedures to which he is subjected in the hospital.

The physician on the hospital staff has an opportunity to press for a review of the oftentimes outmoded rules governing hospital pediatric services which display a lack of understanding of the child's emotional needs. Hospital visiting hours are often rigid; parents may be permitted infrequent brief visits. In some hospitals, at the other extreme, parents are encouraged to remain with their child until he is anesthetized prior to surgery and to be present as the child recovers from the anesthetic.

When time allows, the emotional disturbance entailed in hospitalization may be minimized by proper preparation of the child for the experience. Apart from having a parent present before and after surgery, it has been found possible to reduce the emotional trauma of surgical procedures by simple explanation of what is to follow and by demonstration of the anesthetic procedure and allowing the child to try the mask (4). This has been found to save time as well, by producing a smoother and shorter period of induction and more complete relaxation during the operative procedure. Allowing parents to remain overnight with their children in the hospital and actually assist with routine care are extremely rare policies in the United States, although they have been used in several British children's hospitals for some years. In many countries, especially in Latin America, this has been a long-standing custom, but it has not been subjected to evaluation by modern medical concepts.

In leading teaching hospitals, all children are placed in a separate portion of the hospital, whatever the condition requiring care, under the over-all medical supervision of the pediatric staff, and with nursing care under the supervision of nurses with advanced training in pediatrics. The immediate care of orthopedic and other types of specialized problems is the responsibility of specialists in the fields concerned. Such specialists are also available for consultation about other children, as the need arises. This pattern of care is also being followed in some hospitals not connected with teaching centers.

Under varying patterns of care, it is still essential that physicians and other personnel providing services work together to arrive at and carry out a plan of management for the child. "Teamwork is the present, most vital need of the hospitalized child." (5) This is the opening sentence of a report on a study of actual practices in the main pediatric teaching centers in the country. It was found that, where teamwork of all personnel, professional and otherwise, really existed, children "make satisfactory mental adjustments, their parents understand the complete plan for the child, and the children 'find themselves' at an early date." In institutions lacking understanding of the dynamics of such teamwork, "each worker goes along in his own groove and the child patient and his parents are mentally torn asunder by conflicting impressions or lack of any direction."

Care in Institutions for Convalescent Care. Convalescent care is intermediate between acute care, wherever provided, and return to as normal a state of health as possible. Most of the acute illnesses during childhood go through a short course without aftereffects when given adequate care. Only a brief convalescent period, with attention to diet, rest, and graduated activities, is needed before the child returns to his previous mode of life. When a child has gone through a debilitating illness or major surgery, or when a child whose previous health was poor is recovering from less severe illness, a more prolonged period of convalescent care should be provided to minimize the possibility of permanent damage to the child's health. When conditions in the child's home are not suitable and when facilities for acute care in a general hospital are no longer indicated, the special institution for convalescent care fills an obvious gap. The convalescent institution is of special value to the child who requires prolonged services such as physical therapy when these cannot be provided on an outpatient basis because of the child's condition.

Convalescent care is a continuation of that given during the acute illness. Convalescing children need careful medical and nursing supervision, although not on so intensive a basis as during the acute phase of their illness. A medical, nursing, and technical staff adequate to provide such care in a convalescent institution can be more readily obtained and maintained if the institution is in an accessible location, preferably close to or part of the general hospital or medical center with which it should be affiliated. A large proportion of the children's convalescent institutions in this country, about 100 in all, do not maintain these desirable arrangements; they are not connected, physically or organizationally, with general hospitals, and they are not planned as functional elements in community health programs for children (6).

Children's convalescent institutions offer the possibility of providing prolonged care in a more unhurried and homelike atmosphere than in a general hospital, in which the needs of the whole child can be more readily met. The patients should be considered first as children with the usual range of social and emotional needs for their age and sex, exaggerated or distorted under the stress of prolonged separation from home with superimposed illness or disability. Provision must be made for the educational and recreational needs of the children under care. The nutritional needs of the children require particular attention at this time. For children with specific physical disabilities, a full range of rehabilitative services should be included in the program of the institution, stressing training which encourages participation of the child in daily activities. Older children also should have the benefit of occupational guidance and therapy in keeping with their abilities and disabilities. To accomplish this, the staff of the institution must be a working team of physicians, nurses, nutritionists, medical social workers, and physical, occupational, and other therapists. The child-centered staff conference is a potent tool in achieving the team approach.

In planning convalescent institutions, the advantages and disadvantages of restricting admissions to children with a specific type of condition must be weighed. In the largest metropolitan centers, it may be possible to have convalescent institutions devoted exclusively to the care of children with rheumatic fever or poliomyelitis, permitting concentration on a particular problem. In the vast majority of communities, however, specialization to this degree is not an efficient arrangement. The variation in incidence of poliomyelitis from year to year would result in low rates of occupancy over prolonged periods. With respect to rheumatic fever, the general downward trend in severity and frequency of the condition adds another factor to the expected variations in incidence in different years. A flexible design, permitting conversion of portions of the institution for care of children with various conditions, is therefore desirable. The interest of citizen groups having special concern for a particular condition can be aroused in support of a convalescent institution providing care for a variety of conditions by pointing to the economics in service when institutions operate at or near capacity.

Foster-home Care. The trend in many parts of the country is away from institutional care of any kind when the specific services needed by the child can be provided with reasonable ease in his own home or in a foster home. This trend has been accelerated by the increased costs of all types of institutional care and by the realization that convalescent institutions providing the range of needed services cannot be conducted efficiently in many communities. In general, the younger the child, the greater is the desirability of the foster home when compared to institutional care of any kind. When a choice exists between an adequate convalescent institution and a good foster home, the emotional needs of the child are balanced against the special facilities available in the convalescent institution.

A foster home near a center for outpatient care may also be used to permit a child living at a distance to take advantage of these facilities. The number of suitable foster homes is only a fraction of the demand, especially since foster homes are called upon to assume many functions other than convalescent care. Health agencies may assist in setting up health standards for foster homes, and they may provide health services for children in foster care. Actual selection and supervision of foster homes are usually the responsibility of state or local child welfare agencies.

"Home-care" Programs. Another manifestation of the trend away from institutional care for situations in which the facilities of the institution are not required has been the development of "home-care" programs.

By home care is meant the provision of the full range of medical, nursing, and related services to patients in their own homes who would, or,
at least, should be admitted to a general hospital or a convalescent institution because of the nature of their illnesses (7). Care of children in
their own homes, perhaps with some assistance from public health nursing or social agencies in the community, should not be confused with
home care in the sense used here.

The need for an alternative method of care for patients with prolonged illness is most evident among elderly individuals. The aging of
the population, scientific advances which help the patient survive an
attack of acute illness, the increasing complexity and cost of hospital
care, all point to the need for an adequate substitute for the hospital,
whenever possible. Home care is an extension of the hospital, releasing
hospital beds for those requiring close supervision or complicated diagnostic or therapeutic measures. The patient is seen periodically by the
same types of medical and related personnel who would otherwise provide care in the hospital.

It is essential, however, to remember that its successful application depends
on a high degree of hospital development, in the fields of medical staff,
social service, nursing, physical and occupational therapy. It would be most
unfortunate if so fruitful a concept were to be discredited by wholesale
displacement of patients by hospitals which lack the facilities to carry the
program out successfully. (8)

The home-care plan has also been applied to the care of children,
especially those with rheumatic fever or poliomyelitis. The child is
seen periodically at home by physicians, public health nurses, nutritionists, and medical social workers. Housekeeper service and equipment
are provided to the family if needed. Through arrangements with the
educational authorities instruction is provided in the home, as well as
psychological testing and vocational guidance of older children. This
type of care, despite its complexity, is less expensive than hospital care. It
must still be considered experimental, however, and its adaptation to less
highly developed situations is awaited. It is also limited in geographic
scope, since the economies in home care may be nullified by the time lost
by professional personnel in traveling to and from the homes of patients.

Child-caring Institutions. Various types of institutions not included
in the categories already covered are of importance to the health of children. Residential institutions intended primarily for the education of

handicapped children, such as the deaf, the blind, or the intellectually handicapped, should provide the full range of health services needed by all children as well as the special health services related to the handicaps. Rehabilitation hospitals may combine and go beyond the functions of the general hospital and convalescent institutions for children with physical handicaps, especially those of an orthopedic nature. There are various types of institutions for children with emotional problems, ranging from small boarding homes for children who should be separated for periods of time from the disturbing elements in a home situation to special hospitals for children with manifest psychoses.

Still other institutions provide long-term care of children with progressive or otherwise irremediable conditions. Children with progressive or extreme handicaps have as great a need for warmth and affection as other children, and their social and emotional problems are the more complicated because of the apparent hopelessness of their condition. In deciding upon placement of these children, their need for all that goes with family relationships in the home must be balanced against the possible, adverse effect upon other children in the family. The parents may pour all their love and drain their purse on the severely handicapped child, neglecting the emotional, educational, and even physical needs of his brothers and sisters. Furthermore, the child requiring prolonged care may do better in the noncompetitive environment of a special institution. Health services in these institutions are, however, often handicapped by a feeling of defeatism on the part of the staff and the abandonment of the possibility of improvement even in the light of new advances. The back wards of some institutions probably hide older children and young adults who were admitted as young children. These children may never have had the benefit of psychological testing adapted to their physical disabilities, and they may have been all but forgotten long before modern rehabilitative techniques became available. Whatever types of services are rendered by the institutions, they should be tied in closely with the services in the community in which the child's family resides. Children may shuttle back and forth between institution and the community with no attempt to exchange information between persons responsible for special services in the community and in the institutions.

Large numbers of children are cared for in institutions because of social handicaps. These include children who cannot remain in their own homes because of death or serious illness of one or both parents, or because of serious social problems in the home. Institutions for delinquent children fall in this general group as well. In many instances, the official health agencies are in the best position to maintain health standards and services in these institutions, in cooperation with the agency primarily concerned with supervision of the type of care provided by the institutions.

Chronic Illness. "The term chronic illness refers to illness or disability which is either permanent or recurrent or which requires a long period of supervision or care, as distinguished from illnesses which are short, self-limited in nature, and leave no permanent after-effects." (9) Various forms of care of chronic illness in and away from the home have already been discussed. Convalescent care, for example, is an important element which merges imperceptibly into other phases of prolonged care; in relation to children's institutions particularly, convalescent care is a euphemistic term used to cover chronic care over a period of years. The psychological value of this designation is evident, and even though it may be technically inaccurate, there is some justification for using the term convalescent care as long as there is a possibility of improving the child's condition through medical care or rehabilitative techniques.

The impact of chronic illness in adults on the community is increasing; the reverse is probably the case in childhood, although no reliable information is available to support this contention. The problem of chronic illness is being studied by the Commission on Chronic Illness, established in 1949 through the combined efforts of the American Medical Association, the American Public Health Association, the American Hospital Association, and the American Public Welfare Association, with the support of many official and voluntary health and welfare agencies. The Commission is surveying activities in the field of chronic care throughout the nation; it is supporting intensive surveys in selected communities to obtain data on the prevalence of chronic illness in both children and adults, as the basis for drawing up plans for detailed programs of prevention, treatment, and rehabilitation.

Purchase of Care. Methods of payment for institutional and foster-home care of children are the direct concern of community health agencies. Too often, voluntary hospitals and convalescent institutions are expected to make up the deficit between the actual cost of care and the amount paid by the family or agency, when there is insufficient financial support from the community at large to the institution to make this possible. This problem is accentuated when children from distant communities are hospitalized in institutions supported entirely by local funds. The rapid expansion of voluntary hospital prepayment plans has remedied much of the deficit in acute care, but has barely touched prolonged care or such special problems as the care of premature infants.

Hospitals are reimbursed for services by community agencies in several ways. A common method is the establishment of an arbitrary flat rate to cover all services except physician's fees, with or without regard for actual costs of care. A second method is the setting of a basic rate for bed and board with provision for payment for all additional services rendered, according to a set fee schedule. The latter method greatly increases the amount of accounting in each case. When agreement must be reached on costs in advance of admission of the child, the institution rendering the service tends to request approval for a larger amount of service to avoid the need for revision of the agreement when unexpected services must be rendered.

Use of a daily rate based on the average cost of all the services provided to patients in the institution is a third method of payment. The occasional complicated and expensive case is balanced by the many receiving routine services only, so that the rate tends to be equitable over a period of time. It is generally agreed that the EMIC program, despite its controversial aspects, did much to put hospital administration on a sound business basis by requiring strict cost accounting in the development of the all-inclusive daily rate used under that program. A maximum inclusive daily rate must usually be established to take care of the few hospitals whose costs are sharply out of line with the other hospitals in the area or state. This method of payment benefits the hospital; it costs more for the agency purchasing hospital care because the agency must pay the full costs of care. Its major disadvantage is its tendency to subsidize the inefficiently run hospital.

Regionalization of Hospital Services. Planning for more effective use of hospital and related services on a regional basis has usually developed as part of a more inclusive program, including postgraduate education and consultation services, described in the previous chapter. The movement toward regionalization of hospital services was accelerated by the passage of the Federal Hospital Survey and Construction Act of 1946 (10).

The earliest approach to the problem of bringing better care to children in outlying areas was the "circuit rider," the pediatrician who traveled from place to place holding conferences in hospitals and providing individual consultation to physicians. More elaborate systems have been developed for the interflow of services among hospitals of different types. The primary medical center, usually a group of hospitals immediately affiliated with a medical school, provides a broad range of specialized services and facilities permitting adequate care of highly complicated diagnostic and therapeutic problems. The secondary hospitals are equipped to handle all but the most complicated problems; and the outlying or tertiary hospitals are capable of providing care in uncomplicated cases. The more difficult clinical problems flow into the primary center, while consultants travel to the outlying centers. Several variations of this pattern of medical and hospital services are developing in different parts of the country (11).

CITED REFERENCES

1. HAWLEY, PAUL R., Medicine as a Social Instrument: The Hospital and the Community, *New England J. Med.,* Vol. 244, pp. 256–259, Feb. 15, 1951.
2. "Guide for the Handling of Communicable Diseases in General Hospitals," Bureau of Epidemiology and Communicable Disease Control, New York State Department of Health, Albany, N.Y., 1950.
3. The Hospitalization of Cases of Communicable Diseases, Report of Conference Committee, 1951–1952 Yearbook of the American Public Health Association, *Am. J. Pub. Health.,* Vol. 42, pp. 88–92, Part II, May, 1952.
4. JACKSON, KATHERINE, RUTH WINKLEY, OTTO A. FAUST, and ETHEL G. CERMAK. Problem of Emotional Trauma in Hospital Treatment of Children, *J.A.M.A.,* Vol. 149, pp. 1536–1538, Aug. 23, 1952.
5. LUCAS, WILLIAM P., Communication Presenting Results of Study for National Foundation for Infantile Paralysis, *Pediatrics,* Vol. 5, pp. 741–747, April, 1950.
6. "Convalescent Care for Children, Report of a Study," The National Society for Crippled Children and Adults, Chicago, 1947.
7. SHINDELL, SIDNEY, A Method of Home Care for Prolonged Illness, *Pub. Health Rep.,* Vol. 65, pp. 651–660, May 19, 1950.
8. Home Care at the Montefiore Hospital, editorial, *Am. J. Pub. Health,* Vol. 39, pp. 224–225, February, 1949.
9. LEVIN, MORTON L., "Chronic Illness, Social Work Year Book," pp. 101–109, American Association of Social Workers, New York, 1951.
10. CRONIN, JOHN W., LOUIS S. REED, and HELEN HOLLINGSWORTH, Hos-

pital Construction under the Hill-Burton Program, *Pub. Health Rep.,* Vol. 65, pp. 743–753, June 9, 1950.

11. Regional Planning for Pediatric Education and Services, Chap. V, Report on Better Medical Care for Children, Committee for the Improvement of Child Health, American Academy of Pediatrics, *Pediatrics,* Vol. 6, pp. 532–544, September, 1950.

ADDITIONAL REFERENCES

1. BLUESTONE, E. M., Hospital and Home Care Combine to Close the Gap between the Practice of Medicine and the Social Sciences, *Mod. Hosp.,* Vol. 77, pp. 61–64, December, 1951.

2. WALKER, MILDRED F., "References Useful to Hospital Administrators in Planning and Providing Hospital Services for Mothers and Children," Children's Bureau, Washington, D.C., 1952.

3. VANDER VEER, ADRIAN H., The Psychopathology of Physical Illness and Hospital Residence, *Quart. J. Child Behavior,* Vol. 1, pp. 55–71, January, 1949.

4. "Preventive Aspects of Chronic Disease," Proceedings of Conference Sponsored by the Commission on Chronic Illness, Mar. 12–14, 1951, Health Publications Institute, Raleigh, N.C., 1952.

5. INSLEY, VIRGINIA, Sick Children Benefit from a City's Home-care Program, *Child,* Vol. 17, pp. 78–80, January, 1953.

6. Series of Papers on Home Care, *Am. J. Pub. Health,* Vol. 43, pp. 577–604, May, 1953.

Part II

ESSENTIAL HEALTH SERVICES

9 HEALTH APPRAISAL

An adequate health appraisal is the essential first step in all health services for individual children. This applies equally to presumably healthy children as part of health supervision and to severely handicapped children preliminary to starting complicated rehabilitative services. By health appraisal is meant the evaluation of the total health of the child; attention to the total health of children prevents focusing of attention on the presenting complaint or disability to the neglect of physical, emotional, or social conditions which may be of greater immediate or ultimate significance. Health appraisal is a process in which the observations of parents, teachers, nurses, and others who come in intimate contact with children are used by the physician to supplement the information obtained from his medical examination. Screening examinations of vision and hearing and periodic physical measurements of the child provide additional valuable leads for the physician in the evaluative process.

As part of the medical examination the physician should offer the parent, and the older child as well, the opportunity to talk freely about problems or anxieties bearing on the health of the child. By avoiding a rigid pattern of examination, the physician can obtain vital information on the social and emotional status of the child. The appraisal sets the stage for further health services which may be needed by the child. It may have disclosed conditions due either to hereditary or environmental factors which might affect the child's development. The physician should ask himself, at the end of the health appraisal, what steps should be taken immediately to improve the child's health, and what long-range plans should be recommended for the child.

GROWTH AND DEVELOPMENT

Appraisal of the health status of children differs from that of adults in one major respect: it requires an understanding of the process of growth and development. The child is a growing organism undergoing rapid changes in his total personality and in his physical components. What is beyond the range of normal at one age may be an entirely normal finding at another age. Patterns of growth vary in different children and must be evaluated in determining the health status of a given child. For example,

in boys undergoing a rapid adolescent growth spurt in both weight and height, the degree and rapidity of increase in heart size may closely approximate that seen in a preadolescent boy with progressive cardiac enlargement from rheumatic carditis. It is obvious that the possibility of correctly diagnosing pathologic enlargement of the heart implies an appreciation of these individual variations and growth patterns. (1)

Growth is usually thought of as an increase in size or mass; development is considered as differentiation or change in form. The infant grows in length and weight; his bodily configuration develops into a more linear character after the first birthday. In practice, the phrase "growth and development" is often slurred together; or growth is used alone to encompass both increase in size and differentiation in form. Whatever the definition, what matters is the concept of evaluation of the child going through a dynamic process of growth and development.

Every child is born with a constitutional endowment which sets the broad limits of his physical and mental capacities. The basic fact of constitution must be accepted by the parents and all persons concerned with children. Otherwise children may either be forced to attempt tasks beyond their capabilities, or they may be held back from achieving their full potentialities.

The development of the personality of the growing child, with its inseparable physical, mental, and emotional components, is the result of the interaction of environmental and constitutional factors. No matter how different children may be by heredity, they all go through similar stages of physical and emotional development, unless some grossly pathological condition interferes. The process of development is inborn; the child matures by passing with varying degrees of completeness through each stage to the next. If he is aided by favorable environmental conditions, he will gain the greatest benefits by his experiences and be ready to face successfully the problems at successive stages. Protection against disease, provision of adequate nutrition, meeting emotional needs as they arise are among the factors which encourage the child's development. The physician's understanding of the process of development enables him to help fulfill the child's requirements at each stage within the framework of the family and community.

Physical Growth and Development. The rate of growth of the body as a whole varies with age. Growth is most rapid during the first year after birth when there is about a threefold increase in weight. The first period of rapid growth levels off about the fifth year; from that time until puberty growth is fairly steady. The second period of rapid growth occurs during puberty, after which the rate of growth gradually levels off until maximum growth is reached. Girls go through their pubertal growth spurt earlier than boys, so that girls between eleven and fourteen years of age are taller and heavier on the average than boys of the same age.

The growth of various parts of the body also follows characteristic patterns at different ages. The genital and endocrine tissues shrink in size during early infancy and then grow hardly at all until the sharp prepubertal and pubertal spurt. The brain and other nervous tissue present the opposite type of pattern, with 90 per cent of their total growth occurring during the first six years after birth. The lymphoid tissues have their own distinct pattern of growth; they grow rapidly and fairly steadily from birth, attaining their greatest size during the early school years. Lymphoid tissue normally undergoes spontaneous shrinkage thereafter until, in adult life, its absolute weight is only about half its maximum weight of the early school years.

The varied patterns of growth of tissue systems have many practical implications. For example, the tonsils and adenoids, as lymphoid structures, are normally large at the very time when children first come under health supervision through health services in the schools. Unless the total health status of the children is carefully appraised, a large percentage of children may be referred for medical attention, and possible tonsillectomy, purely because of the size of the tonsils. The rapid growth of neural tissues before six years of age is a possible indication of the extremely rapid development of behavior patterns and the greater emotional stresses during this period of life. The abrupt cessation of the flow of hormones from the mother at the time of birth is probably the chief cause of the shrinkage of the endocrine and sexual tissues during the newborn period; if these are not understood, such conditions as vaginal bleeding associated with these changes may be incorrectly diagnosed and treated.

The growth of children varies not only according to sex; race, nationality, socioeconomic status, and geographic area are also significant factors. Children of Mediterranean or Oriental stock growing up in the United States are generally taller and heavier than their immigrant parents. Negro infants are smaller and more immature on the average at birth than white infants; recent studies have indicated that at least part of the difference is due to socioeconomic factors which influence the nutritional status and adequacy of prenatal care of the mother (2). Growth also varies according to season; the most rapid growth occurs in the fall, with the rate of growth dropping off during the winter and spring (3).

Measurement of Physical Growth and Development. A series of body measurements may be made as part of the health appraisal, including weight, standing and sitting height, circumference of head, chest, and abdomen, and breadth at the shoulders or hips. Measurements of the breadth of the pelvic region and chest circumference for skeletal development, of calf circumference for muscular development, and of thickness of selected skin folds for development of subcutaneous fatty tissue have been proposed as routine procedures in examination of the child of school age (4). While the theoretical desirability of detailed physical measurements is not questioned, practicability precludes all but a few selected measurements except in research situations. In routine practice, height and weight should be measured and recorded periodically throughout infancy and childhood, with the circumference of the head added in children up to about a year of age.

Routine measurement of weight and height is a screening procedure intended to discover children as early as possible when they deviate from normal health. It is not possible to interpret the range of normal in single observations from available height and weight tables because of differences in physique and rates of maturation of children. This difficulty is encountered with the Baldwin-Wood and Woodbury tables, in which weight is given according to sex, age, and height, and to a lesser extent, with the Pryor tables, which present the added relationship of body width at the iliac crest.

Since isolated measurements are of such limited value, increasing use is being made of growth charts which permit recording of a series of measurements of height and weight. Graphic presentation of the series of measurements gives the physician an immediate picture of the progress made by the child over a period of time and places the child in relation to the percentile group above or below the average measurement in which the child falls at a given age. Since a child's body build tends to follow a given pattern between infancy and puberty, any deviation in weight and height from his pattern as established on the chart serves as a signal for further investigation of the child's health. Several growth charts based on a similar principle are available. Those of Jackson and Kelly consist of sets of charts for each sex for infants under one year of age, for preschool children, and for children of school age, each chart having curves for height and for weight by age (5). The Meredith charts are designed for use in children of school age, and present a series of curves showing average measurements and moderately and marked divergence from the average (6). The Boston Children's Center charts cover height and weight for the same age periods as the Jackson-Kelly charts and present, in addition, a means of recording head circumference during the first twenty-eight weeks of life (7). In the Wetzel grids one curve presents the relationship of height and weight, and another the developmental status of the child by showing the height-weight index against age (8). Any of these can be used satisfactorily by a person trained in its use. It bears repetition that, whatever type of graphic aid is used, it is only one tool for bringing children to attention for more detailed medical review and to help in the total appraisal of the child. It should also be realized that the measurements of some children with definite nutritional deficiencies may still appear entirely normal on growth charts over a prolonged period of observation.

Mental and Emotional Growth and Development. Mental and emotional development follows certain general patterns, just as physical development does. The process of development of even the relatively simple behavior patterns is complex but orderly. The fully matured activity is the end result of a series of stages each of which prepared the way for the next. The ultimate ability of the child to run, for example, was heralded in the infant's ability to make a major shift in his body

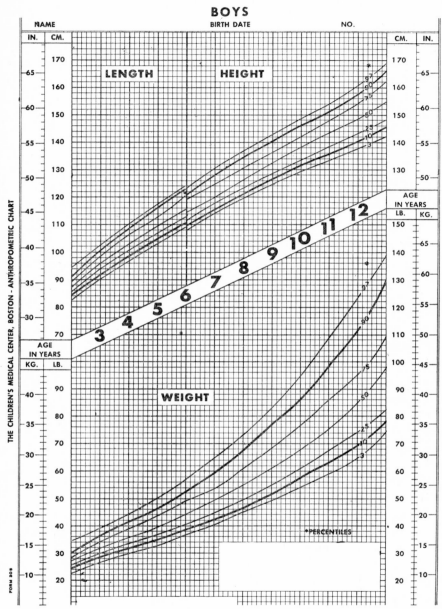

Figure 8. Percentile growth chart prepared by the Department of Maternal and Child Health, Harvard School of Public Health, for use at Children's Medical Center, Boston. (*Reproduced by permission of Harvard School of Public Health, available from Mead, Johnson and Company.*)

posture at about twenty weeks, when the supine infant can roll over on his side. A crawling position is attained at twenty-eight weeks; four weeks later the infant can move about by pivoting on his arms. Finally, at fifty weeks, the infant can creep on hands and feet. Meanwhile, the pattern of stepping movements has been developing, so that he can move about upright with support at about forty-eight weeks of age. Between twelve and eighteen months, creeping is displaced by toddling; by two years of age, well-developed walking is evident and the child takes his first running steps. Thereafter, his walking and running improve in dexterity, but the fundamental patterns have been established (9). Language, responsiveness to other persons, feeding, and sleeping similarly go through a normal evolution which can be predicted in general terms for individual children.

Questions about the most important landmarks in the child's motor development, such as age at holding head erect, standing with and without support, and walking, are included in every medical history. If this information is supplemented by careful observations of the physician at the time of the medical examination, valuable leads can be obtained about the child's general development as well as about the presence of such conditions as cerebral palsy and cretinism. The persistence of certain behavior patterns beyond a given age is an indication for further investigation; for example, the Moro or embrace reflex, elicited by sudden jarring of the infant's crib, should normally be almost gone by about six weeks of age.

While emotional and social development go through stages identifiable in all children, the form the personality takes is dependent to such a large extent upon intimate interpersonal relationships at each stage, and the total personality of the child is so complex, that the variations among children at each stage are great. The following brief presentation only touches on a few of the highlights of these stages, in the concepts of personality development originally elucidated by Freud. The newborn infant can only feel his experiences, and he appears satisfied as long as his immediate physical needs are met. During the first year his feelings of pleasure are largely related to feeding; every new object must be explored with his mouth. His feeling of love for his mother and sense of security are related in large measure to these satisfactions. Individualization of feeding schedules in early infancy and a relaxed approach to weaning and the introduction of solid foods help the infant successfully through this stage. The second year is one of increasing socialization; the young child begins to accept slight delays in having his wants met. He is no longer always at the receiving end, and demands are made upon him. One of the earliest demands by the previously all-giving mother is for bowel control. Coming at a time when the child is in the stress of learning many other activities, and when excretory activities are a source of pleasure to him, the manner of acquisition of bowel control may leave a deep impression upon his immature personality. It is at this time, too, that conflicting feelings toward his mother become more evident.

During the second half of the preschool period the child goes through the difficult process of achieving a degree of independence from his close attachment to his parents. At the start of this stage, the boy's attachment to his mother is very close; seeking her undivided attention leads to hostile feelings toward the father, which may or may not be expressed. Emotional development during this stage prepares the foundation for normal relationships with the opposite sex in later life. The young girl's adjustment during this period is more complicated, since her hostile feelings are directed at the mother, but the stage is equally as important to her emotional development.

It is widely held that the child's personality, his characteristic ways of reacting to life situations, is largely formed before six years of age, although the personality can still undergo significant modifications throughout life. During the early school years, the child learns to depend more upon himself among his age peers and in the school setting, but his basic forms of reactions are mirrors of the ways he learned to react as an infant and preschool child. The period of comparative calm of the early school years is followed by the storms of adolescence, when the child emerging into adulthood establishes his relationships with persons of the opposite sex outside the family circle and when he asserts his independence from his parents while still, in most instances, remaining at home.

Emotional development has been described by Erikson in terms of the child acquiring additive components of a healthy personality, a formulation which was accepted as a basic concept of the Midcentury White House Conference on Children and Youth (10). The infant acquires a sense of trust when his experiences, especially those related to feeding, are satisfying ones, or a sense of basic mistrust when the contrary occurs. At about one year of age he begins to develop a sense of autonomy, when he becomes more self-reliant in his exploration of the environment. This is the period when he first begins to have some freedom of choice and has difficulty in keeping to a straight course because everything about him is distracting. At four or five years of age a sense of initiative develops in the child. The child at this age is guided by his conscience as well as by external admonitions; this sense of initiative must be developed without the sense of guilt becoming too much of a burden. By school age the child begins to have a sense of industry, when the child achieves satisfaction by accomplishing specific tasks rather than simply dreaming about them. The final important component of a healthy personality to be added before adulthood is the sense of identity. During the stormy period of adolescence, the child must clarify in his own mind what his place will be in his social setting. If the adolescent does not get to know himself as a distinct person, he cannot stand independently on his own feet and relate himself well to others.

Measurement of Mental and Emotional Growth and Development. An impression of the child's mental development may be obtained from the history and from observation of the child at the time of the medical examination. Different types of guides have been prepared to help the physician in his evaluation of the child's mental development. Cards may be used for review by the physician immediately before or during an examination, to be sure the salient features of a given stage of development are covered (11). Record forms are often employed for recording the age at which the child performs various activities (Figure 9). When the activities are listed by age in order of their expected appearance, checking on the form the age at which the child performs the activities gives a roughly graphic presentation of his development which eliminates detailed study of the entire medical record of the child to gain the same picture of development. Purely graphic presentation of the child's development, in which the various points representing the relationship of each activity to age are connected in a single line, is undesirable because it tends to make the observer lose sight of the normal range of variation in mental development.

Widely used tools for the measurement of mental development are the many types of intelligence tests. The intelligence quotient, or the relationship of the child's mental age to his chronological age, derived from these tests, should be used as a measurement to be included in the total evaluation of the child, rather than accepting it as a fixed characteristic upon which important decisions, such as educational placement of the child, are automatically based. Intelligence tests measure

Instructions: Check (✔) chronological age at which behavior manifestation first appears. Source of information will be from direct observation in clinic and history from parent.

Item Number	Behavior Manifestations	Behavior Age	0 to 1	1 to 2	2 to 3	3 to 4	4 to 5	5 to 6	6 to 7	7 to 8	8 to 9	9 to 10	10 to 11	11 to 12	12 to 16	16 to 20	20 to 24	24 to 28	28 to 32	32 to 36	3 to 4	4 to 5	5 to 6	Item Number
1	Chin up prone																							1
2	Eyes follow moving objects	0																						2
3	Smiles at person	to																						3
4	Coos	3																						4
5	Head steady	mos.																						5
6	Laughs aloud																							6
7	Grasps and holds toy	3																						7
8	Begins to roll over	to																						8
9	Sits, frog position	6																						9
10	Discriminates strangers	mos.																						10
11	Transfers toy, one hand to other																							11
12	Sits alone	6																						12
13	Vocalizes (da,ma,ba)	to																						13
14	Crawls	9																						14
15	Pulls to standing position	mos.																						15
16	Waves bye-bye																							16
17	Picks up pellet (thumb & index)	9																						17
18	Says one word	to																						18
19	Nursery tricks (pat-a-cake)	12																						19
20	Finger feeds self from tray	mos.																						20
21	Walks alone																							21
22	Uses spoon with some spilling	12																						22
23	Uses phrases	to																						23
24	Follows simple instructions	24																						24
25	Bowel control established	mos.																						25
26	Beginning bladder control																							26
27	Manifests negativism	24																						27
28	Prefers solitary play	to																						28
29	Uses simple sentences	36																						29
30	Runs and climbs stairs	mos.																						30
31	Bladder control established																							31
32	Cooperative play	3																						32
33	Dresses self	to																						33
34	Imagination & exaggeration	6																						34
35	Enjoys motor accomplishments	yrs.																						35

Age groupings under Behavior Age are made to overlap to help stress the wide range of normal variations.

Figure 9. Behavior development chart used by New York State Department of Health. (*Developed by Ruth K. Beecroft, M.D., and Marian Campbell, R.N., reproduced by permission of the New York State Department of Health.*)

only the ability of an individual to answer specific questions or perform specific tasks. The tests are placed in proper perspective when intelligence is defined as "that capacity of the human being which determines his ability to perform certain tasks as set forth in intelligence tests."

(12) The results of a given intelligence test may be influenced by various conditions at the time of the test, such as the child's state of relaxation or fatigue. The existence of only moderate disturbances of vision, of hearing, or of coordination may seriously distort the results of the test, as may a specific reading disability not so readily discovered as the conditions just mentioned. In the presence of more serious physical disabilities, the usual means of testing intelligence are not applicable at all.

Intelligence tests are more difficult to use and are more unreliable in young children. Techniques of developmental diagnosis are available for use at key ages in the infant and young child, to determine not only their over-all mental development but also deviations in behavior patterns due to specific disabilities such as cerebral palsy (13). Development is analyzed in terms of motor behavior, adaptive behavior, and language and personal-social behavior. While theoretically simple to perform, proper use of the tests requires intensive training and considerable experience on the part of the examiner. The tests themselves also are not above criticism, in that the prognoses regarding individual children based on the tests have not been adequately evaluated by long-term studies of the children tested.

Another group of tests, known as projective tests, are used as a means of gaining information about the child's personality (14). The best known is the Rorschach test, in which the person tested is asked to give his reactions to a standard set of ink blots. Others are the thematic apperception and the children's apperception tests in which the person's feelings and interpretations of test situations in pictures are elicited. These tests should be used only by highly trained individuals; they are useful as another tool in evaluation of the child, to determine his need for psychiatric care and to help in school placement.

OTHER SCREENING PROCEDURES

Other screening procedures may be used by nonmedical personnel to disclose suspected deviations from normal development in groups of children. Such procedures spare the physician for functions which only he can perform; at the same time, they help ensure that many more children are tested than might otherwise be possible. Screening tests are used most extensively to detect disturbances in vision and hearing. Certain laboratory tests on blood and urine are used to a lesser extent.

Performance of screening tests and selection of the types of procedures to be used depend upon the situation in each community. There is little point to conducting complicated screening tests which are designed to detect minor degrees of ocular imbalance, for example, if facilities for diagnosis and treatment of such conditions are grossly inadequate. The physicians in the area, and especially the specialists in ophthalmology and otolaryngology, should be consulted before screening procedures are instituted or modifications made in policies for use of these procedures in the various community health services. Physicians differ in their judgment as to what findings on the screening tests are to be considered significant enough for further investigation and follow-up. Overreferral of children with minor or insignificant findings may create antagonism on the part of the medical profession and the public.

Screening Tests of Vision. Tests are available, singly and in combination, for screening visual acuity (both near- and farsightedness), imbalance of the ocular muscles, color vision, and depth perception. No one of these is clearly superior in all or most situations, and care must be exercised in choosing the most suitable tests under given conditions (15).

The Snellen test of visual acuity is based on the ability of the child to read a special eye chart with lines of letters decreasing in size from top to bottom, under standard lighting conditions. Standing at a distance of 20 ft. from the chart, the child reads the letters, one eye at a time, with the other eye covered. If the child can read only as far as the 40-ft. line, his visual acuity is said to be 20/40. A modification of the Snellen letter chart, using the letter "E" pointing in different directions, is available for use with children who are not able to read.

The Snellen test is chiefly of value in detecting varying degrees of myopia. Various other types of screening tests of a more complicated nature have been devised in an effort to discover farsightedness, defects in muscle coordination, and astigmatism. The use of glasses with plus lens is a means of detecting farsightedness in children who have normal or 20/20 vision on the Snellen test. If the child can read the 20-ft. line on the chart with the plus lens glasses on, he is presumed to have some degree of farsightedness.

Imbalance of the ocular muscles in the absence of a frank strabismus may be suspected by use of a simple "cover test." This is performed by covering and uncovering an eye with a card when the child looks at a bright object directly in front of him. In the event the child has any muscular imbalance, the covered eye will shift somewhat when the covering is removed. Other tests for imbalance of the external ocular muscles either are more complicated versions of the "cover test," or else they use glasses with special lenses which produce vertical and horizontal streaks of light. Several types of testing equipment, including the Massachusetts Vision Test and the Keystone Telebinocular Test, combine a battery of eye tests. No group methods of testing the vision of children have been found satisfactory.

Screening Tests for Hearing. The use of audiometers makes possible mass testing for the detection not only of seriously impaired hearing, but also of mild or subclinical degrees of hearing defect in which treatment can most readily prevent the subsequent development of handicapping hearing loss. Of the two types of audiometers in general use for screening purposes, the audiometer using pure tones for testing is gradually replacing the type employing the spoken voice. The group phonograph audiometer, with voice spoken in descending volume, permits testing of 40 children at a time through earphones; the children write on a test sheet as long as they can distinguish what is being spoken. Pure tone audiometers using selected frequencies give a "sweep check" for screening. Several models of both group phonograph and individual pure tone screening audiometers are available and meet accepted standards for their intended purpose. The Massachusetts group test, using a pure tone audiometer to test as many as 40 children at a time, has not been accepted as widely as individual pure tone tests.

The group phonograph audiometer was the pioneer instrument possessing reliability for screening purposes. Its main advantage lies in the fact that it can be used by comparatively untrained personnel. It saves little time as opposed even to the individual pure tone test because of the time required in scoring its test results. "The pure tone testing technique is more efficient because it not only finds more hard of hearing children but all of them in a given school enrollment. The disadvantages of limited (individual) testing by this method may soon be overcome by more extensive use of group, pure tone audiometers which have been introduced since the 1947–1948 survey." (16) The pure tone test is clearly superior to the the phonograph audiometer in another significant respect: it detects the earlier signs of conductive hearing loss manifest first at frequencies above the usual spoken voice.

Laboratory and Other Screening Tests. Urine analyses and complete blood counts are included in the routine work-up of hospitalized children and often also when children are seen because of illness in a physician's office or in a clinic. However, the value of routine testing of urine for screening purposes in questionable. Collection of the specimens, especially in young children, presents obvious difficulties. Determination of the acidity and specific gravity of a single specimen of urine provides no leads for further investigation. The presence of albumin is more often than not finally diagnosed as orthostatic albuminuria, so that the discovery of many children with benign conditions leads to needless apprehension until the nature of the condition is settled. Even routine mass testing of the urine for reducing substances is not productive enough to warrant the effort. Small amounts of sugar may occasionally spill over into the urine, and sugars other than glucose may be present in the urine without adversely affecting the health of the child. Even diabetes mellitus would probably be discovered only rarely in the absence of symptoms, since diabetes in children is usually a more fulminating disease than in adults, presenting symptoms manifest at an early stage to the alert observer.

Complete blood counts are also not practical as a mass screening procedure. The one element in the blood count of value for screening purposes is the hemoglobin determination for the presence of anemia, especially anemia due to iron deficiency. Various types of photoelectric hemoglobinometers are available for rapid testing of hemoglobin levels. The specific gravity method or copper sulfate method, in which drops of blood are dropped in a series of bottles of copper sulfate solution of increasing specific gravity, is simple and reliable, and the results are available immediately (17). One or two levels of specific gravity may be selected for screening individuals for further investigation. The Tallqvist method, in which a drop of blood on blotting paper is matched against a color scale, is unfortunately still used in spite of its gross inaccuracy.

Micromethods of biochemical analyses of various nutrients in the blood are also in use; these are discussed in relation to the appraisal of nutritional status. Other tests in wide use for screening purposes include serological tests for syphilis and various skin tests to determine whether the child has been infected with a given organism, as in the tuberculin test, or whether the child has a certain level of immunity to specific diseases, as the Schick and Dick tests in relation to diphtheria and scarlet fever, respectively. Current opinion about the value of these procedures for screening purposes is presented in the chapter on the prevention of communicable diseases.

Multiple Screening. Mass screening procedures in adults were developed originally for individual conditions. Chest x-rays were taken of groups of the population over fifteen years of age to detect tuberculosis. Suspected cardiac conditions and thoracic neoplasms were discovered incidental to the case-finding efforts to detect pulmonary tuberculosis. Serological tests for syphilis were performed on entire populations. Later, simplified screening tests were developed for sugar in the urine and of elevated blood sugar levels leading to a suspicion of diabetes. The availability of these individual screening tests has suggested the performance of a battery of tests during a single visit, the so-called multiple or multiphasic screening (18). The promotional effort needed to stimulate individuals to submit to a battery of tests is hardly, if at all, greater than for one screening test. The more ambitious projects have included measurement of height and weight, chest x-ray, urine analysis, hemoglobin determination, recording of blood pressure, serological test for syphilis, determination of blood sugar levels, tests of vision and hearing, and measurement of ocular tension.

In spite of extensive trials, multiple screening in adults is still an experimental procedure. Some of the screening tests used are in need of refinement. The question of what to do for the large number of individuals found to have one or another suspected defect remains to be answered. Even though multiple screening in adults is still in a state of flux, the suggestion has been made that the techniques be given a trial in children. It is doubtful that the procedure is adaptable to children. Early discovery in children is an essentially different matter from that in adults, as in relation to diabetes, tuberculosis, and kidney disease. Most types of conditions of importance in children are intimately concerned with deviations in growth and development, requiring individual evaluation rather than a mechanical technical approach. Even if some satisfactory multiple screening method were developed for use in childhood, it probably could not be applied in children under ten or twelve years of age because of the excessive demands it would make on the limited attention span and endurance of younger children. It would be difficult to visualize getting reliable results from having a six- or seven-year-old child submitting in quick succession to even those screening tests which are applicable in childhood.

CITED REFERENCES

1. WASHBURN, ALFRED H., Growth: Its Significance in Medicine Viewed as Human Biology, *Pediatrics,* Vol. 5, pp. 765–770, May, 1950.
2. SCOTT, ROLAND B., M. E. JENKINS, and R. P. CRAWFORD, Growth and Development of Negro Infants: I. Analysis of Birth Weights of 11,818 Newly Born Infants, *Pediatrics,* Vol. 6, pp. 425–431, September, 1950.
3. PALMER, CARROLL E., Seasonal Variation of Average Growth in Weight of Elementary School Children, *Pub. Health Rep.,* Vol. 48, pp. 211–233, Mar. 3, 1933.
4. STUART, HAROLD C., and HOWARD V. MEREDITH, Use of Body Measurements in the School Health Program, *Am. J. Pub. Health,* Vol. 36, pp. 1365–1386, December, 1946.
5. JACKSON, ROBERT L., and HELEN G. KELLY, Growth Charts for Use in Pediatric Practice, *J. Pediat.,* Vol. 27, pp. 215–229, September, 1945.
6. MEREDITH, HOWARD V., A "Physical Growth Record" for Use in Elementary and High Schools, *Am. J. Pub. Health,* Vol. 39, pp. 878–885, July, 1949.
7. STUART, HAROLD C., and ASSOCIATES, "Anthropometric Charts," The Children's Medical Center, Boston, undated.
8. WEITZEL, NORMAN C., (*a*) Assessing the Physical Condition of Children: I. Case Demonstration of Failing Growth and the Determination of "Par" by the Grid Method, *J. Pediat.,* Vol. 22, pp. 82–110, January, 1943, (*b*) The Baby Grid: An Application of the Grid Technique to Growth and Development in Infants, *J. Pediat.,* Vol. 29, pp. 439–454, October, 1946.
9. GESELL, ARNOLD, *et al.,* "The First Five Years of Life: A Guide to the Study of the Preschool Child," Harper & Brothers, New York, 1940.
10. WITMER, HELEN L., and RUTH KOTINSKY, editors, "Personality in the Making," Harper & Brothers, New York, 1953.
11. ALDRICH, C. ANDERSON, and EDITH S. HEWITT, Outlines for Well Baby Clinics: (*a*) I. Recording Development for the First Twelve Months, *Am. J. Dis. Child.,* Vol. 71, pp. 131–137, February, 1946; (*b*) Recording Development for the Second Twelve Months, *Pediatrics,* Vol. 2, pp. 69–73, July, 1948.
12. LEMKAU, PAUL V., "Mental Hygiene in Public Health," McGraw-Hill Book Company, Inc., New York, 1949.
13. GESELL, ARNOLD, and CATHERINE S. AMATRUDA, "Developmental Diagnosis: Normal and Abnormal Child Development," Paul B. Hoeber,

Inc., Medical Book Department of Harper & Brothers, New York, 1947.
14. HALPERN, FLORENCE, Projective Tests in the Personality Investigation of Children, *J. Pediat.*, Vol. 38, pp. 770–775, June, 1951.
15. CRANE, MARIAN M., RICHARD G. SCOBEE, FRANKLIN M. FOOTE, and EARL L. GREEN, Study of Procedures Used for Screening Elementary School Children for Visual Defects: Referrals by Screening Procedures versus Ophthalmological Findings, *Am. J. Pub. Health*, Vol. 42, pp. 1430–1439, November, 1952.
16. GARDNER, WARREN H., chairman, Committee on Hard of Hearing Children of American Hearing Society, Reprint No. 227, from *Hearing News*, February–May, 1950.
17. KOLMER, J. A., and F. BOERNER, "Approved Laboratory Technique," Appleton-Century-Crofts, Inc., New York, 1945.
18. SCHEELE, LEONARD A., Current Experience in Multiphasic Health Examinations: Orientation and Background, *Am. J. Pub. Health*, Vol. 41, pp. 635–639, June, 1951.

ADDITIONAL REFERENCES

1. STUART, HAROLD C., moderator, Symposium on Child Growth and Development, *Child*, Vol. 16, pp. 50–63, December, 1951.
2. PETRIE, LESTER M., C. D. BOWDOIN, and CHRISTOPHER J. McLOUGHLIN, Voluntary Multiple Health Tests, *J.A.M.A.*, Vol. 148, pp. 1022–1024, Mar. 22, 1952.
3. WATSON, ERNEST H., and GEORGE H. LOWREY, "Growth and Development of Children," Year Book Publishers, Inc., Chicago, 1951.
4. STUART, HAROLD C., Normal Growth and Development during Adolescence, *New England J. Med.*, Vol. 234, pp. 666–672, 693–700, 732–738, May 16, 23, 30, 1946.

10 PROMOTION OF MENTAL HEALTH

The emotional well-being or mental health of the individuals composing the community is promoted through the evolution of a family and community setting in which the child's native emotional drives and intellectual abilities are understood and in which the child's increasingly broadening relationships with other persons encourage his fullest development. The promotion of mental health includes, but goes far beyond, merely the prevention of behavior problems in the early years of life and even beyond the prevention of emotionally handicapping conditions in later childhood and in adult life. Every phase of family and community life has some bearing upon the emotional well-being of children. The adequacy of housing, the availability of recreational facilities suitable to each age level, the character and extent of social stratification and antagonisms, economic stresses in the family and community—these are only a few of the environmental circumstances which play their part in influencing the developing personality of the child. How these factors exert their force is a matter of intensive study by sociologists, psychiatrists, epidemiologists, educators, and representatives of other disciplines working as individuals and groups, and many new insights are being gained.

Every institution and agency is involved in the pattern of local relationships in which the children of the community are born and raised. This is so even though no conscious effort has been made to modify the community pattern. Local government, religious bodies, the educational system, and the whole gamut of social agencies form part of this effort, whatever the degree of organization reached in the process.

The practicing physician, whether pediatrician or general practitioner, has two main functions to perform in the promotion of mental health of children within this broad framework. The first is related to his authoritative position as a professional person in the community; his advice is often sought on possible measures for modifying conditions which may have a bearing on mental health. The second function is unique to any physician, whether in private practice or in various community health services; in the course of his routine contacts with patients, he can help allay anxieties and further healthy relationships between parents and children.

Fundamentally, the key to progress in helping parents is the relationship with a non-judgmental, non-critical, accepting person who at the same time is in a position of professional authority. . . . The opportunity the parent is given in her contacts with the medical advisers to the child to assume her natural responsibilities and to exercise her prerogatives as a parent is a therapeutic process in its own right. (1)

Meaning of "Preventive Services." There is especial need in the field of mental health to understand the sense of the word *prevention.* Historically in the child guidance movement, prevention has been thought of as the treatment of emotional disturbances in childhood to avoid more serious and often irreversible disorders of adult life. The early enthusiastic expectations of the exponents of child guidance based on this concept of preventive services have not been borne out in practice (2). This does not imply that adequate psychiatric care of serious emotional disorders in their early stages is not effective in many cases in preventing progress of the condition and even in aiding the individual to attain a higher stage of maturity and social usefulness than before the onset of his emotional illness. This has been amply demonstrated in individual intensive psychiatric treatment based on dynamic principles. Adequate care of all types of emotional problems in childhood is also unquestionably of the utmost value in itself. What has yet to be shown conclusively is that the usual treatment of emotional disorders in childhood prevents incapacitating mental illness in later life.

Care of evident emotional disorders to prevent more serious illness has often been referred to as secondary prevention. Child health services intended for the so-called primary prevention of emotional difficulties are generally understood as those services rendered before pronounced deviations from normal emotional development have called attention to the child. *Anticipatory guidance* is a term used to express this concept (3). The purpose of anticipatory guidance is to reach parents regularly to keep them informed of what to expect at immediately succeeding stages of their children's development. When parents understand the broad range of normal behavior in childhood and are prepared to meet the emotional needs of their children as they arise, the presumption is that parental anxiety due to lack of information or to misinformation will be minimized and favorable parent-child relationships encouraged.

The approach to a mental health program may be clarified by considering four types of services:

1. General education of the public in mental health principles
2. Anticipatory guidance
3. Guidance of persons with general health problems
4. Care of manifest emotional disturbances

This spectrum is suggested merely to place the various services in some sort of perspective. It is artificial in that recipients of services are arbitrarily placed in one or another group according to the intent of the services, whereas several types of services may actually be rendered simultaneously to the same person.

1. *General public health education.* The past few years have witnessed a widespread attempt to educate the public in mental health principles. Motion-picture films, pamphlets, radio broadcasts, and other mass mediums have been used extensively in the traditional pattern of health education. This campaign has brought about increased public understanding of mental mechanisms, and it has begun to remove the social stigma that is still attached to mental illness. It has had further value in promoting more adequate psychiatric services in many communities, but in many others the hopes aroused have been dashed by the impossibility of locating trained personnel to man the desired services.

The approach to the prevention of mental illness through public health education, on the other hand, has marked limitations. Indiscriminate broadcasting of this type of information cannot be expected to have a favorable effect on persons with emotional difficulties.

For persons who are socially well adapted and relatively free of neurotic conflict, the psychiatric information disseminated through mass media channels may be useful in providing reassurance on specific anxiety issues, particularly in relation to child rearing. On the whole, however, the material is so alarmist, places so much emphasis on the prevalence of emotional disturbance . . . and the likelihood and ease of invoking disaster for anybody's future mental health, that the net result may be to produce uncertainty, confusion and distress, even when the gain in sophistication is formidable. (4)

The possibility of arousing anxiety places a heavy responsibility on persons involved in a program of public mental health education. When motion-picture films are used, they should be previewed to be sure they are suitable for their intended audience, and a qualified person should be present at the film showing to guide the discussion. Education in mental health principles may also be restricted to groups having common interests, permitting more careful selection of the material used.

2. *Anticipatory guidance.* This preventive technique aims at reaching the recipient immediately before the information is applicable. For greatest usefulness, the person providing the guidance, whether physician, nurse, or other type of personnel, should have had training in child development and in the emotional needs of children. Much can be accomplished even without such extended training, however, provided the principles are understood and the information given is properly integrated in the total health care of the children. In addition to personal guidance of individual parents, a discussion leader may meet with groups of parents having children of the same age. Individual letters may also be mailed to parents at regular intervals to cover approaching stages of their children's development. Letter services have also been used widely for prenatal instruction.

Special attention should be paid to preparation of parents for situations which most commonly lead to difficulties. The universality of jealousy between siblings and the need for continued attention to the older child should be explained to the parents before the birth of the expected infant. The parents should also be helped to prepare the child for the mother's departure from the home for delivery in the hospital. The mother should have adequte instruction in the introduction of solid foods for the infant. Weaning from the breast or bottle to the cup is another trouble spot which can be smoothed over when the mother is prepared to meet the infant's individual needs in a gradual manner. Not later than a few months after birth of the infant, the mother should be guided in the need for a permissive type of training in bowel and bladder control; this is intended to reduce the possibility of use by the mother of premature or coercive training which might otherwise be more likely to be instituted.

One point to be especially stressed is the psychological preparation of the parents for the child's sharp decrease in appetite and even of total food intake, which occurs so often some time between the twelfth and eighteenth month. If offered in advance of the occurrence, parents will more readily accept the explanation that this is due to the decrease in the rate of the infant's growth and the change in the infant's physique from the pudginess of the infant to the more linear build of the toddler. If the parents face an established feeding problem, the emotional tension already engendered makes it more difficult for them to follow advice based upon the same explanation (5).

Techniques of anticipatory guidance have been developed mainly for parents of children up to six years of age. Beyond the age of school entrance, instruction must be in more general terms and cannot be timed as closely to the expectation of the child's development. Several factors enter into this difference in approach to children from six years of age through adolescence. The emotional development of this age group has not been studied so intensively as that of infants and preschool children. In addition, the variations in personality among children of school age have become more fixed and the emotional characteristics common to the age groups are therefore more difficult to discern. Finally, as age increases, there is a wider range in chronological age at which successive stages in maturity are reached. While the normal variation in age at which the head is held erect is a matter of weeks, and the normal range of age at which the infant first walks a matter of months, the onset of menses normally occurs between about eleven and fifteen years of age, a range of fully four years.

In spite of these differences, preparation of parents for the stages in emotional development of older children is still of decided value. Preparation for satisfactory handling of the child's entrance into school and for possible problems in adjustment in school should be encouraged. Parents should be made aware of such general phenomena as the formation of clubs or gangs of the same sex in the early school period. To minimize the difficulties of adolescence, parents should be helped to give gradually increasing responsibilities to their children in the preadolescent period while continuing to provide the psychological support needed. No later than the preadolescent period, the children themselves should be given the benefits of guidance as well. Girls should be prepared for the onset of menstruation, and both boys and girls for skin changes. The adolescent who appears concerned because he seems different from his fellows needs reassurance about the range of normality. Every attempt should be made to implant an objective attitude toward health in the adolescent (6).

Whatever advice or information is offered must be gauged to the possibility of their acceptance by parents, so as not to arouse anxiety or guilt when it conflicts with firmly fixed attitudes or modes of behavior. It must be realized that, in addition to variation in customs due to different nationality backgrounds, decided swings in recommended methods of child rearing have been characteristic of the American scene from one generation to the next.

The 1890's and 1900's saw a highly sentimental approach to child rearing; 1910 through the 1930's witnessed a rigid, disciplinary approach; the 1940's have emphasized self-regulation and understanding of the child. These sixty years have also seen a swing from emphasis upon character development to emphasis upon personality development. . . . Parents and others in the field of child guidance are warned that, while certain general truths have been discovered, we still do not know the specifics with regard to child training practices. (7)

Anticipatory guidance must, therefore, remain guidance of parents and not become an imperative to be followed at all costs.

3. *Services for persons with general health problems.* Most persons who seek health services for themselves or their children do so because of problems not overtly of an emotional nature. Many of these problems are, however, fraught with anxiety for the persons and families concerned, even though these anxieties may not be expressly verbalized. The presence of a communicable disease, especially tuberculosis or syphilis, the development of any illness having the potentiality for disabling aftereffects even if the acute phase is successfully passed—these are obvious examples of situations in which understanding and warmth on the part of the health worker will pay dividends in better acceptance and use of health services for the greatest benefit to the recipient.

Experiences that are potentially productive of anxiety occur at certain nodal points of stress in the life span of the individual (8). Many of these experiences occur when the person is the recipient of maternal and child health services. Weaning, toilet training, the appearance of siblings in the family group, marriage, and pregnancy may give rise to problems disturbing to the individual and the family. These problems may be the immediate reason for causing the individual to seek help, or they may be discovered incidental to the provision of other services for mother or child. More often than not, they come to light only after a good relationship has been established between the physician or nurse and the person concerned. Fears about the effect of maternal impressions on the unborn child, for example, are very common. The opportunity to express these and other fears to a receptive and noncondemnatory person may be in itself a source of considerable relief to a pregnant woman or a new mother. Having discharged some of her anxiety she is more likely to undertake constructive steps suggested to her, instead of suffering from continued undesirable effects after the fears become firmly implanted.

4. *Care of manifest emotional disturbances.* Emotional disturbances are of all gradations of potential or actual seriousness. Even if it were desirable, it would be clearly impossible to obtain psychiatric help in all these situations. The vast majority of the children with minor deviations from normal emotional development must be handled in the general pediatric setting if they are to be given any help at all. Determination of the limits beyond which specialized psychiatric assistance should be sought in any situation depends upon the understanding and training of nonpsychiatric medical personnel and the availability of specialized psychiatric treatment services. In too many areas of the country this is still an academic question since child guidance clinics and similar facilities are either absent or so limited as to provide only diagnostic services for obviously disturbed children.

The management of the commoner behavior problems of early childhood has always been included in good general pediatric care. A physician who can establish a favorable rapport with parents and who looks beyond the symptoms to the possible causative factors can be very helpful in ameliorating the background conditions in the home leading to the disturbing complaints. If he has a similarly endowed and trained public health nurse working with him, his efforts will be even more effective, since the nurse can further interpret the situation to the parents and follow through in the home. The problems of persistent thumb-sucking or feeding difficulties presented to such a team do not call for pat recommendations but rather a review of the home situation in a search for the causes. This applies to physicians in private practice as well as to professional personnel in public health services.

The physician must first understand and accept the parents and children as they are before he can establish an effective relationship with them. Parents fall into different groups in their ability to function as parents. At one extreme is

the reasonably well-adjusted, reasonably confident, reasonably un-neurotic parent, whose mistakes are due chiefly to "not knowing." . . . With this person, the physician can accomplish a lot in a little time. Then there is the anxious, tense, neurotic parent who may "know" better but who is the victim of her own maladjustment. . . . It is important for the doctor to understand this type of mother so that he will not feel irritated and defeated. (9)

After all, parents do not automatically become mature individuals because they have fulfilled their biological role in producing children. The arrival of children in the household may intensify emotional conflicts which resulted from the experiences of the parents during their own childhood. At times, the depth of the parent's problem suggests referral of the parent and child for specialized psychiatric care, when available, but the parent categorically rejects the suggestion. In such situations, focusing on the relatively minor or early problem of the child may ultimately reduce the resistance of the parent to accepting skilled help for himself.

In this discussion, attention has been centered upon the promotion of mental health and the treatment of emotional difficulties that can be helped to some degree by other than trained psychiatric personnel. The manner of providing specialized services for emotionally disturbed children will be discussed in a later chapter.

Preparation of Personnel. Facts of child growth and development can be taught; attitudes are acquired as a result of experience. Favorable attitudes are essential in services aimed at promoting mental health. The mental health institute or institute in interpersonal relationships is an ambitious technique recently developed for the creation of favorable attitudes on the part of health personnel. "The purpose of the institute is simply to help the students understand, accept and integrate knowledge about human behavior and emotional needs that will enable them to function more effectively as physicians, nurses, teachers, or members of other professions engaged in serving people." (10) Although each institute varies in detail, an essential feature is the free discussion of the social and emotional problems of persons who are run-of-the-mill patients seen by physicians in offices or clinics and by public health nurses on home visits. Psychiatrists and public health personnel form the staff of the institutes. Material from actual interviews of the patients by the "students" in the institute serves as an effective stimulus to discussion and leads to a better understanding on the part of the participant of his own feelings toward his coworkers and toward the recipients of health services.

While a well-conducted mental health institute is rewarding to the agency whose members participate in it, it has, unfortunately, only limited application because of its expense and because so few psychiatrists oriented in public health are available. The more ambitious institutes of several days' to two weeks' duration must therefore be reserved for persons in administrative and supervisory positions. A less ambitious attempt has been the holding of shorter institutes for larger groups of health personnel (11). Psychiatrists, psychiatric social workers, and other members of the staff of local child guidance clinics are helpful in this endeavor when they accept as a responsibility the training in mental health principles of professional personnel in health agencies, especially public health nurses.

Experience leading to formation of favorable attitudes may be provided on the job through a skilled supervisor. This technique has been highly developed in the training of public health nurses and medical social workers. The nurse or other professional person is encouraged to express her own feelings about the patient to the supervisor and to work out for herself, in so far as possible, the reasons for her reactions in different situations.

CITED REFERENCES

1. LANGFORD, WILLIAM S., and KATHERINE M. WICKMAN, The Clinical Aspects of Parent-Child Relationships, *Ment. Hyg.,* Vol. 32, pp. 80–88, January, 1948.
2. ALLEN, FREDERICK H., Developments in Child Psychiatry in the United States, *Am. J. Pub. Health,* Vol. 38, pp. 1201–1209, September, 1948.
3. LEVY, JULIUS, An Experiment in Training Nurses to Help Mothers in Preventive Mental Hygiene, *Ment. Hyg.,* Vol. 23, pp. 99–106, January, 1939.
4. COLEMAN, JULES V., Appraising the Contribution of the Mental Hygiene Clinic to the Community: 2. In the Promotion of Mental Health, *Am. J. Orthopsychiat.,* Vol. 21, pp. 83–93, January, 1951.

5. SPOCK, BENJAMIN, (*a*) Avoiding Behavior Problems, *J. Pediat.,* Vol. 27, pp. 363–382, October, 1945; (*b*) "The Pocket Book of Baby and Child Care," Pocket Books, Inc., New York, 1946.
6. GALLEGHER, J. ROSWELL, Various Aspects of Adolescence, *J. Pediat.,* Vol. 39, pp. 532–543, November, 1951.
7. STENDLER, CELIA B., Sixty Years of Child Training Practices, *J. Pediat.,* Vol. 36, pp. 122–134, January, 1950.
8. ZIMMERMAN, KENT, "Discussion at Conference on State Programs for Mental Health," Milbank Foundation, New York, Feb. 16, 1950.
9. RIDENOUR, NINA, Keystones in Psychological Thinking about Young Children, *New York State J. Med.,* Vol. 47, pp. 277–281, February, 1947.
10. GINSBURG, ETHEL L., "Public Health Is People, An Institute on Mental Health in Public Health," Commonwealth Fund, Harvard University Press, Cambridge, Mass., 1950.
11. HOLLISTER, WILLIAM G., and GRANT W. HUSBAND, Inservice Mental Health Education through Group Experience Workshops, *Am. J. Pub. Health,* Vol. 42, pp. 1071–1077, September, 1952.

ADDITIONAL REFERENCES

1. SENN, MILTON J. E., The Psychotherapeutic Role of the Pediatrician, *Pediatrics,* Vol. 2, pp. 147–153, August, 1948.
2. MERCER, MARY E., The Pediatrician and His Role in Understanding Children's Behavior, *J. Pediat.,* Vol. 38, pp. 525–529, April, 1951.
3. "Healthy Personality Development in Children as Related to Programs of the Federal Government," The Josiah Macy, Jr. Foundation, reprinted by Health Publications Institute, Raleigh, N.C., 1952.
4. FRANK, LAWRENCE K., "The Fundamental Needs of the Child: A Guide for the Rearing and Education of Young Children," The National Association for Mental Health, New York, 1952.
5. WOLFENSTEIN, MARTHA, Trends in Infant Care, *Am. J. Orthopsychiat.,* Vol. 23, pp. 120–130, January, 1953.

11 CONTROL OF COMMUNICABLE DISEASES

The emphasis in the following discussion will be on the contributions which the child health program can make specifically in the control of selected communicable diseases which occur during childhood. Attention will be directed particularly to recent changes in the nature of the problems of communicable disease and in methods of attack upon these problems.

The recurring ravages of yellow fever provided the impetus to the development of the first public health services in the United States. Until fairly recent years, the control of communicable diseases continued to be the greatest single group of activities of most official and many voluntary health agencies, and the treatment of communicable diseases constituted a major portion of the practice of the medical profession. Although the problem of communicable disease is still of importance in certain respects, the size of the problem has receded markedly. The hazard from the so-called communicable diseases of childhood has shown the greatest decline. The mortality rate from the four major diseases in this group, *i.e.,* diphtheria, whooping cough, scarlet fever, and measles, has fallen to less than 2 per cent of its 1900 level (Figure 10).

Factors in Decline in Mortality. The recent decline in the death rate from communicable diseases may be ascribed to specific control measures, to long-term trends in incidence and severity, to increased resistance of children to infections, and to advances in treatment. The role of each factor cannot be fully assessed and varies with each disease. The long-term trend in scarlet fever, for example, has been consistently downward in England and Wales for nearly a century (1). The disease has become much milder, and the severe toxic form of the infection seen so fre-

quently early in the present century is a clinical rarity today. Specific
control measures, apart from prevention of explosive outbreaks due to
contaminated milk or food supplies, have played a comparatively minor
role in this transformation. The advent of effective treatment about 1937

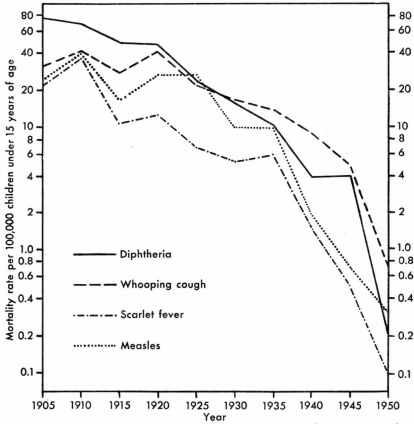

Figure 10. Mortality rates from selected communicable diseases in children
under fifteen years of age, death-registration states of the United States,
1905–1950. Rates per 100,000 estimated midyear population in age groups
(except in 1950, when rate was based on enumerated population as of April
1). (*Data provided by National Office of Vital Statistics.*)

brought about a further sharp drop in the already low death rate from
the disease (2).

No clear long-term decline in mortality is evident in diphtheria,
whooping cough, or measles previous to the present century (1). The

later decline in mortality from diphtheria may be ascribed in large part to specific antitoxin therapy and to progressively improved methods of immunization from the original toxin-antitoxin to present purified toxoids. Even in diphtheria, however, "natural" trends in the disease probably have played an important part in the decline in both mortality and morbidity. In measles, the decline has been more erratic, in accordance with its periodic epidemic character. The impact of temporary passive protection, first with whole blood or convalescent serum, and later with gamma globulin, cannot be isolated from other factors. The consistent flattening of the curve of the death rate since the late 1930's, despite several years of high incidence, may be ascribed mainly to effective treatment of complications of the disease.

In whooping cough, the greater part of the decline in the mortality rate has occurred since 1925. Greater protection of the young child against exposure to whooping cough was probably a factor in the early part of the decline. Effective treatment and active immunization contributed to the later more rapid decline in mortality, and active immunization has probably also played its part in the drop in the reported incidence of the disease.

Changes in Control Measures. Current approved practice in communicable disease control is a far cry from the days of fumigation of the premises and isolation of unfortunate victims in pesthouses. Placarding of the premises has been almost abandoned as waste motion. With decreased severity and vastly improved methods of control and treatment, excessively long periods of isolation of the patient and quarantining of contacts have given way to sounder and more humane methods. This change has been most evident in four common virus diseases of childhood: measles, German measles, mumps, and chickenpox (3). These diseases are widely prevalent and may present special hazards during and after adolescence. The desirability of measures for isolating otherwise healthy children against these diseases in the early school years is certainly questionable. When less stringent regulations concerning these diseases are introduced, a campaign of parent education must be carried out to promote better understanding of their purpose and to quiet the fears that are remnants of former days.

At the same time, the danger of other infections has been more widely appreciated. The anomaly of strict regulations against scarlet fever, while equally serious hemolytic streptococcal infections without a rash

Table 3. SALIENT FEATURES OF SELECTED COMMUNICABLE DISEASES AFFECTING CHILDREN

Disease	Etiological agent	Source of infection	Mode of transmission	Incubation period	Communicability	Methods of control
Chickenpox (varicella)	Specific virus	Virus present in lesions of skin and presumably of respiratory tract	Usually person to person; indirectly by freshly soiled discharges	2–3 weeks; commonly 14–16 days	Highly communicable; probably 1 day before to 6 days after appearance of rash	No immunization Exclusion of patient from school during communicable period Chief importance is possible confusion with smallpox, especially in persons over 15 years of age
Bacillary dysentery (Shigellosis)	Shigella group	Feces of patients or carriers; carriers common	Transfer of contaminated material, hand to mouth, water, milk, flies	1–7 days, usually less than 4 days	Feces usually become negative within few weeks without specific therapy	Safe water and milk supplies, adequate sewage disposal Good infant hygiene No immunization Isolation of infected persons during communicable period
Diphtheria	*Corynebacterium diphtheriae* (Klebs-Löffler bacillus)	Chiefly nose and throat secretions of infected persons and carriers	Person to person or contaminated articles	Usually 2–5 days	Variable period until virulent bacilli have disappeared, usually 2 weeks	Active and passive immunization Isolation until nose and throat cultures negative for virulent bacilli. Concurrent disinfection of soiled articles

Disease	Causative agent	Source	Mode of transmission	Incubation period	Period of communicability	Methods of control
German measles (rubella)	Specific virus	Secretions of mouth and possibly of nose	Direct contact with patient or with freshly contaminated articles	10–21 days, usually about 18 days	From onset of catarrhal symptoms for 4–7 days	Intimate child contacts under surveillance, to be isolated if carriers or having nasal discharge or sore throat. The only measure of value is prevention of exposure of pregnant women to infection, when possible
Infectious hepatitis (catarrhal jaundice)	One or more specific viruses	Probably nose and throat discharges and feces and blood of infected persons	Usual mode not known. Direct contact, contaminated water, food, or milk. Also through blood or plasma, or contaminated syringe	About 15–35 days, average 25 days	Period of communicability unknown	Good community sanitation and personal hygiene. Precautions against possible transmission through blood or blood products or syringes. Isolation of patient during first week of illness. Serum hepatitis almost indistinguishable from infectious hepatitis except for longer incubation period and absence of transmission by natural routes in former

Table 3. SALIENT FEATURES OF SELECTED COMMUNICABLE DISEASES AFFECTING CHILDREN.—(Continued)

Disease	Etiological agent	Source of infection	Mode of transmission	Incubation period	Communicability	Methods of control
Measles (rubeola)	Specific virus	Nose and throat secretions of infected persons	Droplet spread and person-to-person contact; occasionally through freshly contaminated articles	About 10 days to fever; 13–15 days to rash	Highly communicable, usually from 4 days before to 5 days after appearance of rash	Passive immunization with gamma globulin of exposed children under 5 years of age. Education as to special danger of exposing young children to those with fever and acute catarrhal symptoms of any kind. Isolation during period of communicability to protect patient against further infection as well as protection of others
Meningococcal meningitis	Meningococcus (Neisseria meningitidis)	Nose and throat discharges of patients or carriers	Contact with infected persons	2–10 days, usually 7 days	While meningococci are present in throat, usually disappear within	Passive immunization 3–6 days after exposure may avert or modify disease. Prevention of overcrowding, especially in common sleeping quarters

				24 hours under suitable therapy	Isolation of patient until recovery from acute illness; Prompt use of appropriate agent in treatment of patient and administration of similar agent to contacts under medical direction
Mumps (infectious parotitis)	Specific virus	Saliva of infected persons	Droplet spread, direct contact with infected person or with freshly contaminated articles	12–26 days, most often 18 days	Probably from 2 days before symptoms until subsidence of salivary gland swelling	No specific preventive measures; Isolation of patient until subsidence of salivary gland swelling
Poliomyelitis (infantile paralysis)	Viruses of poliomyelitis	Nose and throat discharges and feces of infected persons	Close association with infected persons in large proportion of cases	Usually 7–14 days, may be 3–35 days	Apparently greatest late in incubation period and first week of acute illness	Isolation of patient for 1 week after onset, or for duration of fever if longer; In presence of outbreak, isolation in bed of all children with suspicious illness, pending diagnosis; protection of children against unnecessary contacts; postponement of elective nose or

Table 3. SALIENT FEATURES OF SELECTED COMMUNICABLE DISEASES AFFECTING CHILDREN.—(*Continued*)

Disease	Etiological agent	Source of infection	Mode of transmission	Incubation period	Communicability	Methods of control
						throat operations or dental surgery; avoidance of violent exercise
Smallpox	Specific virus	Lesions of mucous membranes and skin of infected persons	Contact with patients, possible aerial transmission for short distances; contact with freshly contaminated articles	7–16 days, commonly 12 days	From first symptoms to disappearance of all scabs and crusts; highly communicable in early stages	Vaccination Hospital isolation in screened wards for period of infectivity Quarantine of all contacts until vaccinated with a vaccine of full potency
Streptococcal sore throat and scarlet fever	Group A hemolytic streptococci, at least 40 types	Discharges from nose, throat; purulent complications of patients or carriers; contaminated objects	Contact with patient or carrier, or via contaminated floor dust, or clothing or in droplet nuclei from coughing or sneezing	2–5 days	In uncomplicated cases usually for a few days after clinical recovery. Prolonged if even minor discharge persists	No immunization Prompt isolation until clinical recovery or not less than 7 days from onset Pasteurization of milk
Whooping cough (pertussis)	Pertussis bacillus (*Hemophilus pertussis*)	Discharges from laryngeal and bronchial mucous membranes of infected persons	Droplet spread, direct contact with infected person or freshly contaminated articles	Commonly 7 days, not exceeding 21 days	Especially in early catarrhal stage, diminishing until negligible about 3 weeks after start of spasmodic cough	Active immunization Separation of patient from susceptible children during communicable period, especially from young children

Source: "The Control of Communicable Diseases in Man," American Public Health Association, New York, 1950.

were lightly regarded, has almost disappeared. The general trend has been to accept all hemolytic streptococcal infections as of equal significance, whether or not a scarlatiniform rash is present, and to require identical periods of isolation for the group.

Air Disinfection. Of the various techniques of environmental sanitation, air disinfection deserves special mention because of its possible application in places where children congregate. The three methods most widely tried are disinfection by ultraviolet light, disinfection by aerosols, and dust suppression by oiling bedclothes and floors (4). The first two methods are germicidal to pathogenic organisms in droplets and droplet nuclei. Oiling complements the germicidal methods by mechanically collecting dust particles and dried-out particles of secretions from human sources.

Air disinfection by ultraviolet light irradiation has proved helpful as an additional tool in the prevention of cross infection in pediatric wards, especially when children with communicable diseases are being given care. Air disinfection of hospital newborn nurseries is ineffective in controlling spread of infection because direct contact is apparently a more important route than airborne spread (5). Air disinfection in schools and other places of assemblage is still experimental, since the mass of evidence indicates that the expense and effort involved is not justified in terms of illness prevented (6). The use of air disinfection, furthermore, may create a false sense of security against spread of infection. Ultraviolet lamps have been observed in use in more than one hospital newborn nursery in which elementary handwashing techniques were being disregarded by the staff. Whenever air disinfection is employed, it must be only as a possible added factor of safety and not as a major barrier to spread of infection.

DIPHTHERIA

The character of the diphtheria problem has changed qualitatively as well as quantitatively. The decreased prevalence of diphtheria carriers has resulted in a lower level of immunity to diphtheria in older children and adults as disclosed by community surveys of Schick test reactions (7). While this has been accompanied in some areas by the occurrence of an increased proportion of cases in adults, the diphtheria morbidity rate has been declining markedly in all age groups (8).

Active immunization with diphtheria toxoid should be started before three months of age, since reliance can no longer be placed in the transfer of antitoxin from mother to infant *in utero*. This should be followed by stimulating injections about a year later and shortly before the child's entrance into school. Further stimulating doses are recommended by those who emphasize the changed age distribution of diphtheria. Many previously immunized children having low blood levels of antitoxin show a sharp rise soon after a small dose of toxoid (9).

The routine use of the Schick test prior to administration of diphtheria toxoid in children has been discarded in public health practice. The effort involved in giving and reading the test can better be devoted to administration of toxoid to many more children. Even children with negative reaction to the Schick test benefit from a stimulating dose of toxoid by developing a heightened level of immunity against diphtheria. The Schick test is still used in exceptional circumstances in public health practice, as in children suspected of being hypersensitive to toxoid. Its chief value, however, is in epidemiological studies on susceptibility to the disease.

Some public health laboratories prepare diphtheria toxoid for active immunization and diphtheria antitoxin for passive protection and treatment; in other places, health departments purchase and distribute these materials to private physicians and for use in clinics. Antibiotics have no effect on diphtheria toxin and are not a substitute for antitoxin in treatment. Antibiotics are active against the organism itself (10). They are useful in overcoming diphtheria carrier states, particularly in nasal carriers. Removal of the tonsils and adenoids is still necessary, however, in persistent diphtheria carriers.

WHOOPING COUGH

Whooping cough presents a greater hazard in young children than does diphtheria. Not only do 90 per cent of the deaths from whooping cough occur before one year of age, but there is also a greater chance of brain damage or bronchiectasis occurring as sequelae of the disease in young children. The efficacy of pertussis vaccine is now generally accepted. When whooping cough develops in children who have been immunized, the disease tends to be much milder than in nonimmunized children. Since only about one-quarter of newborn infants have passively acquired protective antibodies and these antibodies disappear rapidly during the first three months after birth, it is theoretically desirable to give the vaccine as early as possible. A more prolonged and higher degree of protection, however, is conferred when the vaccine is given after two months of age (11).

Infants should be protected as much as possible from all types of infection, especially when whooping cough is prevalent locally. In non-immunized infants exposed to whooping cough, hyperimmune serum offers temporary protection; in immunized infants, another dose of vaccine will produce a rapid rise in the antibody level. Fortunately, several broad-spectrum antibiotics, effective against gram-negative organisms, provide potent tools in the treatment of children who have either not been immunized or in whom whooping cough has developed in spite of active immunization (12).

Infection with the parapertussis organism produces a mild, pertussis-like disease which may be considered a vaccine failure in children who had received pertussis vaccine. Immunization with parapertussis vaccine is not thought necessary because the disease is mild and the vaccine is not an effective antigen in mice (13). In addition, the organism is highly susceptible to several antibiotics (14).

TETANUS

While tetanus is not, strictly speaking, a communicable disease, it is discussed briefly at this point because of the ease with which tetanus toxoid can be included in the schedule of routine immunizations in childhood. Since tetanus may follow even trivial injuries at any period of life, active immunization against the disease early in life is desirable (15). Once the child has been actively immunized with tetanus toxoid, a stimulating dose given shortly after an injury produces a sharp rise in antitoxin titer in the blood and adequate protection against the disease.

Active immunization with toxoid has several advantages over passive immunization with antitoxin after injury. The horse serum may cause serious anaphylactic reactions. Furthermore, injections of tetanus antitoxin should be repeated at intervals of about two weeks as long as any evidence of a wound exists; this procedure is often neglected, with consequent danger to the patient. Finally, the injury may not be called to medical attention or the wound may appear so insignificant that tetanus antitoxin is deliberately withheld, and the disease may follow. Prior active immunization with toxoid would have conferred a substantial resistance to tetanus even without the administration of a stimulating dose of toxoid.

SMALLPOX

When vaccination against smallpox is required by law, as it is in a number of states, it is mandatory only before the child's entrance into school. Nevertheless, it is desirable that primary vaccination be performed well before the first birthday when there is little danger of infection and multiple inoculations from scratching the vaccination site. Postvaccinal encephalitis is extremely rare after primary vaccination in infants or after revaccination in older persons. The presence of eczema, which predisposes to the development of generalized vaccinia, is the one major contraindication to vaccination in the young child.

The multiple-pressure method is the generally accepted technique of vaccination. The skin over the deltoid region of the arm is cleansed with acetone or some other rapidly drying agent, and the vaccine is applied to the area; the side of the point of a needle is pressed rapidly and firmly a number of times against the skin through the vaccine. With this technique, successful takes are obtained with little or no visible scarring. There is no excuse, even for cosmetic reasons, for using the thigh as the vaccination site. In infants this is likely to lead to infections from soiling of the diapers; in older persons reactions may result from the constant motion of the lower extremities. Immunity against smallpox is maintained by periodic revaccination, using potent vaccine which has been kept well refrigerated until use. Failure of revaccination is often misinterpreted as an immune reaction (16).

IMMUNIZATION PROCEDURES

Diphtheria and tetanus toxoids have been used in combination, as have diphtheria toxoid and pertussis vaccine. The use of diphtheria and tetanus toxoids combined with pertussis vaccine, the so-called "triple toxoid" or "triple antigen," further reduces the number of injections, saving time and effort on the part of professional personnel and decreasing the number of unpleasant medical experiences to which children are subjected.

Table 4. SUGGESTED ROUTINE IMMUNIZATION SCHEDULE

Immunizing Agents	*Age*
1. Diphtheria-tetanus toxoids and pertussis vaccine (combined).................	3 months (or 2–5 months)
2. Diphtheria-tetanus toxoids and pertussis vaccine (combined)	4 months (or 3–6 months, 1 month after first injection)
3. Diphtheria-tetanus toxoids and pertussis vaccine (combined)	10 months (or 3–12 months after second injection)
4. Smallpox vaccine....................	Early infancy
5. Diphtheria-tetanus toxoids and pertussis vaccine (combined).................	Preschool period (single injection)
6. Smallpox vaccine....................	Before school entrance
7. Diphtheria-tetanus toxoids (combined)	During school years (single injection)

Source: Adapted from "The Control of Communicable Diseases in Man," American Public Health Association, New York, 1950.

Reactions to immunization occur frequently. Most of these are local in nature, often accompanied by fever and loss of appetite. These reactions can be minimized by giving the injections intramuscularly in the buttocks in young children and deep in the deltoid in older children. Parents should be warned of the possibility of the reactions and advised in advance of the steps to take should a reaction develop. The rare cases of encephalopathy following administration of pertussis vaccine are more cause for concern. These may terminate fatally, or if the child survives, irreversible brain damage may result. Avoidance of use of pertussis vaccine in children who have a history of convulsions or who show evidence of a respiratory infection are practical steps to reduce the possibility of this serious complication.

Jet injection is a technique developed to minimize the amount of pain caused by the standard type of injection with needle and syringe (17). The material to be injected is forced through the skin under explosive pressure in very thin streams, leaving little or no evidence in the skin of its passage. Although the technique has proved useful in selected clinical situations, it has not been used widely because of cost and the still experimental nature of the technique.

HEMOLYTIC STREPTOCOCCAL INFECTIONS

In discussing trends in mortality from communicable diseases, reference was made solely to scarlet fever among the conditions caused by hemolytic streptococci, because long-term information is not available for the group of hemolytic streptococcal infections as a whole. Scarlet fever is simply a form of hemolytic streptoccal infection in which a characteristic skin rash is present, the rash being due to erythrogenic toxin produced by the particular strain of streptococcus hemolyticus in a susceptible individual. Strains of organism lacking erythrogenic toxin may produce an equally severe pharyngitis or tonsillitis, followed by septic complications or such sequelae as rheumatic fever and acute nephritis. All types of hemolytic streptococcal infections, therefore, deserve the same degree of serious consideration. Barring a possible resurgence in bacterial virulence, continued concern with the hemolytic streptococcal group of infections is motivated chiefly by their intimate association with rheumatic fever.

The need to control hemolytic streptococcal infections in childhood is a pressing one. In contrast to most other communicable diseases of childhood, a hemolytic streptococcal infection confers little or no immunity. Rheumatic fever is more serious in childhood since it is more likely to cause cardiac damage than at later ages. Unfortunately, there are no generally accepted specific measures for the control of hemolytic streptococcal infections spread by direct contact. Prolonged administration of small daily doses of a sulfa drug as prophylaxis against hemolytic streptococcal infections in the community or even within a single school is not a practical procedure because of the difficulty in ensuring regular ingestion of the drugs and the danger of the development of sulfaresistant strains. The use of penicillin for the same purpose is too costly, and it is still experimental. Control measures include careful isolation of infected persons and quarantine of contacts, but the most effective weapon is observation of children for hemolytic streptococcal infections, with prompt and vigorous treatment of the infections as they occur. Education of parents, teachers, and others in intimate contact with children is basic to the success of this approach.

Active immunization against hemolytic streptococcal infections is not advised for general use. The administration of erythrogenic toxin in increasing doses almost uniformly causes a reversal of the Dick test; it protects against the scarlet fever rash, but it probably does not confer any protection against the invasive element in hemolytic streptococcal infections. Use of the immunizing toxin is reserved for groups brought into close and continued contact with these infections (18). This situation would naturally be altered radically if an effective antibacterial immunizing agent were developed.

OTHER COMMON COMMUNICABLE DISEASES

Measles. Measles is of greatest hazard to the young child and to persons in debilitated health. Although the majority of cases of measles occur in children of school age, more than half the deaths occur in children under three years of age. Community efforts must therefore be concentrated upon postponement of the disease until the early school years, when the disease generally occurs in a milder form. This requires intensive public health education to make clear to parents the reasons for contrary attitudes toward the same disease depending on the age of their children. Parents are encouraged almost to welcome the disease if their children are past six years of age while they are urged to do everything possible to postpone the disease if their children are under three or four years of age.

No effective agent is available for active immunization against measles. The preferred agent for passive immunization is gamma globulin, or immune serum globulin, obtained as a fraction of whole human blood. Other agents for the same purpose, now largely discarded, are placental extracts, immune or convalescent human serum, or whole blood. Depending on the individual circumstances, complete or partial protection may be conferred. A large dose may be given to provide complete temporary protection. A smaller, carefully calculated dose may be administered in the hope that a modified, attenuated form of measles will follow. Modified measles has a longer incubation period than the naturally occurring disease, and the clinical picture may be very mild. The modified form confers a high degree of long-standing protection to measles, although a number of cases of measles have been reported in children who had modified measles previously (19).

Minor Communicable Diseases. German measles is a generally mild disease of no public health importance except for its role in the pathogenesis of congenital malformations. Contagious rubella without a rash has been produced experimentally in susceptible human subjects (20). The dramatic impact of the discovery of the danger of the disease during the first trimester of pregnancy was so great that the significance of

German measles in this connection has been somewhat exaggerated. Even in the presence of a large outbreak of German measles, little or no increase in the total incidence of congenital defects can be demonstrated. Gamma globulin has been proposed as a passive preventive measure in pregnant women exposed to the disease, but the efficacy of this procedure has not been clearly demonstrated. Deliberate exposure of girls before puberty to the disease has been advocated in some circles, so that immunity may be developed before the childbearing period. While this may be theoretically desirable, in practice an induced epidemic can hardly be restricted to the age group selected; the result may well be the exposure of pregnant women. In the days of smallpox inoculation, the persons deliberately infected remained on board ship until recovery, for fear of initiating a smallpox epidemic; this is manifestly an impractical procedure to follow in the case of German measles.

Mumps is of importance chiefly because of the high incidence of orchitis in adolescent and older males, whereas this complication is extremely rare before puberty. Measures for the prevention of mumps are still in the experimental stage (21). Deliberate exposure to mumps of boys in their preschool years has the same drawbacks as in the case of German measles, since the disease spreads readily to the high proportion of susceptible adults, with embarassing consequences.

Chickenpox is also of little public health significance, and no effective measures are available to control its spread or alter its clinical course. Regulations regarding isolation of patients with chickenpox are outmoded in many places. Chickenpox is contagious only for a brief period before and after onset of the characteristic eruption; yet much needless school time is lost because the child with chickenpox is not allowed to return to school until all crusts have fallen off. The possible confusion of smallpox with chickenpox, especially in adolescents and adults, is also worthy of note.

POLIOMYELITIS

Poliomyelitis remains a major communicable-disease problem. Only recently has progress been made in the prevention of infection or of initial paralytic involvement, in contrast to the significant developments in treatment and expanded rehabilitation facilities which have greatly lessened residual disability after subsidence of the infectious process.

Gamma globulin from pooled blood containing antibodies to the three major strains of poliomyelitis virus is effective in conferring transient passive protection on the recipient (22). The demand for gamma globulin for this purpose far exceeds the available national supply which has had to be allocated to the various states for distribution. Development of a potent polyvalent poliomyelitis vaccine for active immunization offers the greatest hope for practical control of the disease (23).

Psychologically, poliomyelitis now takes precedence among the communicable diseases; the anxiety engendered in any community in which a few cases occur is out of all proportion to the danger involved. The death rate from poliomyelitis has remained at a fairly even level since 1915. The incidence rate has risen, but at least a portion of the increase has been due to better diagnosis and reporting of nonparalytic illness.

The poliomyelitis virus is probably disseminated widely in the community by the time clinical cases occur. Attempts to erect community barriers to spread of the virus are ineffective. Certain specific measures have been suggested to reduce the extent of paralytic involvement (24). Prompt bed rest is recommended in the event of any febrile illness when poliomyelitis is prevalent.

The hazard of tonsillectomy when poliomyelitis is prevalent has been clearly demonstrated in that there is an increased incidence of bulbar disease if exposure to the virus occurs within a month after operation. The danger of developing bulbar poliomyelitis following tonsillectomy during the poliomyelitis season must be weighed against the risk of postponing the tonsillectomy (25). Highly suggestive evidence has also been adduced that individuals who receive immunizing agents within one month prior to the onset of poliomyelitis are more liable to develop the paralytic form of the disease with increased frequency of paralysis in the injected extremity (26). Elective immunizations for individuals over six months to one year of age may well be suspended temporarily in the presence of poliomyelitis in the community. Pregnancy increases the risk from poliomyelitis, but "there is no evidence of a greater severity of the infection among pregnant women than among a comparable group of nonpregnant married women simultaneously attacked." (27)

The Coxsackie viruses were originally isolated from patients with poliomyelitis, and the viruses were thought to be the cause of a mild poliomyelitis-like disease. Subsequent evidence has shown that this was only a coincidental relationship. Epidemiological studies have since disclosed that the Coxsackie viruses are the cause of herpangina, a specific febrile disease of children, and of epidemic pleurodynia (28).

DIARRHEAL DISEASES

As a world-wide problem, diarrheal disease of infectious origin is still the most important single cause of illness and death in early life. Even in the United States it remains a serious problem in areas with poor sanitation. The dysentery bacilli or Shigella group are the major causative agents in areas of high prevalence of diarrheal disease. The prevalence of Shigella infection, as disclosed by bacteriological surveys using rectal swabs in young children, is closely related to morbidity and mortality rates from diarrheal disease in the group studied (29). The proportion of the population with high prevalence rates of Shigella infection is the major factor determining the over-all morbidity and mortality rates in a given community or area.

Attack on the remaining problem consists in improved sanitation, including fly control, in areas where this is needed, coupled with instruction in personal hygiene which can be done when the public health nurse visits in the home. The infecting organism usually causes illness in a number of members of the household, but children under two years of age are more severely affected. It is important to remember that bacillary dysentery in this country usually manifests itself as an ordinary watery diarrhea rather than by the textbook description of a fecal discharge with blood and mucus. Specific treatment with sulfonamides controls the disease, clears up a carrier state promptly, and helps prevent spread of infection.

Diarrhea in the Newborn Period. Diarrheal disease during the newborn period is a distinct problem and requires a different approach (30). Epidemics of diarrhea in hospital nurseries for newborn infants were reported with increasing frequency during the 1940's. Some of these outbreaks have shown a case fatality of 40 per cent. The patterns of the outbreaks have varied; some have been explosive in character, while others have built up gradually and have extended over a long period when adequate control measures were not instituted. The major reason for the increased frequency of outbreaks is probably the shift from home to hospital deliveries with its attendant congregation of newborn infants in hospital nurseries.

Epidemic diarrhea of the newborn is really a group of diarrheal diseases due to a variety of organisms, including filtrable viruses; recently, the role of certain types of coliform organisms in the causation of outbreaks has been clarified (31). The nature of the offending organism is of little practical importance since similar control measures are employed in any case.

In most institutions in which outbreaks occur, gross errors in technique in the care of newborn infants can usually be demonstrated. Breaches in technique are often multiple so that it is difficult to know just which factors are responsible. Some of the more frequent deficiencies are contamination of artificial feedings, overcrowding, the use of common equipment, inadequate suspect and isolation facilities, and absence or insufficient use of handwashing facilities. Completely or partially bottle-fed infants are affected more often than breast-fed infants in many outbreaks, suggesting a common food source. In a few outbreaks breast-fed infants are found to be affected and the mode of spread may be traced to the common solution used for cleansing the mothers' breasts before feedings.

As in all other phases of the health program, it is of more value to prevent infection whenever this is possible, rather than simply to bring outbreaks under control. Adequate newborn infant care, as described later, will minimize the danger of such outbreaks. There is a general impression that the peak has been passed in the number and severity of outbreaks of epidemic diarrhea of the newborn in many parts of the country. How much of this has been due to improved newborn nursery facilities and techniques is a matter requiring careful evaluation.

OPHTHALMIA NEONATORUM

Ophthalmia neonatorum, or acute infectious conjunctivitis of the newborn, is due to a variety of agents of which the gonoccoccus is the most important. Previous to the use of routine prophylaxis immediately after birth, the condition was a frequent cause of blindness; today impairment of vision from this cause is very unusual. The availability of effective treatment with sulfa drugs and antibiotics has been responsible for much of the recent decrease. Nevertheless, adequate prophylaxis immediately after birth must be continued as a routine procedure.

The Credé method of prophylaxis, consisting of the instillation into each eye of a drop of 1 per cent solution of silver nitrate, has recently been challenged by those who advocate penicillin solution for the same purpose. Penicillin solutions may have an advantage over silver nitrate in being less irritating, and possibly even in being more effective, provided the preparation and maintenance of fresh solutions of penicillin can be assured. However, the use of penicillin leaves too much room for error, and silver nitrate solution in wax ampules distributed by many health departments is still generally favored (32).

TUBERCULOSIS

The control of tuberculosis in childhood is only a small segment of the total community control program, but certain phases of the problem deserve brief review. The total size of the tuberculosis problem has shrunken markedly over the past several decades. The mortality rate has dropped more rapidly among children under fifteen years than among adults, with the greatest decrease among infants under one year of age. The incidence of newly discovered cases is also declining, in spite of intensive case-finding efforts through mass chest x-ray surveys. The favorable picture in childhood is probably due to several factors: general availability of safe milk and the substantial eradication of bovine tuberculosis, the greater ease of contact examination and follow-up among children, and the fact that the higher rates in older persons in part represent a residue of tuberculosis from periods of greater disease prevalence.

Preventive Measures. Protection of the infant or young child from exposure to a known case of tuberculosis can best be secured by hospitalization of the tuberculous patient or by providing care for the infant outside the home. Only when neither measure is possible should BCG vaccine, a living attenuated form of tubercle bacillus, be given in an attempt to protect the infant against the disease. In older children a preliminary tuberculin test should be performed and BCG vaccine given only if the child has a negative tuberculin. In newborn infants preliminary tuberculin testing is not necessary. Ideally the infant should be separated from his household at birth and not be returned for a period of six weeks after immunization. Practically speaking, this cannot be done in situations in which the use of BCG vaccine is most desirable. BCG vaccine gained wide acceptance in European countries immediately after the Second World War when other control measures were all but absent. "It is to be emphasized that BCG vaccination must not be regarded as a substitute for approved hygienic measures or for public health practices designed to prevent or minimize tuberculous infection and disease. Vaccination should be regarded as only one of many procedures to be used in tuberculosis control." (33) Emphasis in control measures must be placed on examination and follow-up of household contacts of persons with tuberculosis, using chest x-rays in the adults and tuberculin testing in the children as the initial procedures.

In former years it was common for summer "health camps," "preventoria," and "fresh-air classes" to be used as measures supposed to build the general resistance of so-called under-par children and of children who had been in contact with tuberculous individuals. It is generally accepted now that these facilities did not accomplish the purpose for which they were established, and most have been discontinued. Many health camps have been converted to frankly recreational purposes under the same auspices under which they were founded.

Case Finding. Although the hazard of tuberculosis is at its lowest ebb during the elementary school years, much effort is still needlessly expended in looking for tuberculosis in this age group. Routine tuberculin testing is certainly not justified prior to the seventh grade, when positive reactors should have chest x-rays taken. Other community chest x-ray facilities may be swamped by requests from school authorities when this is done in the lower grades. Even if tuberculin testing is used for its purported educational value, a few children would serve as well as entire grades. Routine periodic x-raying of the chests of all adults in the school environment, with follow-up of those with suspicious findings, is probably the most productive control measure for the protection of the school child.

The intradermal or Mantoux test, using a purified tuberculin or protein derivative, is the preferred method of tuberculin testing. The scratch or Pirquet test has been almost discarded. While the patch test may be accurate in some hands under carefully controlled conditions, the need to select a suitable hairless patch of skin and the difficulties in avoiding sweating, bathing, or showering during the 96 hours before it is read, make it too cumbersome and inaccurate for a routine procedure, merely to eliminate the needle prick of an intradermal test.

CONGENITAL SYPHILIS

While congenital syphilis is completely avoidable by prevention or discovery and treatment of syphilis in the mother, the number of reported cases of congenital syphilis has fallen only slightly since 1941, in contrast to the sharp decline in syphilis in all stages in adults (34). This probably does not represent the true incidence, since it may be the result of better reporting in areas of comparatively high incidence, but it does indicate that a problem still exists in some places.

If adequate treatment of syphilis in the mother is begun by the middle of pregnancy, there is almost complete assurance that the infant will be born free of the disease. Even if treatment is started much later, the chances are in the infant's favor. If by chance the mother did not report for care or received inadequate care during pregnancy and the infant is born with syphilis, the results of treatment are generally good when treatment is started before the infant reaches the age of three months.

For adequate control of congenital syphilis, the following procedure has been recommended (34*a*):

1. Two serological tests during pregnancy, one early in pregnancy and the other late in the third trimester or at the time of delivery.

2. Immediate treatment of pregnant women who have untreated syphilis.

3. Serological test of pregnant women on admission for delivery when prenatal care was not given previously, and immediate treatment if syphilis is discovered.

4. Serological test for newborn infants of untreated or inadequately treated syphilitic mothers. If the infant cannot be followed adequately for four months, penicillin treatment may be given immediately. Otherwise examinations should be made periodically until the status of the infant is clear (34*a*).

The size of the problem in any area should determine the need for the extensive program to implement these recommendations. Certainly, the problem deserves careful study before it is assumed that no additional effort is required. On the other hand, the cost of the program may be such, especially for the vastly increased number of serological tests to be performed, that carrying out the recommendation regarding two serological tests during pregnancy, for example, may not be warranted.

THE "NUISANCE DISEASES"

Several minor communicable diseases are responsible for considerable absenteeism from school, even though their systemic effects are minimal. They may cause apprehension in the community, and a great deal of effort may be expended by health and school authorities to bring them under control. The chief "nuisance diseases" are ringworm of the scalp, pediculosis capitis, scabies, and impetigo (35).

With advances in treatment of all but scalp ringworm, there is rarely any reason for extended absences from school. For example, DDT powder in talc blown on the scalp has been found safe and effective in destroying head lice (36). Even when the school or health department sets up a special treatment clinic, possibly in a physician's office on a fee basis, an attempt should be made to treat all affected members of the household to prevent an endless cycle of reinfection.

Tinea Capitis. Among the "nuisance diseases," scalp ringworm deserves special consideration. Community outbreaks of scalp ringworm have come to attention with increasing frequency, leading to the belief that nationwide spread, starting in the Northeast, has occurred since about 1940. Scalp ringworm is found exclusively in children, and it disappears spontaneously at puberty. The present epidemic form is difficult to detect in its early stages without the aid of the Wood's lamp, which emits ultraviolet light. X-ray epilation is the most effective form of treatment, but skilled specialists may not be readily available, and resistance may be encountered to what the parents consider a disfiguring procedure. The application of fungicidal ointments to the scalp at frequent intervals in specially established clinics or in the school itself may be the only available alternative. Complicated isolation arrangements may have to be established while this treatment is being used, to avoid prolonged absences by the affected children (37).

CITED REFERENCES

1. GALE, A. H., A Century of Changes in the Mortality and Incidence of the Principal Infections of Childhood, *Arch. Dis. Childhood,* Vol. 20, pp. 2–21, March, 1945.
2. COOKE, JEAN V., The Effect of Specific Therapy on the Common Contagious Diseases, *J. Pediat.,* Vol. 35, pp. 275–295, September, 1949.

3. GELPERIN, ABRAHAM, JOSEPH I. LINDE, and MORRIS A. GRANOFF, Communication to "Trends," *Pediatrics,* Vol. 5, pp. 1039–1041, June, 1950.
4. Progress in the Control of Air-borne Infections, Report of the Subcommittee on Air Sanitation of the Committee on Research and Standards, prepared by Hollis S. Ingraham, Year Book of the American Public Health Association, *Am. J. Pub. Health,* Vol. 40, Part II, pp. 82–88, May, 1950.
5. KRUGMAN, SAUL, and ROBERT WARD, Air Sterilization in an Infants' Ward: Effect of Triethylene Glycol Vapor and Dust-suppressive Measures on the Respiratory Cross Infection Rate, *J.A.M.A.,* Vol. 145, pp. 775–780, Mar. 17, 1951.
6. GELPERIN, ABRAHAM, MORRIS A. GRANOFF, and JOSEPH I. LINDE, The Effect of Ultraviolet Light upon Absenteeism from Upper Respiratory Infections in New Haven Schools, *Am. J. Pub. Health,* Vol. 41, pp. 796–805, July, 1951.
7. COHEN, PHILIP, HERMAN SCHNECK, EMANUEL DUBOW, and SIDNEY Q. COHLAN, The Changed Status of Diphtheria Immunity, *Pediatrics,* Vol. 3, pp. 630–638, May, 1949.
8. DAUER, C. C., Trends in Age Distribution of Diphtheria in the United States, *Pub. Health Rep.,* Vol. 65, pp. 1209–1218, Sept. 22, 1950.
9. JAMES, GEORGE, W. ALLEN LONGSHORE, JR., and JESSIE L. HENDRY, Diphtheria Immunization Studies of Students in an Urban High School, *Am. J. Hyg.,* Vol. 53, pp. 178–201, March, 1951.
10. JACKSON, GEORGE G., SHIH-MAN CHANG, EDWIN H. PLACE, and MAXWELL FINLAND, Sensitivity of Diphtheria Bacilli and Related Organisms to Nine Antibiotics, *J. Pediat.,* Vol. 37, pp. 718–726, November, 1950.
11. MILLER, JOHN J. JR., HAROLD K. FABER, MARY L. RYAN, ROSALIE J. SILVERBERG, and EDITH LEW, Immunization against Pertussis during the First Four Months of Life, *Pediatrics,* Vol. 4, pp. 468–478, October, 1949.
12. HAZEN, LLOYD N., GEORGE G. JACKSON, SHIH-MAN CHANG, EDWIN H. PLACE, and MAXWELL FINLAND, Antibiotic Treatment of Pertussis, *J. Pediat.,* Vol. 39, pp. 1–15, July, 1951.
13. ELDERING, GRACE, and PEARL L. KENDRICK, Incidence of Parapertussis in the Grand Rapids Area as Indicated by 16 Years' Experience with Diagnostic Cultures, *Am. J. Pub. Health,* Vol. 42, pp. 27–31, January, 1952.
14. DAY, ELIZABETH, and WILLIAM L. BRADFORD, Susceptibility of Hemophilus Parapertussis to Certain Antibiotics, *Pediatrics,* Vol. 9, pp. 320–326, March, 1952.
15. PRESS, EDWARD, Desirability of the Routine Use of Tetanus Toxoid, *New England J. Med.,* Vol. 239, pp. 50–56, July 8, 1948.
16. BENENSON, ABRAM S., C. HENRY KEMPE, and RALPH E. WHEELER, Problems in Maintaining Immunity to Smallpox, *Am. J. Pub. Health,* Vol. 42, pp. 535–541, May, 1952.

17. Parenteral Administration by Jet Injection, editorial, *J.A.M.A.,* Vol. 152, pp. 532–533, June 6, 1953.
18. RHOADS, PAUL S., Present Status of Immunization to and Treatment of Scarlet Fever, *Am. J. Dis. Child.,* Vol. 77, pp. 244–252, February, 1949.
19. KARELITZ, SAMUEL, Does Modified Measles Result in Lasting Immunity? *J. Pediat.,* Vol. 36, pp. 697–703, June, 1950.
20. KRUGMAN, SAUL, ROBERT WARD, KATHRYN G. JACOBS, and MARTIN LAZAR, Studies of Rubella Immunization: 1. Demonstration of Rubella without Rash, *J.A.M.A.,* Vol. 151, pp. 285–288, Jan. 24, 1953.
21. HENLE, GERTRUDE, and WERNER HENLE, Studies on the Prevention of Mumps, *Pediatrics,* Vol. 8, pp. 1–4, July, 1951.
22. HAMMON, WILLIAM McD., LEWIS L. CORIELL, PAUL F. WEHRLE, and JOSEPH STOKES, JR., Evaluation of Red Cross Gamma Globulin as a Prophylactic Agent for Poliomyelitis: 4. Final Report of Results Based on Clinical Diagnoses, *J.A.M.A.,* Vol. 151, pp. 1272–1285, Apr. 11, 1953.
23. SALK, JONAS E., Studies in Human Subjects on Active Immunization against Poliomyelitis: 1. A Preliminary Report on Experiments in Progress, *J.A.M.A.,* Vol. 151, pp. 1081–1098, Mar. 28, 1953.
24. Recommended Practices for Control of Poliomyelitis, editorial, *J.A.M.A.,* Vol. 140, pp. 1276–1277, Aug. 20, 1949.
25. GALLOWAY, THOMAS C., Relationship of Tonsillectomy to Poliomyelitis, *J.A.M.A.,* Vol. 151, pp. 1180–1182, Apr. 4, 1953.
26. (*a*) KORNS, ROBERT F., ROBERT M. ALBRECHT, and FRANCES B. LOCKE, The Association of Parenteral Injections with Poliomyelitis, *Am. J. Pub. Health,* Vol. 42, pp. 153–169, February, 1952; (*b*) Relatownship between Inoculations and Poliomyelitis, editorial, *J.A.M.A.,* Vol. 149, p. 170, May 10, 1952.
27. ANDERSON, GAYLORD W., GENEVIEVE ANDERSON, AUDREY SKAAR, and FRANZISKA SANDLER, Poliomyelitis in Pregnancy, *Am. J. Hyg.,* Vol. 55, pp. 127–139, January, 1952.
28. HUEBNER, ROBERT J., EDWARD A. BEEMAN, ROGER M. COLE, PAUL M. BEIGELMAN, and JOSEPH A. BELL, The Importance of Coxsackie Viruses in Human Disease, Particularly Herpangina and Epidemic Pleurodynia, *New England J. Med.,* Vol. 247, pp. 249–256, Aug. 14, 1952.
29. WATT, JAMES, A. C. HOLLISTER, M. D. BECK, and E. C. HEMPHILL, Diarrheal Diseases in Fresno County, California, *Am. J. Pub. Health,* Vol. 43, pp. 728–741, June, 1953.
30. GORDON, JOHN E., and A. DANIEL RUBENSTEIN, Epidemic Diarrhea of the Newborn, *Am. J. M. Sc.,* Vol. 220, pp. 339–354, September, 1950.
31. NETER, ERWIN, CHARLES R. WEBB, CLARE N. SHUMWAY, and MIRIAM R. MURDOCK, Study on Etiology, Epidemiology, and Antibiotic Therapy of Infantile Diarrhea, with Particular Reference to Certain Serotypes of

Escherichia coli, Am. J. Pub. Health, Vol. 41, pp. 1490–1496, December, 1951.

32. Prophylaxis of Ophthalmia Neonatorum, editorial, *J.A.M.A.,* Vol. 148, pp. 122–123, Jan. 12, 1952.

33. The Status of BCG Vaccine, Report of the Council on Pharmacy and Chemistry of the American Medical Association, *J.A.M.A.,* Vol. 144, pp. 1260–1261, Dec. 9, 1950.

34. Congenital Syphilis Issue of *J. Ven. Dis. Inform.,* Vol. 31, No. 7, July, 1950: (*a*) HUSE, BETTY, and W. H. AUFRANC, A Proposal for Joint Action against Congenital Syphilis, pp. 174–177; (*b*) GOODWIN, MARY S., Status of Treatment of Syphilitic Pregnant Women and of Children Who Have Congenital Syphilis, pp. 178–184; (*c*) BUNDESEN, HERMAN N., and HANS C. S. ARON, How to Evaluate Positive Kahn Tests in Infants, pp. 185–190; (*d*) Statistics on Reported Cases of Congenital Syphilis, p. 197.

35. VAN DER SLICE, DAVID, The "Nuisance Diseases," *J. School Health,* Vol. 17, pp. 78–81, March, 1947.

36. EDDY, GAINES W., The Treatment of Head Lice with MYL and DDT Lice Powders and the NBIN Emulsion, *Am. J. Hyg.,* Vol. 47, pp. 29–32, January, 1948.

37. CULBERT, ROBERT W., ANNA E. R. ROBINSON, and MAX N. LERNER, Study in the Reduction of Absences from School of Children with Tinea Capitis, *Am. J. Pub. Health,* Vol. 40, pp. 1089–1095, September, 1950.

ADDITIONAL REFERENCES

1. "The Control of Communicable Diseases in Man, Report of the Subcommittee on Communicable Disease Control of the Committee on Research and Standards," American Public Health Association, New York, 1950.

2. ANDERSON, GAYLORD W., and MARGARET G. ARNSTEIN, "Communicable Disease Control: A Volume for the Health Officer and Public Health Nurse," The Macmillan Company, New York, 1948.

3. "Report of the Committee on Immunization and Therapeutic Procedures for Acute Infectious Diseases," The American Academy of Pediatrics, Evanston, Ill., 1951.

4. OSBORN, JOHN J., JOSEPH DANCIS, and JUAN F. JULIA, Studies of the Immunology of the Newborn Infant: 1. Age and Antibody Production, *Pediatrics,* Vol. 9, pp. 736–744, June, 1952.

5. LINCOLN, EDITH M., chairman, Round Table Discussion, Early Diagnosis and Treatment of Tuberculosis in Children, *Pediatrics,* Vol. 9, pp. 791–800, June, 1952.

6. WRIGHT, JOHN J., CECIL G. SHEPS, EUGENE E. TAYLOR, and ALICE J. GIFFORD, Obstacles to Eradicating Congenital Syphilis, *Pub. Health Rep.,* Vol. 67, pp. 1179–1184, December, 1952.

12 DENTAL HEALTH SERVICES

The status of the teeth and their investing tissues is intimately associated with the well-being of the individual. Inadequate preventive care and dental treatment result in loss of teeth and in disease of the gums and adjacent tissues. The immediate results are pain and dental infection; the ultimate outcome may be total loss of teeth with serious cosmetic effects and interference with nutrition from improper mastication of food. Severe dental malocclusion may be another late result.

The aim of the dental health program is the development of a complete set of healthy teeth in good alignment and the inculcation of habits of dental hygiene and dental care which will maintain these benefits throughout adult life. The dental profession cannot achieve this goal singlehanded. Community-wide preventive services, accompanied by a program of public health education and organized treatment services, are needed. The medical profession, by lending its support to the initiation of such a program, can make a valuable contribution to total child health. In addition, the practicing physician can promote improved dental health of children under his immediate care (1).

Attainment of the ultimate objective requires not only the full application of preventive techniques, regular dental examination, and treatment of dental caries, but also a range of other dental treatment services, such as the use of space retainers and other prosthetic devices, corrective orthodontic care, treatment of periodontal disease and mouth infections, and treatment of the tooth pulp, as indicated. While these services are provided as part of the best type of individual dental care, they are included only partially, if at all, in a community program for all children at the present time. The size of the problem is too vast for the situation to be otherwise. Public attention has, therefore, been focused upon the prevention and treatment of dental caries, because this condition constitutes the bulk of the dental problem, and control of dental caries would prevent some of the other oral conditions for which more complicated dental services are required. While the problem of dental caries should receive major attention, it should not be to the complete exclusion of consideration of malocclusion and conditions of the soft tissues of the mouth.

DENTAL CARIES

Dental caries is the most common chronic ailment in the nation, so common as to be almost universal. The statistics of selective service examinations from two world wars are often cited in proof of this contention. Although the requirements in number of serviceable teeth were minimal, dental defects constituted the largest single cause of rejection in the First World War. Dental defects resulted in rejection of 4.3 per cent of men called up for examination before Pearl Harbor in the Second World War, although the regulations required only six opposing posterior teeth and six opposing anterior teeth for acceptance for service (2). Later, these requirements were lowered sharply, and inducted men, who would otherwise have been rejected, were given dental care after entrance into service.

To measure the size of the dental caries problem and provide methods of evaluating the results of dental health programs, several indices have come into general use (3). The measure of prevalence having most general application is the DMF rate, or the number of decayed, missing, and filled permanent teeth per person, usually stated by age group; it may be broken down further by sex, race, or other factors for more detailed study. Analysis of each component of the total DMF rate gives a fairly accurate picture of the amount of treated and untreated dental caries and the dental needs of each age group of the population.

A closely related index is the rate of tooth loss, or the number of missing permanent teeth per person; this is essentially a measure of neglected dental caries in childhood. The DMF rate can also be used to give a rough estimate of the incidence of dental caries, or the number of new cavities per child each year. The technique used must be known when comparing data from various surveys. Reliable data can be obtained only by skilled examiners using a dental explorer and mouth mirror. Use of a tongue depressor and light discloses only gross caries and actual tooth loss. The x-ray provides a more refined technique by revealing the presence of cavities inaccessible to the dental explorer.

Numerous surveys of the dental status of children have revealed the extent of the problem of dental caries. Most of these surveys have shown that at least 90 per cent of children in the lower elementary school grades have already experienced caries. Typical of the surveys are the ones made in Maryland (4). These revealed an average DMF rate of 4.0 per child, with the rate ranging from 0.3 at six years of age to 3.7 at twelve years of age, rising to 9.2 at nineteen years of age. Except when some specific factor, such as the presence of fluoride in the drinking water, is operative, the prevalence of caries has been found to be fairly uniform in different localities. The extent to which the problem has been met has, of course, depended upon many factors, including social and economic conditions, the availability of dentists providing care for children, and the presence or absence of an organized local dental health program. Until techniques of caries prevention became available, only a very rare, favorably situated community could have hoped to meet effectively the total problem of dental caries in childhood.

Mechanism of Dental Caries. While knowledge of the pathogenesis of dental caries is still incomplete and controversial in some aspects, enough is understood and generally accepted to provide a reasonably sound basis for program planning (5). The initial phase is probably decalcification of the enamel by acid produced by lactobacilli and other bacteria acting on carbohydrates in the mouth. Decalcification is followed by breakdown of the organic portion of the tooth. Dental caries tends to occur first in pits and fissures in the teeth. Dental plaques adhere to these pits and fissures and can be removed from them only with difficulty.

What effect diet has upon the development or prevention of dental caries, apart from the role of carbohydrates, is still controversial; the single generally accepted concept is the increased susceptibility to caries of teeth formed during periods of inadequate vitamin D intake. No clear-cut evidence has been presented that other vitamins or minerals in the diet have any influence on the incidence of dental caries.

Preventive Measures. Until the advent of fluoride on the dental scene, no measures were available for the prevention or retardation of dental caries. One of the great fiascos of public health education, and one not to be laid at the door of the health educator, was the campaign based on the slogan, "A clean tooth never decays." Experience sadly showed that clean teeth decayed, just as teeth in the poorest state of hygiene did. While more recent evidence has shown that toothbrushing carried out meticulously after each ingestion of food by cooperative young adults does reduce the incidence of caries (6), the intensive educational effort needed to duplicate these results on a mass scale would hardly be justified by the benefits produced. The reported beneficial effect is apparently due to prompt removal of food particles from the mouth before acid production can be initiated, rather than to mouth cleanliness as such.

There is no evidence that periodic dental prophylaxis retards the development of dental caries. Proper cleaning and scaling of the teeth have cosmetic benefits and are important in promoting health of the soft tissues; the latter ultimately helps prevent tooth loss, but not by altering the caries process. Ammonium-ion and penicillin dentifrices have been widely promoted to the public. Ammonium-ion dentifrices have been shown to be ineffective in preventing dental caries (7). Adequate control studies have not been reported on the use of penicillin dentifrices upon which judgment as to their place in inhibiting dental caries can be based.

Reduction of Dietary Carbohydrate. Decreasing the amount and frequency of ingestion of free sugar exerts a markedly favorable influence on the rate of dental decay. It has been common experience in children's institutions, in which only small amounts of candy and other sweets are eaten, to find a low prevalence of dental caries, whatever the adequacy of the diet in other respects. Certainly the effort to reduce children's consumption of sweets and soft drinks is based on sound scientific grounds. Even a minor success in eliminating lollipops and other between-meal sweets is worth while from the viewpoint of promoting dental health.

The immediate outlook for the reduced ingestion of free sugars for the country as a whole is discouraging; long-term trends in carbohydrate consumption show a steady increase. The pressures for further increasing the consumption of soft drinks far exceed the comparatively feeble efforts of the health professions to counteract them. On the other hand, the physician should at least set a good example. The candy-coated tongue depressor, even assuming its debatably increased acceptability to the child, is hard to reconcile with a warning against between-meal sweets; nor does a lollipop proffered as a good-will offering by the physician after a painful injection make the task of the conscientious mother any simpler. The physician can take positive measures as well, by parent education and adequate control of diets of hospitalized children (1).

Topical Application of Fluoride. Fortunately the efficacy of caries-preventive measures is greatest in those procedures requiring the least motivation to individual action. The application of fluoride solution to the teeth, which requires only that the parent be convinced of the value of a painless procedure for the child, is decidedly effective. The most effective procedure of all, the addition of fluoride to the drinking water supply, necessitates no individual action beyond that required for any community function.

The application of fluoride solution to the teeth for the partial prevention of dental caries was accepted as a routine clinical and public health procedure within six years of its introduction in 1942, and a standardized technique was evolved (8). The teeth are first cleaned thoroughly. One quadrant of the mouth is isolated and dried; a 2 per cent solution of sodium fluoride is applied to the tooth surfaces, and the teeth are allowed to dry in air for three minutes. The other three quadrants of the mouth are similarly treated in turn. This procedure, without initial cleaning of the teeth, is repeated three times at intervals of two to seven days. A procedure has been developed which reduces the time per child, by having one person handle four children simultaneously, taking advantage of the time that must be allowed for drying of the solution after application.

With this technique of application, an average reduction of 40 per cent in the amount of new dental caries may be expected on examination a year after the procedure. The protective effect lasts at least three years; the first series of applications should be given at three years of age, and the applications should be repeated at seven, ten, and thirteen years of age. This spacing ensures that newly erupted teeth receive prompt attention. Application of the sodium fluoride solution to the teeth soon after eruption, especially in the deciduous teeth, apparently also increases its effectiveness (9).

Fluoridation of Water Supply. Although this procedure is technically the responsibility of the environmental sanitarian, its promotion and over-all supervision is intimately connected with the dental health and general child health programs. The low prevalence of dental caries in areas served by drinking water containing fluoride ion has been known for some time (10). Reports have been accumulating on the effects of fluorine artificially introduced into the community's drinking-water supply (11). Seven years after the introduction of 1.2 parts per million (1.2 mg. per 1,000 ml.) of fluoride ion into the drinking water of Newburgh, N.Y., for example, the DMF rate in the permanent teeth of children nine years of age was 52 per cent less than among children of the same age at the time fluoridation was instituted, whereas no decline occurred in the control city. At the same time, careful medical and x-ray examinations have disclosed no systemic effects from ingestion of the fluoride (12). If the full effects of fluoride artificially introduced into the water supply is the same as that in areas in which fluoride is found naturally, a decrease of 60 per cent in the prevalence of dental caries may be anticipated.

Fluoridation of water has received the unqualified endorsement of leading national health agencies and professional organizations (13). Fluoride has been introduced into the water supplies of several major cities and many smaller municipalities. Nevertheless, the opposition has become more vociferous as the fluoridation movement spreads. The active support of the local medical and dental societies helps swing the balance in favor of fluoridation as the question is raised in additional communities.

Fluoridation of drinking water is limited to communities having communal water supplies served by competent water-treatment plant operators. Topical application of fluoride must be used elsewhere; it so happens that fluoridation of drinking water cannot be used in rural and semirural areas, which are poorly served by dentists providing dental care for children. In communities in which the water supply has recently been fluoridated, topical application of fluoride should be used until a significant reduction in dental caries has been achieved by the former means. Once the full effects of water fluoridation have been obtained, no further protection can be gained from application of fluoride solution to the teeth (14).

CORRECTION OF DENTAL CARIES

The universality of the problem of dental caries is aggravated by the limited amount of dental services available for its correction. There is, in addition, an extreme maldistribution of those dental treatment services for children which are available; the rate of children's visits to dentists is seven times greater in some states than in others (15). Even if all children could be given the full benefit of known preventive measures, a large residue of dental caries requiring correction would still remain. Some communities most favored with children's dental services would probably be in a position to develop an adequate program for treatment of the residue. In most areas, the total number of hours of dental treatment services available would still be far short of the amount needed.

Admittedly, solution of the problem of providing dental treatment must be of a long-range nature. To make the greatest inroads on the total problem, it is essential that organized community programs be developed. Accumulated experience has shown the futility of attempting to promote or provide dental care for all children in need of treatment at the start of a program. New dental decay develops at a faster rate than existing caries can be corrected. As a result, comparatively few children have the benefit of complete dental correction and programs become an endless treadmill of activity productive of few demonstrable results. Many so-called programs have been of an essentially emergency nature, restricted almost entirely to the extraction of teeth so decayed as to cause persistent pain or infection.

Incremental Care. Programs of incremental care of dental decay have been suggested as the best organized method of making significant inroads on the problem of dental caries in the space of a few years in communities in which a fair amount of dental treatment can be provided. In the first year of this type of program, all children of a given age receive complete dental examinations and treatment through whatever resources are provided in the local plan. In the following year, any new decay developing in these children is corrected, and an additional group of children, which has reached the age of the first group when originally enrolled, is given complete care. The same pattern is followed in succeeding years, the care of incremental defects being carried to higher age levels as far as finances and facilities permit.

Programs of incremental care have the dual purpose of saving essential permanent teeth, while it is still possible to do so, and of developing good health habits in children so that they will later cooperate with their parents in having continued care after the age limit of the formal program has been passed. The approach used in incremental care frankly acknowledges that many children with existing caries will have to go without treatment other than what they would have obtained in the absence of the organized program. Even though these older children would have had to go without care in any case, it is sometimes necessary to include provision of a limited amount of emergency dental care for them for conditions seriously detrimental to their general health and to avoid community criticism.

Motivation of children and their parents to seek periodic dental care, preferably from family dentists through their own resources, is an important part of any community dental health program. With progress in preventive techniques, treatment of dental caries should become less painful and prolonged, since fewer cavities must be prepared and filled and those which occur will tend to be in accessible sites. This should help reduce fear of dental treatment and resistance to regular dental care.

It is useless to arouse a desire for dental care unless dentists, when available, are willing to devote sufficient time to children's dentistry. The problem is most acute in the care of young children.

It is not the inability of the dentist to restore deciduous teeth, nor is it his inability to manage his child patient that prevents his rendering an adequate service for children. More realistically perhaps, it is the difficulty encountered in receiving for that service a fee which compares favorably with that received for restorative and prosthetic dentistry. (16)

The dental health education program must, therefore, be accompanied by efforts, through dental organizations, to encourage dentists to set apart a larger segment of their time for the provision of dental care for children. Provision of postgraduate training of children's dentistry may solve part of the problem. Scheduling of dental care for children at a time when dentists are generally not occupied with adult patients may also help; special arrangements may have to be made with the school authorities for this.

For care of children whose parents cannot meet the costs themselves, dentists may be reimbursed for services rendered in their own offices on a fee-for-service or time basis. Dentists may also be employed full-time or part-time for work in special dental clinics. For small communities or rural areas, it may be simpler to have the dentist and his staff use portable equipment set up in a location convenient to the children, rather than transporting the children long distances. When portable equipment cannot be used for lack of needed facilities, use may be made of dental trucks or trailers, which are complete diagnostic and treatment centers within themselves.

Standards should be established for a community program which will cover in some detail the services to be rendered. Such standards can best be worked out by the health agency sponsoring the program with the aid of an advisory group from the local dental profession. The standards can be maintained most readily by having a group within the local dental profession work with a supervising dentist employed by the agency. Periodic spot checks may be made of children cared for under the program. The results of these checks may be made available to the advisory group from the dental profession to use as the basis for periodic meetings of the entire dental group providing services under the program; more rapid progress and more favorable relationships may be anticipated through this approach than if the data were discussed directly with the dentists concerned.

MALOCCLUSION

Some degree of dental malocclusion or "crooked teeth" is present in about 50 per cent of all children of school age. In half of these the condition is severe enough to produce secondary effects. It may adversely affect the health of the soft tissues of the mouth or interfere to some degree with adequate mastication. Possibly even more serious in some instances are the social and emotional effects. Dental malocclusion may interfere with educational or vocational opportunities either because of the appearance of the condition, or because of emotional reactions of the individual, which may be out of proportion to the actual physical condition.

Some of the factors influencing teeth to grow in good alignment are well understood; others, especially those related to size of the jaw, are poorly understood. Maintenance of deciduous teeth until the normal time of exfoliation and preservation of the first permanent molar teeth have been mentioned as important factors in promoting normal occlusion of the teeth. Appliances to retain the spaces formed by prematurely lost deciduous teeth or by loss of permanent teeth are a phase of preventive care.

Less emphasis is placed now upon the role of thumb-sucking and similar habits in causing displacement of the teeth than in former years. Little permanent effect will remain if thumb-sucking ceases before the child reaches about six years of age (17). Thumb-sucking after infancy is looked upon as a symptom for which the causes must be sought and treated rather than as a vicious habit to be "broken" at all costs. The latter approach may not only be ineffective, but it may fix the habit.

Orthodontics is the branch of dentistry concerned with preventing and treating conditions which affect the masticating system, in which proper occlusion of the teeth is an important part. Although the size of the malocclusion problem is well recognized, programs of orthodontic care have been developed in only a few areas. When developed, they have been included in or associated with the program for physically handicapped children. Prosthetic appliances for children to replace missing teeth and to produce better function may also be included in these programs.

Orthodontic treatment is prolonged and expensive, often requiring several years for adequate correction, and the number of orthodontists available is very limited. For these reasons, children with the more severe cases of malocclusion must be selected from the very large number with varying grades of malocclusion if the greatest returns are to be attained. Because of the great discrepancy between the need for orthodontic care and the number of orthodontists available, it is advisable to have orthodontists set apart special sessions for children whose care is paid for under an organized program whenever this arrangement is possible. This type of arrangement, whether in the orthodontist's own office or in a clinic, makes possible treatment of larger numbers of children at smaller cost.

PARTICIPATING PERSONNEL

The dentist must obviously provide the professional services for the prevention, diagnosis, and treatment of dental disease, for which only he has been specifically trained. A logical function of the dentist is the prevention of dental handicaps, such as loss of many teeth or severe malocclusion, by treatment of early dental disease. In view of the shortage of dentists, they should not be called upon for services which can be performed by less skilled personnel. Routine dental prophylaxis and topical application of fluoride do not require the professional skills of the dentist. It is also a waste of the dentist's time to have him perform routine dental examinations of children, if correction of any defects is to be carried out by another dentist after notification of the family. It is more reasonable to promote regular dental supervision in the first place. Exceptions to this policy would, of course, be made for research purposes or, occasionally, as a means of demonstrating a need and promoting dental health services in the community.

In state dental health programs and in larger local programs, a dental director is needed for planning and administration. He advises the health officer on all aspects of dental health, especially upon technical aspects of the program with which the health officer, as a physician, would be least acquainted. He may be personally responsible for supervision of dentists employed full-time or part-time in the program, or he may have supervising dentists within the organization for this function.

Dental Hygienists. The first dental hygienists were trained to perform dental prophylaxis shortly before the First World War in a direct effort to prevent dental caries by promoting dental hygiene, in accordance with the general teaching of the time. When it became apparent that clean teeth continued to decay, the dental hygienist's functions developed in two divergent directions. On the one hand, she became more of a dental assistant, helping the dentist while he worked at the chair; she continued to perform routine dental prophylaxis, but from the viewpoint of relieving the dentist of this chore rather than of preventing tooth decay. On the other hand, she was given an educational function, teaching children good toothbrushing techniques and promoting regular dental care through lectures and demonstrations. In some places she even made home visits to encourage correction of known dental defects following school dental examinations.

The availability of a caries-preventive measure by topical application of fluoride solution has brought the role of the dental hygienist under critical reappraisal. She has come full circle to her original function of performing a definite procedure for the prevention of dental decay.

To be really effective, the private practitioner has much to gain from promoting and encouraging the application of the drug to school children under conditions which stimulate interest in the total health problem. Specifically, topical application programs in schools where nearly all children can be reached not only permits the procedure to reach more children but it can be done with less expense if carried out by a dental hygienist. (18)

Most states now permit dental hygienists to perform topical application of fluoride, and others are falling into line. Administrators of dental health programs and school authorities must decide how large a segment of the dental hygienist's time should be devoted to the procedure. The trend in communities without fluoridated drinking-water supplies is toward allocating an increasing amount of time for this purpose, allowing health educators and public health nurses to perform some of her educational and follow-up functions.

Another category of auxiliary dental personnel is the dental assistant. The dental assistant does not have uniform functions but, in general, helps the dentist by performing routine activities such as sterilization of instruments, passing instruments to the dentist, and obtaining supplies. While dental hygienists often function as dental assistants in the private offices of dentists, the tendency is for the routine functions of the dental assistant to be performed by a person who is trained by the dentist on the job. The use of auxiliary personnel for simple treatment procedures in children, such as uncomplicated fillings and extractions, has not been attempted in the United States (19).

CITED REFERENCES

1. ROVELSTAD, GORDON H., The Pediatrician's Responsibility in the Prevention of Dental Caries, *J. Pediat.*, Vol. 36, pp. 687–696, June, 1950.
2. GOLDSTEIN, MARCUS S., Physical Status of Men Examined through Selective Service in World War II, *Pub. Health Rep.*, Vol. 66, pp. 587–609, May 11, 1951.
3. KNUTSON, JOHN W., Simplified Procedure for the Collection of Basic Data for Dental Program Planning and Appraisal, *Am. J. Pub. Health*, Vol. 37, pp. 1439–1448, November, 1947.
4. KLEIN, H., C. E. PALMER, J. W. KNUTSON, Studies on Dental Caries: I. Dental Status and Dental Needs of Elementary School Children, *Pub. Health Rep.*, Vol. 53, pp. 751–765, May 13, 1938.
5. EASLICK, KENNETH A., editor, "Dental Caries, Mechanism and Present Control Technics as Evaluated at the University of Michigan Workshop," pp. 201–224, The C. V. Mosby Company, Medical Publishers, St. Louis, 1948.
6. FOSDICK, L. S., The Reduction of the Incidence of Dental Caries: I. Immediate Toothbrushing with a Neutral Dentifrice, *J. Am. Dent. A.*, Vol. 40, pp. 133–143, February, 1950.

7. HAWES, R. R., and B. G. BIBBY, Evaluation of a Dentifrice Containing Carbamide and Urease, *J. Am. Dent. A.,* Vol. 46, pp. 280–286, March, 1953.

8. KNUTSON, JOHN W., Sodium Fluoride Solutions: Technic for Application to the Teeth, *J. Am. Dent. A.,* Vol. 36, pp. 37–39, January, 1948.

9. AST, DAVID B., Sodium Fluoride Dental Caries Prophylaxis, *New York State Dent. J.,* Vol. 16, pp. 441–448, October, 1950.

10. "Fluoridation in the Prevention of Dental Caries," a manual prepared by the Council on Dental Health, American Dental Association, Chicago, February, 1951.

11. AST, DAVID B., and HELEN C. CHASE, The Newburgh-Kingston Caries Fluorine Study: IV. Dental Findings after Six Years of Water Fluoridation; *Oral Surg., Oral Med. and Oral Path.,* Vol. 6, pp. 114–123, January, 1953.

12. SCHLESINGER, EDWARD R., DAVID E. OVERTON, and HELEN C. CHASE, The Newburgh-Kingston Caries Fluorine Study: V. Pediatric Aspects— Continuation Report, *Am. J. Pub. Health,* Vol. 43, August, 1953.

13. Fluoridation of Public Water Supplies, Statement of the Inter-Association Committee on Health, *Am. J. Pub. Health,* Vol. 42, pp. 338–339, March, 1952.

14. DOWNS, ROBERT A., and WALTER J. PELTON, The Effect of Topically Applied Fluorides in Dental Caries Experience on Children Residing in Fluoride Areas, *J. Dentistry for Children,* Vol. 18, pp. 2–5, Third Quarter, 1951.

15. "Child Health Services and Pediatric Education, Report of the Committee for the Study of Child Health Services," The American Academy of Pediatrics, Commonwealth Fund, Harvard University Press, Cambridge, Mass., 1949.

16. LAMONS, FRANK F., and MARY L. MORGAN, Overcoming Physiological and Psychological Blocks in Dentistry for Children, *J. Am. Dent. A.,* Vol. 44, pp. 15–21, January, 1952.

17. SILLMAN, J. H., Thumb-sucking and the Oral Structures, *J. Pediat.,* Vol. 39, pp. 424–430, October, 1951.

18. FORSYTH, BRUCE D., and WALTER J. PELTON, Dentistry for Children, *J. Dentistry for Children,* Vol. 19, pp. 15–19, First Quarter, 1952.

19. FULTON, JOHN T., New Zealand's School Dental Nurses, *Pediatrics,* Vol. 8, pp. 438–445, September, 1951.

ADDITIONAL REFERENCES

1. PELTON, WALTER J., and JACOB M. WISAN, editors, "Dentistry in Public Health," W. B. Saunders Company, Philadelphia, 1949.

2. KNUTSON, JOHN W., "Dental Caries," The C. V. Mosby Company, Medical Publishers, St. Louis, 1948.

3. PRICE, WALTER C., P. A. SCIULLO, and VIRGINIA STILLEY, Dental

Health Service as a Function of Preventive Pediatric Care, *J. Pediat.,* Vol. 39, pp. 206–210, August, 1951.

4. GRABER, T. M., Orthodontic Problems in Pediatric Practice, *Pediatrics,* Vol. 9, pp. 709–721, June, 1952.

5. HEYROTH, FRANCIS F., Toxicological Evidence for the Safety of Fluoridation of Public Water Supplies, *A. J. Pub. Health,* Vol. 42, pp. 1568–1575, December, 1952.

6. PHAIR, W. PHILIP, and MARIAN F. DRISCOLL, The Status of Fluoridation Programs in the United States, Its Territories and Possessions, *J. Am. Dent. A.,* Vol. 45, pp. 555–582, November, 1952.

7. A Survey of the Literature of Dental Caries, Prepared for the Food and Nutrition Board, National Research Council, under the supervision of the Committee on Dental Health, Publication 225, National Academy of Sciences, National Research Council, Washington, D.C., 1952.

13 NUTRITION SERVICES

Nutrition education, stemming from the pioneer milk stations, was one of the earliest activities in the field of child health. New knowledge in the science of nutrition was quickly applied in the child health program. Formerly so prevalent, rickets and scurvy have become clinical rarities in many parts of the country. Along with increased public interest in nutrition, the per capita consumption of dairy products, citrus fruits, and green and yellow vegetables has risen significantly (1). There can be little doubt that mothers and children have better diets and are in better health because of this than a few decades ago.

These solid accomplishments in themselves justify the efforts which have been expended to improve the nutritional status of the American people. A constructively critical approach, with careful testing of new information obtained from the laboratory and with proper evaluation of programs based on the body of nutrition knowledge already available, will assure further rapid progress. This has been the case in clinical medicine where, for example, thorough testing of the important role of dietary protein before and after surgery and during convalescence from illness preceded general acceptance of this concept by the medical profession. Just as in clinical medicine, a more balanced approach to the community nutrition program is replacing the swings of feeling about nutrition that have characterized the recent past.

Diet, Nutrition, and Nutritional Status. By *nutrition* is meant the complete physiological process of digestion, absorption, utilization for growth and energy needs, and finally breakdown and elimination of the various nutrients or food factors in the diet, or the body of knowledge relating to these processes. *Diet* or *dietary intake* is the actual food ingested, regardless of its ultimate use in the body economy. *Nutritional status* is the end result of the utilization of nutrients in the diet in meeting the nutritional needs of the individual, including such special demands as growth, physical activity, pregnancy and lactation, and disease processes.

The term *optimum nutrition* has been another source of confusion (2). Optimum nutrition suggests that amounts of the various nutrients above the level needed to maintain a person in good health will result in additional measurable benefits in growth or endurance or in ability to perform special functions. No clear-cut clinical evidence has been presented that additional food or supplements of nutrients, beyond that found in an adequate diet, will produce any beneficial effects in a healthy person. On the contrary, dietary excess may be detrimental to general health. Obesity, resulting from excessive caloric intake, is probably the most common form of malnutrition in the United States, predisposing to several of the more serious chronic diseases in adult life. Vitamin A intoxication is an example of dietary excess in infancy (3). It results from the feeding of large doses of vitamin A by parents to infants, often in the belief that, if a little vitamin A is good, a great deal is so much better.

The concept of levels or zones of nutritional status merging into one another provides a sound basis for understanding nutritional problems. Five such zones have been suggested by Dann and Darby (2):

1. Saturation, in which no further nutrient can be stored in the body, except in excess and as a detriment to the individual.

2. Unsaturation, but without functional impairment, with no actual or potential deficiency.

3. Potential deficiency disease, "regarded as existing when in the absence of clinical evidence of a deficiency (*a*) a new stress on the organism will cause a rapid development of the clinically manifest disease or (*b*) a suitable physiological or biochemical test yields evidence of decreased reserve capacity."

4. Latent deficiency disease, the mildest form detectable clinically, "characterized by vague, indefinite, non-specific symptoms."

5. Clinically manifest deficiency disease, which may be mild or severe, depending on whether the disease can be readily diagnosed by clinical means alone.

Clinically manifest deficiency disease may be the end result of a progression from the higher levels of nutritional status, or a person may never have been above the level of potential deficiency disease from birth and may have adjusted at that level. The degree and chronicity of food deprivation, in relation to the person's previous condition, are important factors in determining the resulting nutritional status of the individual.

Dietary Needs. The daily dietary allowances recommended by the National Research Council are used generally in this country in nutrition education and in assessing the adequacy of diets (4). These are allowances rather than standards, to avoid the implication that they are the minimum amounts of nutrients required to prevent the development of deficiency states. Actually, a certain excess has been allowed above the required minimum for each nutrient, as based on experimental and clinical evidence, to take care of expected individual variation, but generally not enough to meet unusual demands such as illness or environmental stresses. In translating the allowances into everyday foods, seven major food groups have been suggested. These so-called basic-7 food groups are leafy green and yellow vegetables; citrus fruits, tomato, and raw cabbage; potatoes and other vegetables and fruits; milk, cheese, and ice cream; meat, fish, eggs, and beans; bread and cereals; and butter and fortified margarine.

Mass self-medication with vitamins and other concentrated nutrients is a recent phenomenon on the American scene. This has extended in places to the routine administration of these food elements to factory workers and even to school children on the theory that this will ward off infections and increase efficiency. There is no reliable evidence that these practices are of any value. "If a person takes a good diet, he will not benefit from vitamin supplements, and . . . if the patient does not take an adequate diet, the treatment is a good diet, not vitamins." (5) The major exception to this principle is vitamin D supplementation throughout the period of growth. It may also be desirable to employ dietary supplements for poorly nourished pregnant women and for patients with clinical deficiency states in order to overcome any deficiencies rapidly (6).

Factors in Nutrition. The availability of enough foods of good nutritional content is obviously closely related to the economic status of the family. Within various economic levels, however, there is a broad range of diets favorable or unfavorable to health. Poor food selection may be due to ignorance of the rudiments of good nutrition. It may also be the result of firmly established dietary patterns related to ancestral nation-

Table 5. RECOMMENDED DAILY DIETARY ALLOWANCES, FOOD AND NUTRITION BOARD, NATIONAL RESEARCH COUNCIL

	Calories	Protein, gm.	Calcium, gm.	Iron, mg.	Vitamin A, I.U.	Thia-mine, mg.	Ribofla-vin, mg.	Niacin, mg.	Ascorbic acid, mg.	Vitamin D, I.U.
Children up to 12 yr.*										
Under 1 yr.†	110/2.2 lb. (1 kg.)	3.5/2.2 lb. (1 kg.)	1.0	6	1,500	0.4	0.6	4	30	400
1–3 yr. (27 lb., 12 kg.)	1,200	40	1.0	7	2,000	0.6	0.9	6	35	400
4–6 yr. (42 lb., 19 kg.)	1,600	50	1.0	8	2,500	0.8	1.2	8	50	400
7–9 yr. (58 lb., 26 kg.)	2,000	60	1.0	10	3,500	1.0	1.5	10	60	400
10–12 yr. (78 lb., 35 kg.)	2,500	70	1.2	12	4,500	1.2	1.8	12	75	400
Children over 12 yr.										
Girls 13–15 yr. (108 lb., 49 kg.)	2,600	80	1.3	15	5,000	1.3	2.0	13	80	400
16–20 yr. (122 lb., 55 kg.)	2,400	75	1.0	15	5,000	1.2	1.8	12	80	400
Boys 13–15 yr. (108 lb., 49 kg.)	3,200	85	1.4	15	5,000	1.5	2.0	15	90	400
16–20 yr. (141 lb., 64 kg.)	3,800	100	1.4	15	6,000	1.7	2.5	17	100	400
Woman (123 lb., 56 kg.)										
Sedentary	2,000	60	1.0	12	5,000	1.0	1.5	10	70	
Moderately active	2,400	60	1.0	12	5,000	1.2	1.5	12	70	
Very active	3,000	60	1.0	12	5,000	1.5	1.5	15	70	
Pregnancy (latter half)	2,400‡	85	1.5	15	6,000	1.5	2.5	15	100	400
Lactation	3,000	100	2.0	15	8,000	1.5	3.0	15	150	400

Further recommendations

Fat. Fat allowances must be based at present more on food habits than on physiological requirements. There are several factors which make it desirable (1) that fat be included in the diet to the extent of at least 20 to 25 per cent of the total calories and (2) that the fat intake include essential unsaturated fatty acids to the extent of at least 1 per cent of the total calories. For children and for adolescent persons, it is desirable that 30 to 35 per cent of the total calories be derived from fat. Since foodstuffs such as meat, milk, cheese, nuts, etc., contribute fat to the diet, it is necessary to use separated or "visible" fats such as butter, oleomargarine, lard, or shortenings to supply only one-third to one-half the amounts indicated.

Iodine. The need for iodine is met by the regular use of iodized salt; its use is especially important in adolescence and pregnancy.

Phosphorus. Available evidence indicates that the phosphorus allowances should be at least equal to those for calcium in the diets of children and of women during the latter part of pregnancy and during lactation. In general it is safe to assume that, if the calcium and protein needs are met through common foods, the phosphorus requirement also will be covered, because the common foods richest in calcium and protein are also the best sources of phosphorus.

Copper. Infants and children require approximately 0.05 mg. for each kilogram of body weight. The requirement for copper is approximately one-tenth that for iron. A good diet normally will supply sufficient copper.

Vitamin K. The requirement for vitamin K usually is satisfied by any good diet except for the infant *in utero* and for the first few days after birth. Supplemental vitamin K is recommended during the last month of pregnancy. When it has not been given in this manner, it is recommended for the mother preceding delivery or for the baby immediately after birth.

Folic acid. There is evidence that folic acid (pteroylglutamic acid) is an essential human nutrient. The quantitative requirement cannot be closely estimated from evidence now available.

SOURCE: Adapted from "Recommended Dietary Allowances," revised 1948, National Research Council Reprint and Circular Series, No. 129, Washington, D.C., October, 1948. Reproduced with permission of National Research Council.

* Allowances for children are based on the needs for the middle year in each group (as 2,5,8, etc.) and are for moderate activity and for average weight at the middle year of the age group.

† Needs for infants increase from month to month with size and activity. The amounts given are for approximately 6 to 8 months. The dietary requirements for some of the nutrients such as protein and calcium are less if derived largely from human milk.

‡ During the latter part of pregnancy the calorie allowance should increase to approximately 20 per cent above the preceding level. The value of 2,400 calories represents the allowance for pregnant, sedentary women.

ality or to local habits. Methods of food preparation may lead to destruction or discarding of valuable nutrients. Isolation of the community may limit the variety of foods available, but this factor has become less important as a result of improved methods of transportation and food preservation.

Emotional factors in feeding have a profound influence in determining the adequacy of dietary intake. While these are most obvious in infancy and early childhood, when so-called feeding problems are matters of intense concern to parents and their professional advisers, feeding patterns and food likes and dislikes developed in childhood carry over into adult life and ultimately affect the dietary habits of succeeding generations. Food fads, in themselves an emotional abberation, may give rise to severe deficiency states. Feeding problems and food fads are not respectors of economic status. On the contrary, it may well be that feeding difficulties in early childhood are more common in those groups in the population in the best position to provide an adequate diet for children.

Other factors also play their part in determining the nutritional status of the child and his family. Overcrowding in the home or a disordered household in general may produce chronic fatigue in the child and result in diminished appetite. Insufficient time may be allowed for meals, or entire meals may be omitted. Dietary surveys among school children usually disclose a varying proportion of children who have missed breakfast. Chronic low-grade infections also cause a reduction in the child's appetite, and these infections may be perpetuated by poor nutrition.

Conditioning factors may lead to deficiency states in the presence of otherwise adequate dietary intake. Some of these (growth, pregnancy and lactation, and moderate physical activity) are taken into account in the recommended allowances of the National Research Council. Acute and chronic illness may also produce unusual nutritional demands. Nutrients may not be absorbed adequately because of diarrheal conditions. Celiac disease, a common syndrome producing nutritional deficiencies in infancy and early childhood, is probably the result of poor absorption of essential nutrients from the gastrointestinal tract. Other conditions, such as glycogen-storage disease, may interfere with proper use of nutrients through disturbances of internal metabolism.

Appraisal of Nutritional Status of Population Groups. Much of the controversy in the nutrition field has been due to imperfect development of tools for measuring nutritional status. Confusion has also resulted from use of the same tools to study the nutritional status of individuals and of large groups, without interpretation of the differences in approach.

Children and pregnant and lactating women are often selected as subjects for the study of nutritional status (7). These groups provide a sensitive index of the nutritional status of the community as a whole since the nutritional demands of growth and of pregnancy and lactation tend to change potential or latent deficiency to clinically manifest disease if the diet is inadequate to meet the added demands. Signs of nutritional deficiency in children are also less apt to be confused with changes due to aging.

Several types of tools are available for appraising the nutritional status of groups. Chief among these are dietary histories, laboratory tests, and medical examinations.

1. *Dietary history.* Dietary intake is often used loosely as the equivalent of nutritional status, whereas it is only a single factor, although the major one, influencing the state of nutrition of population groups. Dietary histories vary widely in content and complexity. Use of a check list of a good diet to record the foods generally eaten is the simplest method. Dietary histories may include the kinds and amounts of foods eaten on a single day or those eaten during a period of a week or more.

The desire to obtain a sample of a typical diet over a period of time must be weighed against the increasing inaccuracy of the data as the time period is lengthened. The most reliable diet history is probably a recording covering three days, preferably during the middle of a week in which no holidays occur. The history may be recorded on a special form by the persons studied, to be checked and supplemented in interviews by trained persons, or it may be obtained entirely by interview. In any event, reliable information on details of food intake should not be expected after the lapse of a day from the time the food is eaten.

Dietary histories for research purposes require an entirely different approach from those used to obtain a general picture of the food habits of a community and require even more cautious interpretation. The effect of the manner of food preparation on the nutrient quality of the food may not be fully evaluated. Long-term dietary intake may be quite different from that recorded during the period of study, and various conditioning factors influence the actual nutritional status of the persons under investigation. In spite of these drawbacks, a carefully conducted and interpreted dietary survey probably provides the most convenient and reliable index of nutrition problems in a community.

2. *Laboratory examinations.* Simple laboratory tests, such as determination of the hemoglobin level, have long been used as aides in appraising nutritional status. Tolerance tests and other biochemical methods have also been used to measure the level of various nutrients in the blood or the degree of their saturation in the body. These more cumbersome methods were applicable only to limited research studies prior to the development of simplified microtechniques. A widely applied method, using not more than three drops of blood, permits measurement of the levels of vitamin A, carotene, ascorbic acid, riboflavin, serum protein, alkaline phosphatase, and hemoglobin (8).

The significance of the blood levels of various nutrients differs with each nutrient. The plasma level of water-soluble nutrients such as ascorbic acid is a reflection of recent dietary intake; the level of the fat-soluble nutrients, which are readily stored in the body, is related more closely to long-term intake. The serum protein determination is of little practical help, since it is lowered only in extreme deficiency states. The significance of the alkaline phosphatase after infancy is not clear.

3. *Clinical appraisal and physical measurement.* A complete medical examination is not a practical procedure in studying the nutritional status of large population groups. Instead, inspection of selected tissues has been used extensively as one phase of nutrition surveys, on the assumption that deficiencies of various nutrients give rise to recognizable changes in these tissues early in the clinical stage of deficiency disease (9). Deficiency in vitamin A, for example, manifests itself as hyperkeratosis follicularis, or chronic "gooseflesh," which is most marked on the thighs. Lack of niacin or riboflavin gives rise to recognizable changes in the tongue, and chronic inadequacy of ascorbic acid to sponginess and redness of the gums.

Conclusions regarding the prevalence of clinical deficiency states in a given population based on these findings must be accepted with marked reservations. Variation in judgment of different observers, which exists in any type of clinical appraisal, is enhanced by the nonspecificity of the lesions used as evidence of deficiencies in various nutrients. " 'Corneal vascularization,' once regarded as a definite physical sign of riboflavin deficiency, has subsequently proved valueless for assessment of the nutritional level of this vitamin. . . . Animal experimentation has demonstrated that corneal vascularization may result from a wide variety of dietary deficiencies." (10) The technique of biomicroscopy, which magnifies the lesions and presumably permits earlier diagnosis, has been discarded largely for these reasons. Color photography is also used to record the lesions for objective study, since the picture may be evaluated without the bias due to knowledge of the individual photographed (11). The value of this more objective method is limited by the degree of specificity of the lesions studied.

4. *Combination of methods*. Because of the deficiencies noted in each of the techniques for appraising the nutritional status of population groups, surveys combining and correlating the several methods are superior to any single method. A survey team of skilled personnel, consisting of a physician, a biochemist or a technician under the supervision of a biochemist, a nutritionist, and a public health nurse, aided by a clerical staff, can obtain information rapidly either for epidemiological purposes or for field research in connection with a basic nutritional research program (12). The Public Health Service had several such teams operating in different parts of the country prior to discontinuance of its special nutrition program in 1950. Grants for correlated studies have since been administered on a regional basis by the Department of Agriculture.

Appraisal of Nutritional Status of Individuals. The methods used in epidemiological studies of population groups are properly screening techniques of only limited value when applied to individuals. Even the results of careful physical examination, including evaluation of skin turgor, muscle tone, and color of skin and mucous membranes, as well as a search for lesions presumably due to nutritional deficiencies, are widely divergent in the hands of different medical examiners. The experience of the examiner and the character of the group examined explain many of these discrepancies. A well-nourished child of Scandinavian stock may appear thin and pale to an observer whose experience has been with children of South European background. Conversely, a poorly nourished child may be overlooked by an observer whose standards have been formed in a situation in which a poor state of nutrition is a common condition.

No one body measurement or group of measurements can be relied upon as an index of nutritional status. Measurements made only once fail to reveal the majority of children in obviously poor condition on clinical appraisal. Even serial measurements have limitations in the study of the individual child. There is considerable overlapping in the schedules of development in groups of children with clear-cut nutritional deficiencies as compared with children in an apparent good state of nutrition who come from families with sufficient income to provide an adequate diet (13).

It is clear that accurate methods for the appraisal of the nutritional status of individuals are not available. For practical help to the child, however, the situation is less discouraging. The obviously undernourished or obese child is readily discovered by medical examination, or the presence of malnutrition may be suspected by a teacher or public health nurse and the child brought to medical attention by follow-up services. Serial charting of height and weight is useful as a screening device by giving an added indication of something amiss in a child who had been doing well previously; it also points to the need for close attention to children whose measurements deviate persistently from those expected for age and sex. Even a short dietary study will disclose children whose food habits predispose to poor nutritional states and, therefore, point them out for individual follow-up.

Even though the individual child with potential or latent deficiency disease cannot readily be singled out by available methods applicable on a broad scale, awareness of the child's background may help disclose the possibility of the existence of nutritional deficiency. Beyond that, knowing the characteristics of the group from which the child comes raises the examiner's index of suspicion so that attention can be focused on these children and their parents. In short, an adequate health appraisal, taking into account the social and emotional factors in the life of the individual mother and child, remains the most reliable means of determining the state of nutrition of the individual.

Nutrition clinics have been developed in a few localities to serve as a central place in which persons suspected of nutritional deficiencies may be examined carefully, combining the various techniques described for mass studies. These clinics may be associated with school health services, in which case the majority of the children seen are referred by school personnel. Children referred by private physicians may also be seen in consultation on request. Even though located in a hospital, a nutrition clinic may serve the community as a whole. Most nutrition clinics are really integral parts of the outpatient departments of teaching hospitals and serve only the patients referred from other clinics in the hospital.

Promotion of Improved Nutrition. Many programs have been conducted to improve the dietary habits of the entire community by promoting wiser selection and preparation of available foods in relation to the income of various population groups. Brief dietary surveys may be used to gain community interest by disclosing dietary lacks, even though these lacks may not be associated with manifest deficiencies. The principles in such community-wide efforts are similar to those of other types of public health education. Mothers and children benefit from such programs as members of the community. Of more direct concern to the maternal and child health program is the teaching of selected groups such as pregnant women or parents of preschool or school children. These groups share common interests and problems which make them more receptive to instruction, and they are more likely to be influenced in making desirable changes in their food habits. The effectiveness of group teaching is enhanced if persons of the same nationality background are brought together, since suggestions made within the framework of traditional dietary patterns are more likely to be accepted than are unfamiliar food practices.

Groups of women with similar interests and health needs can be assembled in several ways. Pregnant women can be reached in outpatient departments of hospitals or health department clinics, or through parents' classes to which pregnant women under the care of private physicians may be referred. Efforts may be made to bring together mothers of infants and preschool children in connection with clinics and other health services for the group or through day-care centers or nursery schools. Parents of school children are assembled with relative ease through organizations associated with the schools. Nutrition instruction of children is given as part of the organized educational program (14). Such instruction benefits the family as a whole, as well as the children, since the teaching should carry over into the home.

School Lunch Programs. The few limited municipal school lunch programs soon after the First World War were started following the disclosure of widespread malnutrition among school children. With the economic depression of the 1930's, the existence of food surpluses in the face of widespread dietary inadequacies led to distribution of some of the surplus foods to schools. The nutritional benefits were so evident that the program steadily expanded even when the food surplus no longer existed.

Major emphasis upon nutrition, rather than upon use of surplus foods, was formalized in the National School Lunch Act of 1946. The greater part of the appropriation under this Act is used by the Department of Agriculture for grants-in-aid to states for state-administered school lunch programs; the Act required that a gradually increasing proportion of state funds be made available to match the Federal funds. This has stimulated the development of school lunch programs throughout the country, and some states have spent far more than the matching funds specified in the law. Three types of meals are specified under the law for varying amounts of financial aid. Type A is a complete meal for which the maximum amount of aid is granted. Type B is intended as a supplement for food brought to school by the child. The type C supplement consists of only a glass of milk.

A well-conducted school lunch program provides a hot meal of high nutritional value to the portion of the student body whose dietary intake is otherwise inadequate. Effort should be concentrated in enrolling school children in poor or borderline nutritional status in the program. Perhaps more important in the long run is its educational value in providing a practical demonstration of what constitutes an adequate diet. Lunches can be made attractive and children allowed ample food choices. The force of example in seeing other children eat a variety of foods in adequate amounts encourages the child whose food selection is limited to broaden his choice of foods. Type B or C school lunch programs can be useful to a lesser extent, since even the provision of milk is a gain for the child. On the other hand, school lunch programs that are poorly managed may be a negative force in the school and community setting, since they present bad examples of food selection and preparation.

Feeding in Institutions. The nutritional needs of children in institutions, along with the methods of food preparation and service, require special attention. Children under medical care in hospitals or convalescent institutions are liable to develop nutritional deficiencies as a result of their illnesses, unless their special needs are met. Children institutionalized because of neglect or other social reasons have often been on inadequate diets for long periods before admission to the institution. Any feeding problems present may be accentuated by the emotional reactions to institutionalization. On the other hand, the new situation may have positive values if these are exploited properly. Feeding the children in small groups, rather than from individual trays at their bedside at one extreme to regimented dining halls at the other, and encouraging the child to participate in preparation of the table may help create a favorable attitude toward food which will persist after discharge.

Physicians who administer or staff institutions should promote adequate dietary standards and desirable food service practices. Health departments, departments of social welfare, and voluntary agencies often provide consultant or supervisory services in developing and maintaining such standards. Consultant services are particularly valuable in those institutions, generally smaller ones, which do not have trained dietetic personnel on their own staffs. Even larger institutions benefit from consultant service from an outside observer who can study the food practices of the institution without being enmeshed in the daily round of activities and personnel problems.

These consultant services often prove acceptable, after initial resistance on the part of the institution, when palpable gains are demonstrated. Reduced waste both in the kitchen and in rejected food savings by wiser food purchases and heightened staff morale by better work organization are primary benefits. More complete consumption of food at mealtimes also results in less demand for between-meal feedings, with consequent release of nursing time for other functions.

PROFESSIONAL PERSONNEL

A well-rounded community nutrition program, which includes studies of the nutritional status of the population and educational and follow-up services, requires the services of physicians with special training in nutrition, nutritionists, and biochemists or technicians, in addition to generalized public health nurses and other public health personnel. Programs of this broad nature are still in the early stage of development. Most nutrition programs are far more limited, placing primary emphasis upon education of the general public and of special groups, with secondary stress upon the discovery and correction of malnutrition.

Physicians. "A physician with thorough training in both public health administration and clinical nutrition is preeminently qualified to be the director of the nutrition unit in a State health department." (15) This ideal has been achieved in only one or two states. The medical nutritionist would plan and direct the program, working out cooperative relationships with other agencies concerned with nutrition. He would also supervise teams studying the nutritional status of the population. Physicians with some special training in nutrition are also needed to perform clinical appraisal in special studies or as a part of the general child health program. The nutrition director supervises or provides the direct training of such physicians. Few local health departments can justifiably employ a full-time medical director for their nutrition programs at the present stage of development. His functions are usually carried by the director of the maternal and child health or other full-time program.

Nutritionists. Nonmedical nutritionists carry the brunt of existing nutrition programs and have immediate responsibility for the content of the services. Traditionally, nutritionists devoted most of their attention to direct services to individuals and groups. They worked with individual recipients of health services in clinics and even in home visits. It is now widely accepted that the nutritionist functions more effectively in an indirect capacity, by reaching larger segments of the population through consultant and advisory services to public health nurses and others whose work brings them in immediate contact with the public and through assistance in the preparation of material for purposes of professional and public health education.

Even though the nutritionist may function chiefly as consultant to other personnel, some complicated services continue to require her direct attention. Detailed dietary analyses demand specifically trained personnel; so does consultation service to institutions, especially when consultation is provided regarding food service practices. The nutritionist may also serve physicians in clinics and in private practice by assisting patients with the practical details of the general dietary instructions given by their physicians.

The fields of activity of the dietitian and the nutritionist overlap in a well-developed program. The dietitian is mainly concerned with the preparation of food for either group feeding or for individual patients requiring special diets. She is generally employed in institutions or in school lunch and other group feeding programs, although she may also function as a field consultant to institutions.

The nutritionist is primarily concerned with the promotion of improved nutrition of the community and is more concerned with community agencies, but she also gives detailed instruction to meet individual needs, and as time has gone on, she has become increasingly involved in detailed dietary problems of special groups such as the obese or cardiac patients seen in special clinics. The work of nutritionists with institutions and other group feeding situations is largely within the original field of the dietitian. Actually, many nutritionists have come to public health nutrition from hospital backgrounds in dietetics and have found their previous experience invaluable in their new work. Rather than attempt to set up a rigid wall between the two groups, the tendency is to utilize well-trained individuals from each category to best advantage in the public health program.

CITED REFERENCES

1. PHIPARD, ESTHER F., and HAZEL K. STIEBELING, Adequacy of American Diets, in "Handbook of Nutrition, American Medical Association," 2d ed., pp. 599–617, The Blakiston Company, New York, 1951.
2. DANN, W. J., and WILLIAM J. DARBY, The Appraisal of Nutritional Status (Nutriture) in Humans, with Especial Reference to Vitamin Deficiency Diseases, *Physiol. Rev.*, Vol. 25, pp. 326–346, April, 1945.
3. FRIED, CHARLES T., and MILTON J. H. GRAND, Hypervitaminosis A, *Am. J. Dis. Child.*, Vol. 79, pp. 475–486, March, 1950.
4. "Recommended Dietary Allowances, Revised 1948," National Research Council Reprint and Circular Series, No. 129, Washington D.C., October, 1948.
5. CULVER, PERRY J., Vitamin Supplementation in Health and Disease, *New England J. Med.*, Vol. 241, pp. 970–977, 1011–1017; 1050–1057, Dec. 15, 22, 29, 1949.
6. POLLACK, HERBERT, and SEYMOUR L. HALPERN, Therapeutic Nutrition, Publication 234, National Academy of Sciences—National Research Council, Washington, D.C., 1952.
7. GOLDSMITH, GRACE A., Relationships between Nutrition and Pregnancy as Observed in Recent Surveys in Newfoundland, *Am. J. Pub. Health,* Vol. 40, pp. 953–959, August, 1950.
8. BESSEY, OTTO A., and OLIVER H. LOWRY, Biochemical Methods in Nutritional Surveys, *Am. J. Pub. Health,* Vol. 35, pp. 941–946, September, 1945.
9. Vitamin Deficiencies: Stigmas, Symptoms and Therapy, Council on Foods and Nutrition, American Medical Association, *J.A.M.A.,* Vol. 131, pp. 666–667, June 22, 1946.
10. Evaluation of Signs of Deficiency Diseases, editorial, *J.A.M.A.,* Vol. 145, p. 826, Mar. 17, 1951.
11. BROWE, JOHN H., and HAROLD B. PIERCE, A Study of Nutritional Status

among School Children and Their Response to Nutrient Therapy, *Milbank Mem. Fund Quart.,* Vol. 28, pp. 223–237, July, 1950.

12. SINCLAIR, HUGH M., Nutritional Surveys of Population Groups, *New England J. Med.,* Vol. 245, pp. 39–47, July 12, 1951.

13. MANN, ARVIN W., SAMUEL DREIZEN, TOM D. SPIES, and S. IDELL PYLE, The Determination of Status and Progress in Children with Nutritive Failure, *J. Pediat.,* Vol. 31, pp. 161–171, August, 1947.

14. ROWNTREE, JENNIE I., The Place of Nutrition in the Health Education Program, *Am. J. Pub. Health,* Vol. 42, pp. 293–298, March, 1952.

15. Nutrition Programs in State Health Departments, Report Prepared by a Subcommittee of the Committee on Diagnosis and Pathology of Nutritional Deficiencies for the Food and Nutrition Board, National Research Council, *Pub. Health Rep.,* Vol. 65, pp. 411–445, Mar. 31, 1950.

ADDITIONAL REFERENCES

1. SMITH, CLEMENT A., and HAROLD C. STUART, Appraising the Nutritional Status of Mothers and Children, *Am. J. Pub. Health,* Vol. 38, pp. 369–373, March, 1948.

2. "Nutrition Surveys: Their Techniques and Value," National Research Council Bulletin No. 117, Washington D.C., May, 1949.

3. SPIES, TOM D., SAMUEL DREIZEN, GEORGE S. PARKER, and DONALD J. SILBERMAN, Detection and Treatment of Nutritive Failure in Children: Recent Observations, *J.A.M.A.,* Vol. 148, pp. 1376–1382, Apr. 19, 1952.

4. LEICHSENRING, JANE M., and EVA D. WILSON, Food Composition Table for Short Method of Dietary Analysis (2d revision), *J. Am. Dietet. A.,* Vol. 27, pp. 386–389, May, 1951.

5. JOLLIFFE, NORMAN, Critical Evaluation of Public Health Programs in Nutrition, *J.A.M.A.,* Vol. 147, pp. 1411–1413, Dec. 8, 1951.

6. WHITEHEAD, FLOY E., Dietary Studies of School-age Children in Ascension Parish, Louisiana, *Am. J. Pub. Health,* Vol. 42, pp. 1547–1551, December, 1952.

14 PROMOTION OF CHILD SAFETY

Temporary or permanent disability following an accident is as real to the individual and society as disability following illness. Yet, until recent years, the seriousness of the problem of accidents has met with public and professional apathy. With the emergence of accidents as the leading cause of death in childhood after the first birthday, due to the rapid decline in mortality from other causes, many groups have become aware of the problem. Increasing numbers of physicians are becoming interested in making their potentially valuable contributions to the prevention of accidents among the families in their practices. "As one pediatrician has recently expressed it: 'With one-third of all children who died dying in accidents, I have come to the conclusion that as long as I work only on the prevention of disease, I am only partly serving my patient's interest.' " (1)

The initially disjointed efforts by various public and professional groups are being replaced by more effective action on a national, state, and local scale (2). The primary interest of the various groups naturally differs according to their specific areas of responsibility. Accidents occurring in the streets or in motor vehicles are a major concern of police and other agencies responsible for traffic control. Fire departments take the lead in the elimination of hazards which may result in conflagrations. School authorities bear the responsibility for safety of the child in the school and on the school grounds. Architects, engineers, recreation groups, and agencies concerned with the development and maintenance of building codes all have their special fields of interest.

Individual parents and local groups of citizens are also usually more aware of specific hazards to which their own children are exposed. Dangerous street crossings and hazardous conditions on school grounds are more likely to arouse the interest of parent groups than more wide-spread hazards such as potentially dangerous situations in their own homes. Certain correctable hazards are too often accepted as inevitable parts of daily living. This attitude affects the work of the agencies having official responsibility for preventing or correcting hazardous conditions within their sphere of activity, since those bearing legal responsibility for safety measures must ultimately report to the community on their work. An alert citizenry not only will support them with sufficient funds for their work, but it will call them to task if proper safety services are not being provided.

As members of the community, physicians are interested in the prevention of accidents wherever they occur, whether in the schools, in motor vehicles, in public places, or in the home. Because of their prestige in the community, they may be able to stimulate agencies having specific responsibilities to institute adequate preventive measures. However, the major contributions of physicians, and of health agencies as well, can be made in promoting child safety in and about the home, and it will be on home safety that the greater part of the following discussion will be focused.

The Public Health Problem. The size of the problem of accidental death at different ages is fairly clear (Table 6). Similar data are avail-

Table 6. MORTALITY RATES IN VARIOUS AGE GROUPS FROM ALL CAUSES, FROM ALL ACCIDENTS, AND FROM SELECTED ACCIDENTS, PER 100,000 ESTIMATED POPULATION, UNITED STATES, 1949

Age group	*1–4 years*	*5–14 years*	*15–24 years*
All causes	150.	60.	130.
All accidents	37.8	22.5	51.6
Motor vehicles	11.6	8.8	30.3
Poisonings by solids or liquids	2.9	0.2	0.4
Falls	1.8	0.8	1.6
Burns and scalds (other than fire or explosion)	1.9	0.2	0.1
Fire or explosion	7.4	2.4	1.7
Drowning	5.5	4.5	5.0

Source: "Accident Fatalities in the United States," Vital Statistics—Special Reports, Vol. 36, No. 19, National Office of Vital Statistics, July 8, 1952.

able by geographic areas. The rates of nonfatal accidents and the extent of disability resulting from them are less well understood. The generally used index of approximately 150 nonfatal accidents for every accident having a fatal outcome is based on data from the National Health Survey of the 1930's. The index is subject to the limitations of the Survey which covered only urban situations at a time when environmental conditions were quite different from subsequent periods. The index also fails to take into account any differences between age groups. A more recent local study of nonfatal accidents in children from one through fifteen years of age, for example, revealed about 230 nonfatal accidents for every fatality, even though the study did not tap all possible sources of information (3).

The problem of accidents can be attacked logically only if the dissimilar nature of accidents at different age levels is understood. During the school years, deaths from accidents in public places, mostly due to motor vehicles and drowning, outnumber home accidents three to one. Accidental death from firearms stands high on the list, whereas poisonings are far behind in this age group. The child of school age spends much of his time away from home, but he has not learned to master the hazards of the outside environment as well as he has those more familiar to him in and about the home. Some of this difference may be explained by the more lethal character of the hazards outside the home during the school years. The first accidental submersion during swimming or the first careless running in front of a speeding car may be more likely to end fatally than a tumble or scald at home.

The accident fatality picture is different in the preschool group. Among children from one through four years of age, deaths from home accidents outnumber all other accidental deaths and, by themselves, constitute the leading cause of death. Among home accidents, falls, burns of all kinds, and poisonings are the major offenders. The young child has not had enough experience to face the hazards of the home and requires a greater degree of protection even within this circumscribed environment.

The recorded death rate from accidents among infants is more than twice as high as among children over one year of age. Home accidents constitute the greater part of the total. Even so, home accidents are well down on the list of causes of deaths among infants, largely because neonatal factors are far more important. The recorded mortality rate from accidents in infancy, however, cannot be accepted without marked reservations. Many of the deaths ascribed to mechanical suffocation in bedclothes or from aspiration of vomitus, reportedly causing two-thirds of all fatal home accidents to infants, are probably due to other causes (4). Evidence of overwhelming infection, such as mononuclear pneumonia, is found on careful postmortem study of infants dying suddenly, supposedly from mechanical suffocation (5). A healthy infant can readily turn his head to obtain air even when his face is in a pillow; those who cannot avoid suffocation are probably already seriously ill. If deaths reported as due to suffocation are eliminated, the size of the mortality rate among infants is about the same as in the preschool group. Since deaths from mechanical suffocation are counted in the reported data, it is misleading to lump infants and preschool children together in studying accident fatalities in young children.

Although the mortality rate from all accidents has declined more slowly than other causes of death in childhood, an encouraging feature has been the more rapid decrease in fatal home accidents as compared with other types of accidents. This decline has been particularly marked in the preschool period; in this age group the thirty years between 1920 and 1950 have seen a drop of 60 per cent in the rate from poisonings, 80 per cent from burns and scalds, and 55 per cent from falls (Figure 11). Improved medical and nursing care of traumatic conditions accounts for only a portion of this decline. The major drop in mortality from burns and scalds occurred between 1921 and 1935, before sulfa and antibiotic drugs were available and before modern methods for combating shock were used. Similarly, only a small part of the decline in deaths from poisoning can be ascribed to improved treatment especially since the major decline occurred prior to 1930. This decline lends weight to the possibility of further reduction of death and disability through parent education and similar techniques, as well as through medical care and rehabilitative procedures.

Community Patterns of Home Accidents. The variation in types of home accidents in different communities is sufficiently great to warrant study of each local situation. Lye and kerosene poisonings are common in young children in some areas and very rare in others, depending upon the types of cleaning agents and fuel used in the household. The incidence of burns from unprotected heating equipment or accidents due to defective electric wiring may likewise show considerable geographic variation. Knowledge of these facts guides the development of a community home accident prevention program. Physicians called upon to treat accidents in children are in an excellent position to call attention to the local problems and to suggest broader surveys which then serve as a means of arousing interest in a control program.

In studying deaths from home accidents, detailed information must be obtained to supplement data from death certificates. Even so, there are too few deaths from accidents in any community to permit detailed analysis of causative factors. "Only a concerted study of all accidents—

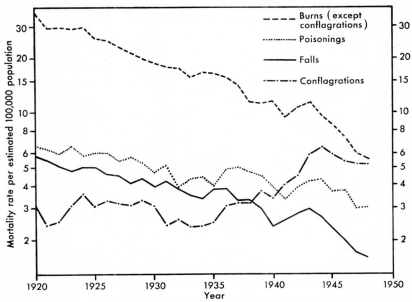

Figure 11. Mortality rates in children one through four years of age from selected accidental causes, United States, 1920–1948. Years following 1948 are not comparable because of change in method of listing. (*Data provided by National Office of Vital Statistics.*)

those resulting in minor injuries as well as those with major sequelae —will permit a real knowledge of cause." (6) Prior to such a study, the injuries to be included in the study must be defined. The National Safety Council has suggested that injuries causing interference with usual activities for at least twenty-four hours be included. This definition is often difficult to apply in the case of young children. An additional criterion, particularly useful in the young, may be medical attention for the injury.

A detailed survey of home accidents over a prolonged period is possible only when a special source of funds and personnel is available. In the usual situation, a less ambitious approach must be used. Information on all injuries requiring hospitalization is a first step. Trained volunteers may be used in spot house-to-house checks of accidents during a selected period prior to the visit. Public health nurses or sanitarians may obtain information on accidents in their routine visits to homes.

Environmental and Personal Factors. The growing child handles objects, moves about and explores his environment, and runs and climbs as he reaches the stage in his development which enables him to do so. The potentialities for getting into dangerous situations increase progressively as he grows older. The number of situations in which the young infant can accidentally harm himself is limited. He can roll off a bed or table if left momentarily untended. He will reach for an open safety pin when his eye-hand coordination has matured sufficiently. During the crawling stage he may tumble down an unprotected stairwell; or he may pick up and swallow lye or other poisonous material on the floor. When somewhat older, he may climb and fall from an unprotected window or porch or get to toxic materials in the medicine chest.

At first, the young child must be the passive recipient of protective measures. Soon he is expected to participate to a limited degree in ensuring his own safety. A child of three or four can be taught to keep his toys off stairways and out of lines of household traffic. As the child grows, he gradually takes on added responsibility for his own safety and the safety of others. This gradual change from passive protection to active participation has been expressed as the reciprocal relationship between protection and education of children in the prevention of accidents (7). Parents and other adults responsible for children are intermediaries in this process. At first they must be encouraged to make all necessary environmental changes for fullest protection of the child; later, while eliminating needless hazards to the child, they must allow the child the opportunity to learn from hazards of a minor nature to protect himself against more serious dangers later in life.

Through his knowledge of child growth and development, the physician can help prevent many accidents. "It is important to *anticipate* with the child's parents some of the accident situations which are likely to arise as the child grows and develops. Handled in this way, it becomes a natural part of the child-rearing program, and will not be likely to produce attitudes of anxiety, fear and overprotection in the parents." (8)

Accident-proneness. Much is being written about the accident-prone person who, by definition, has repeated accidents because of emotional factors of which he may be only dimly or not at all aware. Investigations of groups of adults have shown a concentration of accidents in a relatively small proportion of the persons studied. Further inquiry strongly suggested that many of the accidents in the group of repeaters were the result of otherwise unexpressed feelings of resentment or hostility. A few studies indicate that a somewhat similar situation may exist even among young children. In a relatively safe nursery-school environment, it was found that a small group of children with the most vivid personalities suffered the greatest number of injuries (9). Even the most confirmed skeptic of the role of emotions in producing accidents must accept the fact that a child may inflict "accidental" injuries on others during a display of jealousy or temper. The same course of events may take place when the emotional basis of the action is less evident.

Although not included technically in the definition of accident-proneness, physical abnormalities should be considered when a child has more than one accident not clearly due to environmental factors. Orthopedic difficulties such as knock knees and flat feet, or disturbances in muscular coordination in a child with previously unsuspected cerebral palsy, may be the cause of repeated tumbles. Undiagnosed impairment of hearing or petit mal epilepsy may also be causative factors. The occurrence of one or more accidents may, therefore, be a significant lead toward the discovery of some underlying physical or emotional condition, the correction of which will lead not only to the prevention of further accidents but to improvement in the child's health.

The relative importance of environmental and personal factors in the causation of accidents is difficult to assess. Whatever the role of accident-proneness is ultimately found to be, a public health approach requires that factors amenable to correction in the environment be corrected first, or at least not neglected, while searching for any emotional factors involved. It should be remembered that even repeated accidents to the same child are not necessarily due to purely personal factors. They may simply be the result of continued exposure to uncorrected hazards or to a succession of new hazards.

The Role of Health Agencies. National health organizations and medical groups can contribute to the program of home accident prevention by promoting higher safety standards in home equipment, children's clothing and supplies, and similar matters. They can also stimulate their local affiliates or counterparts to participate in community programs, where the essential work must be done.

While a local program can be developed on the basis of general experience, a survey of the local problems, as outlined previously, helps spotlight the problems that should be attacked first. Based on this information, health education to promote child safety in and about the home may be readily incorporated in the total health program. In a cooperative program with medical organizations, physicians in private practice caring for children can be alerted to accident hazards in the homes of their patients. Physicians can suggest correction of these hazards, especially when they have been called to give medical attention to an injured child. Interested physicians may distribute check lists of accident hazards to their patients to encourage correction of any found to be present. The in-service training of professional personnel working in various clinics should include an awareness of the seriousness of the home accident problem. Possible hazards to the growing child may be pointed out to the mother by the public health nurse in the course of her home visiting. Advice in the prevention of home accidents can also be included in booklets on the care of the infant and preschool child and in general films and radio broadcasts.

A final word may be offered as a caution against undue emphasis upon prevention of home accidents as an isolated activity. Workers concentrating on this field may neglect the many other factors in the home which may hinder their work or actually make their work harmful. The presence of young children in the home, with their constant demand for attention, often results in physical fatigue and emotional strain in the adults of the household. In none of the educational material or in direct work with parents should there be any hint of blaming the parents. Only by first giving parents support in their difficulties will they become receptive to further ideas. If the prevention of home accidents is not presented to the parents in a positive fashion, it may increase nervous tension in a household and precipitate rather than prevent accidents. Fear is a two-edged sword, and extreme care should be exercised in its use as a motivating mechanism in the home accident prevention program.

CITED REFERENCES

1. WHEATLEY, GEORGE M., chairman, Round Table Discussion, Prevention of Accidents in Childhood, *Pediatrics,* Vol. 9, pp. 237–242, February, 1952.
2. See, for example: "Accidents: Childhood's Greatest Health Hazard, Addresses Presented at Joint Meeting of the American Academy of Pediatrics and National Safety Council," reprinted by Metropolitan Life Insurance Company, New York, 1951.
3. BUCKNALL, NATHALIE, Home Accident Prevention: The Home Safety Program of the Los Angeles City Health Department, *Am. J. Pub. Health,* Vol. 41, pp. 959–962, August, 1951.
4. WERNE, JACOB, and IRENE GARROW, Sudden Deaths of Infants Allegedly Due to Mechanical Suffocation, *Am. J. Pub. Health,* Vol. 37, pp. 675–687, June, 1947.
5. GRUENWALD, PETER, and MENDEL JACOBI, Mononuclear Pneumonia in Sudden Death or Rapidly Fatal Illness in Infants, *J. Pediat.,* Vol. 39, pp. 650–662, December, 1951.
6. ROBERTS, HELEN L., JOHN E. GORDON, and AUTINO FIORE, Epidemiological Techniques in Home Accident Prevention, *Pub. Health Rep.,* Vol. 67, pp. 547–551, June, 1952.
7. DIETRICH, HARRY F., Clinical Application of the Theory of Accident Prevention in Childhood, *Am. J. Pub. Health,* Vol. 42, pp. 849–855, July, 1952.
8. "Rx, Are You Using the New 'Safety Vaccine'?" Presented by the Committee on Accident Prevention of the American Academy of Pediatrics, Metropolitan Life Insurance Company, New York, 1952.
9. FULLER, ELIZABETH M., Injury-prone Children, *Am. J. Orthopsychiat.,* Vol. 18, pp. 708–723, October, 1948.

ADDITIONAL REFERENCES

1. "Accident Facts, 1952 ed.," National Safety Council, Chicago, 1952.
2. ARMSTRONG, D. B., and W. GRAHAM COLE, Can Child Accidents Be Prevented in Your Community? *Am. J. Pub Health,* Vol. 39, pp. 585–592, May, 1949.
3. KENT, FREDERICK S., and MADELINE PERSHING, Home Accident Prevention Activities, *Pub. Health Rep.,* Vol. 67, pp. 541–546, June, 1952.
4. "Home Accident Prevention: A Guide for Health Workers," Public Health Service Publication No. 261, Public Health Service, Washington, D.C., 1953.
5. LANGFORD, WILLIAM S., RODMAN GILDER, JR., VIRGINIA N. WILKING, MINNIE M. GENN, and HELEN H. SHERRILL, Pilot Study of Childhood Accidents: Preliminary Report, *Pediatrics,* Vol. 11, pp. 405–415, April, 1953.

Part III

HEALTH SUPERVISION

15 PRINCIPLES OF HEALTH
SUPERVISION

Health supervision is the mechanism through which basic health services are brought to bear upon the presumably normal individual during the maternity cycle and from birth through adolescence. Regular health supervision is the final common pathway through which services for the promotion of positive health and the prevention of ill health most readily reach the individual in the form suited to his needs at the moment. The physician is the central figure in health supervision, providing its various elements simultaneously, and giving one or the other element greater emphasis as indicated by the needs of the individual served.

This highly individual character is the major feature which distinguishes health supervision from other health services of a preventive nature. It is essentially the difference between individual or personal hygiene and community or mass hygiene. The two preventive approaches are complementary, not antagonistic; both are needed to raise the health of the entire community to the highest possible level. For example, milk and food that are sanitary on delivery must be further protected by the consumer; community efforts to promote better mental health through more recreational facilities and reduction in tensions between groups are nullified if unsound parent-child relationships in the home have an overwhelmingly adverse influence on the emotional development of children.

In care of the individual, health supervision merges imperceptibly into remedial services. As pointed out earlier, a clear dividing line cannot be drawn between preventive and therapeutic services. At the very minimum, health supervision must include follow-up so that any suspected deviations from normal health or expected growth and development are adequately diagnosed and so that needed remedial services are available either from the family's own resources or through community effort. This concept of mass and individual hygiene and their relationship to remedial services is expressed in graphic form in Table 7.

Table 7. EXAMPLES OF HEALTH SUPERVISION OF THE INDIVIDUAL IN THE SPECTRUM OF HEALTH SERVICES

Community hygiene (mass measures)	*Health supervision (individual or personal measures)*	⟶	*Remedial services (through family physicians supplemented by community services)*
	Periodic health appraisal		
	Early detection ⟶ of abnormal Follow-up conditions services		More complete diagnosis, with treatment as indicated
Protection of milk and water supplies	Immunizations against communicable diseases		
Social measures to promote favorable emotional climate in community	Promotion of sound interpersonal relationships within family		
Reduction of accident hazards on public thoroughfares	Education of individual parents in child safety		
Use of fluoride in water supply to prevent dental caries	Individual dental health services		

Health supervision of the presumably healthy individual is of comparatively recent origin and is still evolving in content and methods of application. Historically, health supervision evolved from concern for preventable mortality, when pioneers in the fight against infant mortality realized they were on an endless treadmill in their efforts to ferret out and treat sick infants. Similarly, prenatal care sprang from efforts to reduce the excessive number of maternal deaths in all parts of the nation. With increased knowledge of nutritional needs of mothers and children and the availability of immunizing agents against some of the major communicable diseases of childhood, new elements were added and there was a further trend in the direction of universal health supervision before the occurrence of known deviations from good health. More recently, increased understanding of the emotional needs of children and of methods of meeting these needs has resulted in a further broadening of the concept of total health supervision.

Elements of Health Supervision. The components of skilled health supervision are so intermingled in practice that a person observing a visit for well-child care has difficulty in defining them as entities. The promotion of physical and mental health certainly cannot be separated; malnutrition on an emotional basis cannot be overcome unless the possibility of disturbed parent-child relationships is investigated preliminary to remedial measures. If health supervision is accepted as a total process which is more than simply the sum of its component parts, its various elements can be analyzed without diluting the concept of care of the child as a whole.

The various elements of health supervision apply from the time of conception through adolescence. Although the same general principles hold throughout the maternity cycle, and through infancy and childhood, the emphasis upon one or another element changes and methods of applying the principles vary. The peculiar features of health supervision in each period will be explored in succeeding chapters.

1. *Periodic health appraisal and follow-up services.* The nature of an adequate general health appraisal of the child has been discussed at some length, and the special features of medical examinations during the maternity cycle will be presented in the next chapter. Periodic health appraisal is a basic case-finding mechanism. The development of many new programs concerned with specific disease states has resulted in many parallel and duplicating services for the prevention and early discovery of these conditions in children. A universal system of health supervision would automatically take care of the preventive and case-finding aspects of these diversified programs, in so far as health services for individuals are involved.

When deviations from good health or expected growth and development are discovered as a result of health appraisal, follow-up services are required to see to it that indicated diagnostic and remedial measures are taken. The effectiveness of follow-up depends, to a great degree, upon the adequacy of the health appraisal itself. The parent should be present at the time of the medical examination, and the physician should discuss with the parent the findings upon which the recommendations for follow-up are based. A careful medical examination impresses the parent with the soundness of the recommendations being made for follow-up.

When the medical examination is performed by the family physician, he should call upon community health agencies for assistance for follow-up if the child should lapse from care or conditions be found requiring health services which are beyond the family's ability to obtain for any reason. If the examination is performed under the auspices of a community agency, the objective of follow-up should be to get the child under the care of a family physician or, when this is not possible, under the care of agencies acting in lieu of the family physician. Follow-up service does not end with referral to the physician or agency concerned; it seeks to be sure that the child is actually brought for care, that the physician or agency is adequately informed of the reasons for referral, and that all concerned are aware of community facilities pertinent to the health problem underlying the referral.

2. *Promotion of mental health.* Since the mother and child are already under care, full advantage should be taken of the opportunity presented to apply the techniques of anticipatory guidance to prepare parents for the successive stages of the child's development. Through the welter of propaganda about infant and child care emanating from commercial sources, as well as from various health agencies, parents still seek guidance in the emotional aspects of child care from the physician who is seeing her child periodically for other reasons. A small amount of time allowed for the mother to express her feelings, and reassurance freely given by the physician when the anxiety of the parent is found to be out of proportion to the actual emotional problem, will go far in mitigating these problems.

The physician should work closely with any local efforts being made to reach groups of parents and children, to supplement and reinforce his own services to individuals. He may participate in group education himself; or he may encourage persons under his care to join the proper group and provide information or leads to the group leader for the benefit of his patients.

When mild problems, usually based on interpersonal factors within the family, are found in the course of health supervision, the physician should be prepared to offer guidance in their management. For more serious problems, referral should be made to whatever private or community services are available, and the use of these services should be interpreted to the parents.

3. *Meeting nutritional needs.* Since the nutritional status of the mother or child is known in general terms from the health appraisal, and the presence or absence of any conditioning factors determined as well, advice on nutrition given as part of health supervision is more

soundly based on the needs of the individual. Guidance is thus offered to parents regarding nutritional needs when they are most receptive. This carries from the prenatal period, when preparation must be made for breast feeding and when the mother's diet directly influences the health of the offspring, through infancy and childhood and the special needs of the adolescent period.

4. *Protection against communicable diseases.* A schedule of initial and booster injections against diphtheria, whooping cough, tetanus, and smallpox can be fitted easily into routine visits for health supervision, rather than requiring special visits to the family physician or to an immunization clinic. Education of parents in the nature of communicable diseases should also be considered as a routine part of health supervision, with due emphasis upon protection of young children against measles and whooping cough in particular, and upon the importance of hemolytic streptococcal infections throughout childhood. If anything, various immunizing procedures tend to preempt too prominent a place in many health supervision programs. Unless the mother appreciates the other values of health supervisory visits, she may well discontinue these visits altogether as soon as the initial series of immunizations is completed.

5. *Promotion of dental health.* The physician should urge regular dental care for children, starting as soon as possible after three years of age, depending upon the availability of facilities in the community. The physician should not wait until the presence of obvious cavities before referring a child to a dentist although, of course, he must urge immediate dental care when serious dental conditions are discovered. Efforts to limit the frequency and amount of free sugar in the diet, apart from mealtimes, should also be included in health supervision.

There is little point to an examination by a dentist or a dental hygienist simply to disclose the presence of dental caries, preliminary to referral to a dentist for treatment. The practical universality of dental caries makes this a useless step, except possibly during the preschool period when the demonstration of the presence of cavities may convince the parents of the need for early dental care.

6. *Promotion of child safety.* Instruction of parents and children in methods of preventing accidents can also be provided most readily as part of health supervision. This is really only one aspect of anticipatory guidance since the parents should be helped to understand that successive stages of growth and development require appropriate meas-

ures to promote the child's safety, with increasing stress on the child's own experience in encouraging the child to assume more responsibility for his own safety.

Provision of Health Supervision. Ideally, the physician taking care of the child during illness should also have full responsibility for health supervision when the child is presumably well. The advantages of continuing care of the child through illnesses and periods of presumed health are self-evident. Through periodic health appraisal, the physician obtains a picture of the child when well and so has a baseline against which to judge the seriousness of apparent abnormalities when the child is ill. It also furthers better relationships between the physician and the child and parents, since the confidence developed in the physician during periods of good health carries over into the more disturbing situation when illness strikes. Conversely, a physician who has seen the child during an acute illness can better provide aftercare and obtain cooperation of the family in follow-up examinations for the presence of possible complications.

If the premise is accepted that a well-qualified and interested physician should unquestionably provide care for the child during health as well as illness, and if it is further granted that this care should be financed from the family's own resources when this is not too great a burden, it follows that care of the child by the same physician during apparent good health and during frank illness should be promoted as an ultimate goal by all those interested in the improvement of child health. This goal of continuing care by the same physician is still far from being achieved for large segments of the population for a number of reasons. Many parents are still ignorant of the value of regular health supervision for their children and make no attempt to obtain this service. Other parents who take their infants to their physicians regularly during the first ten or twelve months after birth neglect further care during the preschool period. In many areas of the country the services are not available where the children live and adequate transportation is not available to reach distant centers. Lack of financial means presents an obstacle for a varying proportion of parents; parents also tend to stop health supervisory visits for their children at the first sign of economic stress, even though they continue to finance care of acute illnesses. Finally, as the American Academy of Pediatrics study of child health services so clearly showed, there are not enough physicians well trained in child health supervision, especially in rural areas, to provide the necessary services. Even when physicians have had some training in care of the presumably normal child, they often retain primary interest in frank pathological findings; or they may not have the time to devote to health supervision because of the many serious problems of acute illness faced in daily practice.

Maternal health supervision is probably being provided more adequately by the physician who performs the delivery and who manages complications of pregnancy than is the case with continued health services for children. Although this is only an impression, it is probably true that prenatal care, even in a presumably normal pregnancy, is accepted by a greater proportion of physicians as an integral part of their practices than is health supervision for children. There is little question that the techniques of health supervision during pregnancy are closely related to care of the sick patient, but the intensive campaign of education carried out by the medical profession and by health agencies must be given its due share of credit.

Promotion of Health Supervision. Since the goal of having complete health care for every child by a single physician is still far from attainment, active measures are needed to bring this goal closer. Governmental and voluntary agencies, including professional organizations of physicians, dentists, nurses, and other groups providing health and related services, can make significant contributions to the promotion of adequate health supervision. Their efforts may be considered in two complementary parts:

1. The promotion of adequate health supervisory care by the family physician through the family's own resources is the basic activity. This is done by providing opportunities for postgraduate professional education to physicians and related groups, and by demonstration services in the community having both public and professional educational functions. Related to this promotional activity must be the provision of the services of public health personnel to the family physician. "Even when (the physician) is not working in a clinic setting, ways must be found to make more readily available to him the services of the public health nurse, nutritionist, social worker . . . and all necessary consulting services. The fact that families may find it possible to pay for a portion of these services should not deprive them of services available to those considered indigent." (1)

2. Health supervisory services must be provided for those portions of the population to whom these services are not otherwise readily available.

Each of these functions will be expanded in the discussion of health supervision during the age periods to which they are relevant.

Continuity of Services. Although health supervision is valuable even when rendered only for brief periods during the development of the child, its value is increased more than proportionately if a continuity of service is maintained and if records of services rendered at an earlier age are carried over to later stages in the child's development (2). Again this can best be achieved when the child is kept under the care of a physician adequately trained and interested in providing child health supervision from birth through adolescence. The difficulties facing physicians in the provision of continued care throughout childhood are most marked for the groups in the population having the greatest need for such services, especially in children from low-income families. When migrant labor is involved, continuity of services becomes an impossibility.

Every effort should be made, particularly within a given community, to transfer pertinent information from one agency to another in successive phases of the child's development or when the child moves. Health data on preschool records should be made available to health personnel in school health services. While there is general agreement on the desirability of this procedure, the transfer is rarely accomplished in practice, even when the child received health supervision during infancy and the preschool period under the auspices of a public agency.

CITED REFERENCES

1. RICHMOND, JULIUS B., Health Supervision of Infants and Children, *J. Pediat.,* Vol. 40, pp. 634–650, May, 1952.
2. "Child Health Record from Infancy to Adulthood," American Academy of Pediatrics, Evanston, Illinois, 1945.

ADDITIONAL REFERENCE

1. STUART, HAROLD C., Meeting the Health Needs of the Child, *Pub. Health Rep.,* Vol. 67, pp. 1076–1079, November, 1952.

16 THE MATERNITY CYCLE

In some oriental cultures it is customary to calculate a child's age by including the period of gestation. This practice indicates acceptance of the fact that the infant is not a fortuitous new product at birth. The fetus grows at an awe-inspiring rate, and developmental changes during fetal life are of a degree of complexity not remotely approached at any later age. Any changes within the uterine environment, whatever their nature, may exert a profound influence on the sensitive fetus. Health services during the maternity cycle help ensure survival of the fetus and the birth of an infant free of conditions which will interfere with sound development. Maternal health supervision is, therefore, the common denominator in preventive programs relating to fetal and neonatal mortality, and to premature birth, congenital malformations, cerebral palsy, and a number of other conditions, in so far as scientific knowledge makes this possible.

The importance of maternal health services in the later development of the offspring must be stressed as a counterpoise to an older view which treated the infant almost as a by-product of pregnancy. In addition, preservation of the best possible state of health of the mother is a basic need if the newborn infant and growing child are to have the benefit of adequate maternal care in its physical and emotional aspects during the whole span of development. In placing such great emphasis upon the direct and indirect value of maternal health services to the offspring, it is with full realization that such services would be justified in terms of health benefits to the mother alone.

Services Prior to Pregnancy. The entire previous life of expectant parents forms the physical and emotional groundwork for parenthood. Attitudes toward reproduction are determined by earlier emotional experiences. The realization is growing that a healthy attitude toward sex can be promoted if parents answer the child's questions naturally to the extent of his interest and his ability to absorb such information. More formal instruction in the facts of human reproduction, whether given in the schools or under the sponsorship of church or parents' groups, can only supplement information and modify attitudes previously acquired. Some secondary schools help prepare adolescent boys and girls for parenthood through courses in family life or as part of home economics instruction.

Many community agencies are taking an active part in assisting in preparation for marriage, pregnancy, and child rearing. Churches and social-work agencies have shown an increasing willingness to provide premarital guidance as well as guidance in problems arising after marriage. Most states have laws requiring premarital serological tests for syphilis, and many go further in calling for evidence of a medical examination. Measures designed to bring the woman to conception in favorable physical and mental condition, having the support of a husband who has a good understanding of his role in the family, are as important as care during the maternity cycle.

Control of conception also has a bearing on maternal health in certain instances. In only two states, Massachusetts and Connecticut, are there legal prohibitions against giving advice on this subject even when the health of the mother is at stake. In most other states, advice on methods of child spacing or total avoidance of conception is given by physicians in private practice, in hospital gynecological services, or in special clinics conducted by voluntary health agencies. In a few Southern states, state and county health departments conduct clinics in which the simplest forms of contraception are usually recommended. The laws of the various states differ markedly with respect to sterilization. In some states sterilization is carried out for reasons other than health of individual women; extreme mental deficiency or psychosis may be used as justification for compulsory sterilization under the supervision of the state (1).

PRENATAL CARE

Pregnancy has been called a physiological or normal process. While this statement is literally true, and while it is helpful in furthering a more favorable attitude toward childbearing, it must still be realized that in no other so-called normal process is the balance so delicately poised. Under the best of conditions, pregnancy produces a strain on the entire organism; when a woman has been in poor health prior to pregnancy, childbearing may be the trigger mechanism precipitating a serious outcome. The need for adequate and continued care throughout the maternity cycle is self-evident.

Health supervision during pregnancy is usually referred to as prenatal care. It is essential that women be brought under medical care as early as possible in pregnancy to achieve the full benefits of prenatal care. Education of the public in the value of early prenatal care has been one of the major contributions of the maternal health program. Public health nurses have emphasized this point in their home visiting and through other educational activities. A generation ago, a woman rarely sought medical attention much before the expected time of delivery; today, the opposite situation exists at least in those areas of the country in which health services and medical care even approach minimum standards of adequacy. The experience in Philadelphia, in which 85 per cent of women were found to be under care before the beginning of the fifth month of pregnancy, is probably duplicated in many large cities throughout the country (2). This degree of care is not generally found in rural areas and in cities lacking adequate medical facilities. The improvement in care allows little room for complacency, however, since the groups most vulnerable to complications because of previous poor health are the ones who may not have adequate prenatal care available or who ·may fail to take advantage of available facilities. An objective set some years ago that "in the United States *all* maternity patients should have advice and treatment throughout the maternity cycle by or under the immediate supervision of a doctor of medicine recognized as a specialist in obstetrics" (3) still remains a distant goal.

1. *Medical appraisals.* Adequate prenatal care requires periodic medical examinations at monthly intervals during the first six or seven months of pregnancy, with visits every two weeks thereafter, and visits every week during the month before expected term. At the initial visit a medical history is taken, with a detailed review of the course and outcome of any previous pregnancies. The first day of the last menstrual period is recorded and the expected date of delivery calculated from it. Measurement of weight and blood pressure is made as part of a complete physical examination; the pelvic examination should include vis-

ualization of the cervix through a speculum. At each subsequent visit, starting at about four months, an abdominal examination is made to determine the height of the uterine fundus and the character of the fetal heart sounds. At about the eighth month of pregnancy, the abdominal examination is used to obtain information about the position and presentation of the fetus.

Pelvic measurements are made on the initial or second visit to determine the adequacy of the birth canal for delivery of the infant. Internal measurements are used routinely; these should be supplemented by x-ray pelvimetry when manual measurement is not conclusive or when difficulty in a previous pregnancy suggests the possibility of an inadequate pelvis. Although some obstetricians have advised routine x-ray pelvimetry in every first pregnancy, the more widely held opinion is that it should rather supplement clinical measurements in selected cases (4). External pelvic measurements have been discarded in many places as not providing reliable information.

Laboratory examinations should supplement the physical examination. Analysis of the urine is routine starting with the first visit, and examination of the blood, at least for hemoglobin level, should be performed early in pregnancy. A serological test for syphilis is essential and is required by law in most states. The blood groups of the pregnant woman, including her Rh status, should be determined. The husband of an Rh-negative woman should also be tested and, if he is found to be Rh positive, more careful follow-up of his wife instituted. A routine x-ray of the chest for possible tuberculosis is desirable; if an x-ray is not readily obtainable, tuberculin testing, followed by x-ray of positive reactors, may be substituted as second choice to initial x-ray.

The pregnant woman is warned to report any untoward symptoms, such as headaches or edema, which may be early manifestations of a complication of pregnancy (5). On each subsequent visit the weight, blood pressure, and urine are checked. Suspicious symptoms and signs should be investigated and treated promptly.

2. *Emotional aspects of pregnancy.* While great strides have been made in the care of pregnancy as a biological process, comparatively little has been done in promoting mental health during this climactic life experience. A pregnancy has a great emotional impact upon both parents, intensifying feelings and changing relationships previously existing in the household. Even in a wanted pregnancy, there may be

considerable anxiety. An unwanted pregnancy, whether or not acknowledged consciously by the mother, produces a variety of mixed emotions, which may result immediately in poor cooperation on the part of the parent in carrying out recommendations for her prenatal care and, more remotely, in difficulties in future pregnancies (6). An out-of-wedlock pregnancy has emotional implications which need particular attention. Expectant parents should be given an opportunity to express their anxieties stemming from attitudes prior to pregnancy or deriving from superstitions or horror tales of neighbors and friends.

3. *Nutrition services during pregnancy.* Recent years have seen a decided shift from the commonly accepted concept that the fetus, as a parasite of the mother, has its nutritional needs met at the mother's expense. Restriction of diet to prevent excessive weight gain received major emphasis. Diet during pregnancy is now thought of as the total nutritional value of the pregnant woman's food intake to meet the needs of mother and fetus, rather than simply a matter of caloric limitation.

Studies of the outcome of pregnancy in European women suffering dietary deprivation during the Second World War and recent investigations in the United States and Canada have brought the subject of maternal nutrition to the fore (7). Groups of pregnant women initially on good or excellent diets, or receiving diets supplemented to correct any deficiencies, have been compared with groups of women on inadequate dietary intake. In the former group, the incidence of toxemia has been lower and the general well-being of the mothers better than in the other group. The studies also suggest that the condition of the infant at birth is affected by the maternal diet. A lower late fetal and neonatal mortality rate, with a decreased incidence of premature birth, was observed in infants whose mothers received an adequate diet. One of the more recent studies points to the increased incidence of toxemias of pregnancy in women who are overweight at the start of pregnancy, while markedly underweight women have more premature labors and toxemias than women of average weight (8). Although no single study has covered a large enough group of women and infants to be conclusive, the trend of the combined studies is sufficient to justify major efforts in promoting more adequate nutrition during and before pregnancy to further the health of mothers and infants.

In addition to the needs of the fetus, there is often impairment of digestion and absorption of food early in pregnancy, as well as the loss of food from vomiting. If a pregnant woman's diet is found to be inadequate by accepted standards, every effort should be made to persuade her to change her dietary habits in a favorable direction (9). If lack of financial means prevents her from purchasing enough foods of nutritive value, supplementation of her food budget should be sought from public or voluntary welfare sources. Great Britain, in the midst of a war for survival, markedly improved the diets of pregnant women and children by alloting to these groups of the population sufficient quantities of its limited supplies of food of high nutritive value (10).

Supplementation of the diet by vitamins and other nutrients in pure form has been suggested as an additional routine dietary measure. Routine dietary supplementation is opposed by most nutritionists since no permanent change in dietary habits is effected, even if the supplements are known definitely to have the same value as the original food. However, provision of an adequate diet during pregnancy at times may be thought of as a medical emergency. When an adequate diet cannot be provided because of insufficient funds or when there is lack of time or personnel to educate the pregnant woman, supplementation by other than complete food may justifiably be used as a last resort.

If breast feeding is to be successful, adequate preparation must be made for it during the prenatal period. The use of soap and alcohol on the nipple should be avoided since these agents make the nipples more easily traumatizable by sucking (11). Equally important is the investigation of any emotional blocks to breast feeding which may be present; these blocks may resolve themselves if the subject of breast feeding is discussed freely, provided the aversion is not due to deep-seated emotional factors. It has been shown that a high proportion of mothers who had expressed positive feelings toward breast feeding during pregnancy had enough milk shortly after delivery to make supplementation with artificial feedings unnecessary, in contrast to the inadequacy of lactation in mothers with doubtful or negative feelings toward breast feeding (12). If the expectant mother is told that lactation does not become fully established for a period of about a week after delivery, this should also help reduce the difficulties with the first few days of breast feeding.

4. *Prevention of communicable diseases.* The communicable diseases of greatest hazard to the pregnant woman or her offspring are syphilis and tuberculosis. Diagnosis of preexistent syphilis early in the prenatal period and prompt diagnosis of syphilis acquired during preg-

nancy, followed by an adequate course of treatment, will give practically complete protection to the fetus. In most cases of tuberculosis, the pregnancy may be carried through to term, provided the pregnant woman is under close medical supervision; the infant should be separated from the mother immediately after birth. "The bad results of pregnancy associated with tuberculosis are very often due to poor or inadequate medical treatment." (13)

Every effort should be made to protect the pregnant woman against other communicable diseases as well. The role of German measles early in pregnancy in the genesis of congenital malformations in the offspring has been discussed. Influenza was an extreme hazard to pregnant women during the pandemic of 1918 and 1919, but this disease or group of diseases has not been dangerous in its milder form since then.

5. *Dental health.* Dental examinations and treatment should be provided early in pregnancy wherever local facilities permit. The idea that dental decay progresses more rapidly during pregnancy—for every child a tooth—is no longer held; factors operating during pregnancy may actually retard caries (14). Nevertheless, any cavities present should be filled and any local infection eliminated as an aid to better general health. Care of the soft tissues of the mouth is especially important since the gums tend to become spongy and swollen during pregnancy.

6. *Prevention of accidents.* If anything, curtailing of physical activities to avoid interruption of pregnancy has been overemphasized in the past. Pregnant women must still be cautioned against climbing ladders and undue fatigue, but squatting and other activities which limber the muscles should be encouraged.

Provision of Prenatal Care. Continuity of care by a single physician is basic to adequate maternal health supervision. During the prenatal period, the delicate balance of normality makes it essential that any deviation be discovered and treated promptly. Details of the pregnant woman's condition which bear on the conduct of labor and delivery are known intimately to the physician who provided prenatal care. A satisfactory relationship between physician and patient furthermore breeds confidence in the patient. For all these reasons, health agencies have promoted early prenatal care by physicians and have provided follow-up services to ensure the provision of such care throughout the maternity cycle.

To assist the practicing physician in providing adequate care, medical consultant services have been offered by or through many health agencies. One method is through payment of a fee to a qualified consultant selected by the physician from a panel of specialists. This type of service was made available throughout the country under the EMIC program. Another approach is through a full-time or part-time consultant on the staff of the health agency who may round out his consultative functions with administrative or direct clinical responsibilities for a prenatal clinic program.

Prenatal clinics are still necessary in different situations to supplement services rendered by private physicians. Most prenatal clinics in the larger cities function as outpatient obstetrical services of hospitals in which medically indigent patients who will be delivered in the hospital are given prenatal care. This theoretically provides continuity of care throughout pregnancy and delivery. Usually, however, the pregnant woman is seen by different physicians on successive visits, and still another physician attends the delivery. The clinics themselves are often overcrowded and the clinic surroundings unattractive. Under these circumstances, it is impossible to develop a sound physician-patient relationship. Some leading university-hospital clinics are attempting to overcome these deficiencies by providing a pleasant atmosphere and using an appointment system to prevent undue waiting by patients. Above all, by assigning a physician, generally a hospital resident, to carry a given patient through pregnancy and delivery, it becomes possible to develop the positive aspects of care, and to orient the physician in the type of care desirable in his own practice later.

Hospital clinics are not generally financed or supervised by outside health agencies, although there are many instances of clinics conducted by health departments using hospital quarters through special financial arrangements, and a great many more in which the services rendered for individual patients are financed through health or welfare agencies. Even when hospitals retain full administrative and financial control over prenatal clinics in their outpatient departments, health agencies can still make use of the more adequately run clinics for postgraduate professional education.

In years past, state and local health departments and voluntary health agencies often conducted prenatal clinics in areas in which the number of practicing physicians was adequate to meet the community's needs for prenatal care. It was common for physicians to permit or even encourage routine prenatal care for all their patients in these clinics, reserving only the provision of delivery and immediate postpartum care for themselves. Partially as a result of the educational impact of these clinics, care during the entire maternity cycle is now generally provided by the practicing physicians in many of these communities. Even when the fee for the services may be met by a community agency, continuity of services is ensured.

Areas still needing special clinic services are mostly of a rural character, where the ratio of physicians to population is low and where delivery by untrained midwives may also be common. In these areas, the clinics provide prenatal care for women to whom this service would not otherwise be available, even though delivery care may be obtained at a hospital some distance away. Prenatal care may also be provided at the clinics to women who will be delivered by midwives. Such clinics may also serve a useful consultative function when a well-trained obstetrician either conducts the clinic or visits it periodically to review unusual problems with the physician in charge.

Parents' Classes. Group instruction for pregnant women in the form of mothers' classes is an extremely valuable method of education in the hygiene of pregnancy and in fostering sound relationships later between mother and infant (15). Often the husbands are included in the group process, either in separate classes for fathers or in joint sessions with their wives. The parents' classes may be conducted by hospital personnel as an adjunct to a clinic service, thus providing unhurried instruction of a kind that can rarely be given in a clinic setting. More often, they are led by public health nurses employed by health departments or visiting nurse services. When adequate precautions are exercised in maintaining the patient-physician relationship, practicing physicians make full use of these community parents' classes for their patients, either by direct referral or by granting permission upon request of a public health nurse or of the patient herself. When any abnormalities are disclosed during the classes, the woman concerned is urged to see her physician immediately.

The general content of parents' classes is fairly uniform, and is usually covered in 6 to 10 sessions lasting two hours each. A description of the normal maternity cycle is presented, along with a simple picture of growth and development of the fetus. The nutritional needs of the pregnant woman and actual diets fulfilling these needs are presented as early as possible. Other subjects covered are preparation for breast or artificial feeding, care of the newborn infant, and psychological preparation of other children in the family for birth of the new baby. Parents' classes often include a tour of the hospital obstetrical suite in which delivery is to take place.

The parents' class is the method of choice in reaching pregnant women, supplemented by individual visits by public health nurses in the presence of special needs. The inherent values of group discussion are equally as important as the economy of effort achieved in dealing with a group as compared with individual instruction in the physician's office, in the clinic, or on a home visit. The pregnant woman realizes that many of her problems are common to others as well; each member of the group is encouraged to air her anxieties and doubts so that, in the interplay of feelings, each becomes a source of insight and of help to the others. Husbands can participate in at least some of the sessions and contribute to this group feeling. The few expectant fathers who attend either joint sessions with their wives or special sessions of their own constitute a group not ordinarily reached; and they serve as a focus for the dissemination of information to other fathers in the community.

Hospitalization during Pregnancy. Hospital care under qualified medical and nursing supervision should be available for women with various intercurrent conditions and complications of pregnancy. Pregnant women with rheumatic heart disease may require hospitalization to carry them safely through to term (16). Increasing use has been made of expectant treatment in cases of toxemia of pregnancy and placenta previa (17). The patient is kept under close observation in a well-equipped hospital, sometimes for prolonged periods. Even if pregnancy is not carried fully to term, the infant is considerably larger and more mature at birth and therefore has a better chance of survival.

In several maternal health programs about the country, emphasis is placed upon the discovery of pregnant women with conditions requiring this type of care, with the costs of hospitalization financed either directly by the health agency when the family cannot bear the cost or through an arrangement with a welfare agency. Housekeeper services may be provided as an adjunct to hospitalization, when needed. This type of program is not to be embarked upon lightly, since it requires fine obstetrical judgment to select the patients for expectant care and to weigh the relative dangers and potential benefits for each patient. In severe cases of premature separation of the placenta, for example, a defect in blood clotting may develop which may cause intractable hemorrhage (18). Of the utmost importance is careful supervision of such patients if they are discharged from the hospital before delivery. Follow-up services to be sure that this is done may be provided by the health department even if the latter does not meet the costs of hospitalization itself.

Priorities in Nursing Services. Individual public health nursing services obviously cannot be provided for all pregnant women, and some method must be developed in every community to select those women most in need of such services. When practicing physicians appreciate the public health nurse's contributions and call upon her services for their patients as needed, reliance can be placed on the physicians' referrals to determine priorities. Even under these favorable circumstances, however, a very important group of women does not come to attention; these are the women who fail to report for care until they are close to term or in labor. Public health nurses are in the best position to discover women who neglect themselves through ignorance or through a wish to conceal their pregnant state.

The following order is suggested as a guide in setting up priorities in nursing services: Women in their first pregnancy, especially those at extremes of the childbearing period; pregnant women discharged from the hospital prior to term after treatment for a complication of pregnancy; those bearing children out of wedlock, especially adolescent girls; women who have suffered serious complications or unfortunate outcomes of previous pregnancies, such as fetal or neonatal deaths or markedly premature deliveries; and, finally, those who have had a large number of pregnancies and who are approaching the end of the childbearing period. All these women face greater hazards during childbearing than do other pregnant women.

DELIVERY AND POSTPARTUM CARE

Hospital care during delivery and the immediate postpartum period has become the accepted and preferred method of care in the United States only during the past few decades. From 1935, when statistics on place of delivery first became available on a national scale, to 1949, the proportion of hospital to home deliveries rose from 38 to nearly 90 per cent. The highest proportion of hospital births, 98.5 per cent, took place among the white population of the Pacific states. The lowest proportion was found among the nonwhite population of the East South Central states in which only 28 per cent of the births occurred in hospitals (19). However even this represented almost a threefold increase in a decade, since the corresponding figure was 10.6 per cent in 1940.

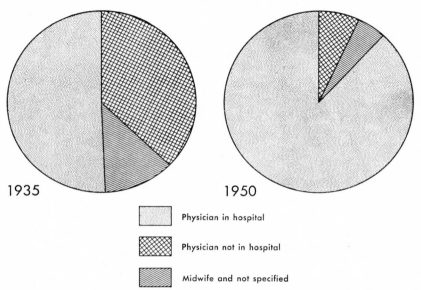

1935   1950

☐ Physician in hospital

▨ Physician not in hospital

▨ Midwife and not specified

Figure 12. Percentage distribution of live births by persons in attendance and place of delivery, United States, 1935–1950. (*Data provided by National Office of Vital Statistics.*)

This trend toward hospital deliveries will probably continue in those sections of the country in which the proportion is not already approaching 100 per cent. The inadequate number of hospital maternity beds, which has been the chief deterrent to hospital delivery in these areas, is being overcome by the nationwide hospital building program aided in part by Federal funds under the Hospital Construction Act.

Arguments occasionally advanced in favor of home delivery are no longer valid. The danger of serious infection in a hospital situation is minimized by aseptic techniques and by effective therapy. The cost of hospitalization has not risen in proportion to the increase in daily rates since the length of the postpartum hospital stay has been markedly reduced. In favor of hospitalization are the immediate availability of blood in case of hemorrhage, the ease of obtaining consultant services when needed, and the intensity and quality of nursing care. The argument that it is possible to provide more easily for the individual needs of the patient in the home situation is rapidly losing force as hospital personnel become more interested in the psychological aspects of maternity care.

Since hospital care during delivery and the early postpartum period has become the accepted practice in the United States, all persons and agencies concerned with maternal health are vitally concerned with the facilities and type of care provided for the purpose. The medical profession has assumed primary responsibility for improving the medical aspects of obstetrical care; indeed no other group could legitimately or effectively do so. The functions of regional hospital planning and of consultation services through physicians employed by health departments have been discussed.

Standards of hospital obstetrical care, especially in hospitals markedly deficient in this regard, have been vastly improved through the advisory and supervisory services of the more highly developed health departments (20). For national use, suggested standards and recommendations have been prepared by the Children's Bureau aided by some of the nation's leading obstetricians (21). These set forth suggested qualifications of medical and nursing personnel, number of nurses needed, and physical and auxiliary facilities, including an isolation unit and provisions for immediate availability of blood for transfusion. It recommends general principles for medical and nursing care of maternity patients and the proper maintenance of hospital records. Minimum and recommended standards established by state and local departments of health, some antedating publication of the Federal recommendations, have followed the same type of pattern.

There is general agreement of the desirability of physical separation of the maternity service from other services in the hospital. The delivery suite should be a distinct unit within the maternity service, with at least one labor room in which women in labor can be kept under constant supervision. An adequately equipped recovery room is being included more frequently in the maternity suite. The newborn nurseries should be conveniently arranged in relation to the rooms for the mothers, to encourage maximum participation of mothers in the care of their own infants. A room or at least some convenient space should be set apart for demonstrations to mothers in infant care. These and other features of newborn care are discussed in some detail in the next chapter.

Hospital Nursing Services. Nursing care given during labor and the early postpartum period is felt intimately by maternity patients and is, therefore, an important factor in the formation of maternal attitudes. Progressive health departments work closely with hospital nursing staffs to help improve these services. Consultant services provided by specially trained public health nurses are well accepted by hospital nursing staffs, especially if the element of compulsion is absent or minimal. Nursing services are also reduced more readily to routine techniques which tend to become fixed over the years, even though they have outlived their usefulness. The consultant nurse can demonstrate that simplified methods of breast and perineal care, for example, not only save nursing time and energy but are to be preferred for reasons of safety. Hospital nursing staffs have also made liberal use of training opportunities in maternity care provided by health departments.

Early Postpartum Care. Care during the early postpartum period has also undergone striking changes since 1940. As part of the general appreciation of the abuses of excessive bed rest, early progressive activity and ambulation following delivery have become general practice. The wave of births during the 1940's, accompanied by a greater proportion of hospital deliveries, was a situation providing fertile soil in which the idea of early ambulation could germinate. The average postpartum hospital stay of ten to twelve days was cut in half. In many places the period of hospitalization was further reduced, as an emergency measure, because of the overcrowding of maternity services.

The suggestion has even been advanced in some quarters that maternity patients in rural areas lacking hospital facilities be admitted to a special obstetrical room in a physician's office suite and discharged home in an ambulance with the infant within a few hours of delivery. There is no question of this method of delivery being more convenient for the physician, but it presents obvious gross disadvantages to the mother and infant, not the least being the trauma from excessive handling before they have had a chance to recover from the birth process. In any case, the earlier discharge of the mother and infant to her home, for whatever reason, necessitates close working relationships between the hospital and community health services.

Home Delivery. Although home deliveries constitute an increasingly small proportion of total deliveries, problems of a medical and social nature are concentrated in this group. In areas in which hospital facilities are available, women choosing delivery at home, often of foreign birth, may not have obtained prenatal care. In other areas the lack of hospital facilities is just one indication of the inadequacy of local health services in general. The contribution to be made by community health agencies is relatively greater in these situations. These services improve the care at delivery and are at the time of great assistance to the physician providing obstetrical care. In the case of home deliveries by midwives, which constitute somewhat less than 40 per cent of the total number of home deliveries, this contribution is even more significant.

The services rendered by public health nurses may be divided into preparation for delivery and assistance at delivery and during the postpartum period. Preparation for delivery must go beyond the usual elements of prenatal care since it must include preparation of the home for the actual delivery and for aftercare. The provision of sterile obstetrical packages is a direct service needed in many such situations. The assembling of such packages is often done by volunteers. Such groups may also prepare and maintain a loan closet of equipment and supplies for use in home deliveries. Nursing assistance to physicians at home deliveries is provided much less frequently than prenatal supervision. It is time-consuming and constitutes a serious drain on public health nursing services that might better be devoted to other activities, especially since nursing services are generally meagre in areas in which home deliveries are common. Postpartum visits are in a different category and are usually provided independently of assistance at delivery.

Midwives and Nurse-Midwives. In many countries with modern health practices, the midwife is an accepted part of the prevailing system of medical care. She provides care during the maternity cycle unless some significant abnormality supervenes. Her training prepares her specifically for this function since emphasis is placed upon early recognition of abnormalities requiring the services of a physician. In the United States, on the other hand, the midwife has been at the periphery of accepted health services. Even in the exceptional instances in which she has been adequately trained for her role, she has been looked upon as a necessary evil when medical care has been lacking.

As women of foreign birth have passed out of the childbearing age, the demand for services of midwives has all but disappeared among groups of recent foreign extraction, even though a number of physically fit midwives might still be available. In the South, particularly among rural Negroes, and in the Southwest, among Spanish-speaking and Indian groups, a different situation prevails. The low ratio of physicians to population among these groups makes it impossible for obstetrical care to be provided by physicians under prevailing conditions. The untrained "granny" midwife of the South and her counterpart among the other groups mentioned is the only resource to whom the pregnant woman can turn.

The usual approach to this problem has been the training of the midwife to any extent possible, with supplementation of the midwife's services through prenatal clinics and other methods. Licensing has played a secondary role in these endeavors since the lack of a substitute made it impractical to prohibit practice by untrained midwives. By appealing to the pride of the midwives, local departments of health have been able to instill elementary ideas of cleanliness and of the desirability of noninterference in the management of labor. Above all, the midwives have been impressed with the need to call for medical help at any evidence of difficulty. When prenatal clinics are conducted, midwives are encouraged to accompany their patients for medical examination early in pregnancy and periodically thereafter. Under such circumstances, midwives become case-finding agents for women with complications of pregnancy. A number of state and local health departments employ consultant nurses who have had advanced training in midwifery; these nurse-midwives supervise the instruction of midwives and assist in other phases of the maternal health program.

One factor in the declining proportion of midwife care has been the aging and retirement of untrained midwives while few young women are entering the field as replacements. Most practicing midwives are well over fifty years of age, and many can care for only a limited number of patients because of physical infirmity. In some of these rural areas, the number of practicing physicians is also declining. To fill the vacuum, voluntary and official health agencies have occasionally resorted to the use of nurse-midwives for direct maternity care, in addition to their supervisory functions. Most of the deliveries managed by nurse-midwives occur in the home, although an attempt has been made in at least one area to have the nurse-midwife continue care of her patient through delivery in a hospital. Obstetrical care by nurse-midwives is intended purely as a stopgap solution, in the absence of medical care for the uncomplicated pregnancy. Nurse-midwives are assuming important functions in nursing education, but these are apart from their participation in community health services.

Natural Childbirth. Active, conscious participation of women in childbirth has been stressed recently as an important factor in the early establishment of desirable relationships between mother and infant (22). "Natural childbirth" was first proposed in Great Britain as a method of reducing fear and pain to a minimum (23). The theory upon which this method is based is that fear, from ignorance or superstition, causes muscular spasm at the uterine outlet, requiring excessive contractions of the remainder of the uterus, and hence severe labor pains, to overcome this. Although the theoretical basis of this method has never been established experimentally, the method itself has been successfully adapted for use in this country (24).

Active participation of the mother at delivery is the culmination of a training program carried through pregnancy. The pregnant woman is helped to rid herself of misconceptions and fear through group instruction. She prepares herself physically for delivery by learning and practicing relaxation exercises, and she is taught what to do to help at each stage of labor. The patient is given support and encouragement throughout delivery, and anesthesia is provided to the woman at her request, although it is used for only brief periods in most cases.

In many respects, natural childbirth is simply good prenatal and delivery care since essential parts of the process are instruction of the pregnant woman, obtaining her cooperation through understanding, and providing psychological support throughout delivery. If the promises of natural childbirth are borne out with wider experience, it should favor the physical condition of the offspring because of the reduction in the amount of sedation, as well as in the establishment of favorable parent-child relationships.

Natural childbirth cannot be used when any significant abnormalities are present, nor are all women otherwise suitable subjects. It is still too controversial for broad use (25). Furthermore, it requires more concentrated medical and nursing care than other methods. Even with these objections, natural childbirth deserves the close attention of workers in the field of maternal and child health. As time goes on, there may be increasing demands upon community health agencies by hospitals and private physicians for assistance with prenatal preparation in instruction and exercises. In meeting such requests, a piecemeal approach should be avoided; there is little use in conducting exercise classes unless proper care can be provided through delivery.

POSTPARTUM EXAMINATION AND TREATMENT

It is generally accepted that a postpartum medical examination should be provided at about six weeks after delivery, and it is conceded as a desirable goal that additional postpartum examinations should be performed between six months and one year following delivery. These should be complete medical examinations including an adequate pelvic examination with direct visualization of the cervix with the aid of a speculum (26). Abnormalities discovered on these examinations should be treated promptly. If the treatment required is beyond the capacity of the physician giving the obstetrical care, every effort should be made for the community to arrange or provide these services. The importance of these examinations and treatment is demonstrated by citing the one fact that cancer of the cervix occurs several times more frequently in women who have borne children and that this form of cancer can be virtually eliminated in this group by proper treatment of postpartum cervical infections or lacerations discovered by visualization of the cervix.

SPECIAL PROBLEMS

Evidence previously presented indicates that serious disturbances during the maternity cycle and abnormalities of the offspring tend to occur more frequently in certain groups of the population, and in a relatively small proportion of women within those groups. More exact definition of the extent of concentration of these problems awaits further study. Enough is known to indicate that women who have suffered one complication, such as toxemia of pregnancy, or who have given birth to stillborn infants or to infants who died shortly after birth, whether or not the birth was premature, are several times more vulnerable to difficulties in subsequent pregnancies. The later disturbances may appear to be of a different nature, but they are really expressions of the same fundamental difficulties. For example, a woman of borderline fertility may finally conceive after several years, only to have the pregnancy terminate spontaneously after a few months gestation; subsequent pregnancies may end in premature deliveries resulting in the birth of infants who die in the early neonatal period.

With the problem of maternal mortality essentially conquered, it is possible to pay more attention to the smaller group of women in whom maternal and fetal complications appear to be concentrated. Current clinical studies hold out hope of more specific measures, some involving hormonal therapy, in preventing a recurrence of serious outcomes of pregnancy in these women and even of preventing initial difficulty (27). While better tools would permit a more effective attack on this problem, this should not be used as an excuse for postponing more vigorous and widespread application of measures already available.

Except under very favorable conditions of medical care, women who have experienced one or another of the serious outcomes of pregnancy tend to be lost from sight until a new pregnancy occurs. With an effective system of interagency referral, such women could be readily called to the attention of the public health agency; even without a referral system, review of the live and stillbirth certificates would quickly bring many of these women to light. Through a cooperative program with the medical organizations and the health agencies of the community, these vulnerable women may be examined either by their own physicians or through public facilities and arrangements made for the correction of obvious physical disturbances when this is possible. Measures to make the dietary intake more adequate, when the nutritional status appears to be a factor, can be readily incorporated in the community program. Conversely, an attempt should be made to correct any obesity present. Public health nurses should work directly with this group of women to help them improve the hygienic conditions of their home and to be sure that they report immediately for the more intensive care they require as soon as they suspect the presence of a new pregnancy.

Infertility. Infertility is at one extreme of the spectrum of maternal health problems. It constitutes a major form of wastage of the reproductive capacity of potential parents, depriving the community of useful citizens and creating serious problems in the interpersonal relationships of married couples. Marriages productive of only one child, in spite of the desire of the parents for more children, also have a bearing on the emotional development of the only child. Infertility is a relative matter. Three years of childless marriage has been generally accepted as a criterion for evaluation of the size of the problem of infertility. It has been pointed out, however, that a period as long as this should not be allowed to elapse before the situation is investigated in individual cases, especially when the wife has passed the age of thirty, since the chances of conceiving and carrying through to term decrease with advancing age (28). About 50 per cent of infertile women become pregnant after adequate medical evaluation and treatment. Similar services must be provided for the husband, since abnormalities in the male are responsible for a high proportion of infertile marriages.

The provision of such services has not been generally accepted as a function of official health agencies; almost all existing infertility clinics are conducted as part of the outpatient departments of general or specialized maternity hospitals or are sponsored by voluntary health agencies in the community. When such services are available in the community, the public health nurse can serve a valuable function by discovering married couples in need of services and interpreting the services to them after clearance with the family physician concerned.

Other Problems. The reduction of fetal mortality is a function of the maternal health program. Fetal mortality may be divided into two main parts, depending upon whether fetal death occurred before or during delivery. At the present time, deaths occurring during birth are in general of a more preventable nature, traceable to such factors as avoidable trauma, poor judgment in the use of operative procedures, and improper anesthesia or analgesia of the mother. Viewed in another way, the most rapid gains are being made in reducing late fetal mortality, but the bulk of fetal deaths after the early weeks of gestation nevertheless still occurs at or near term (29). The greater part of fetal salvage in the future must, therefore, be achieved in the group having the best prognosis for ultimate sound health if their lives can be saved before birth.

Fetal mortality is also closely related to conditions such as congenital malformations, premature birth, and erythroblastosis fetalis. Discussion of the preventive aspects of programs bearing on these conditions will be deferred for the section on special problems of the newborn period. This is not intended to deprecate in any way the vital role of the physician providing obstetrical care in the prevention of death or disease in the offspring. The emphasis is rather the reverse, that the greatest future gains are to be anticipated in the emergence of the maternal health program as the basic preventive service relating to the health of children.

CITED REFERENCES

1. BUTLER, FRED O., Sterilization in the United States, *Am. J. Ment. Deficiency,* Vol. 56, pp. 360–363, October, 1951.
2. KANDLE, ROSCOE P., and HENRY GOETZ, A Method to Determine Levels of Immunization, Medical, and Nursing Services in Prenatal and Infant Care, *Pub. Health Rep.,* Vol. 65, pp. 315–330, Mar. 10, 1950.
3. DAILY, EDWIN F., Maternity Care in the United States—Planning for the Future, *Am. J. Obst & Gynec.,* Vol. 49, pp. 128–143, January, 1945.
4. SAVAGE, JOHN E., Clinical and Roentgen Pelvimetry: A Correlation, *Am. J. Obst. & Gynec.,* Vol. 61, pp. 809–820, April, 1951.
5. For fuller listing, see "Standards of Prenatal Care: An Outline for the Use of Physicians," Children's Bureau Publication No. 153, Washington, D.C., 1940.
6. PARKS, JOHN, Emotional Reactions to Pregnancy, *Am. J. Obst. & Gynec.,* Vol. 62, pp. 339–345, August, 1951.
7. "Maternal Nutrition and Child Health," Bulletin of the National Research Council No. 123, Washington, D.C., November, 1950.
8. TOMPKINS, WINSLOW T., and DOROTHY G. WIEHL, Nutritional Deficiencies as a Causal Factor in Toxemia and Premature Labor, *Am. J. Obst. & Gynec.,* Vol. 62, pp. 898–918, October, 1951.
9. BERRY, KATHERINE, and DOROTHY G. WIEHL, An Experiment in Diet Education during Pregnancy, *Malbank Mem. Fund Quart.,* Vol. 30, pp. 119–151, April, 1952.
10. JAMISON, WILSON, The Place of Nutrition in a Public Health Program, *Am. J. Pub. Health,* Vol. 37, pp. 1371–1375, November, 1947.
11. NEWTON, NILES R., Nipple Pain and Nipple Damage: Problems in the Management of Breast Feeding, *J. Pediat.,* Vol. 41, pp. 411–423, October, 1952.
12. NEWTON, NILES R., and MICHAEL NEWTON, Relationship of Ability to Breast Feed and Maternal Attitudes toward Breast Feeding, *Pediatrics,* Vol. 5, pp. 869–875, May, 1950.
13. COHEN, JACK D., ELIZABETH A. PATTON, and THEODORE L. BADGER, The Tuberculous Mother: A Five- to Twenty-year Follow-up of 149 Women with 401 Full-term Pregnancies, *Am. Rev. Tuberc.,* Vol. 65, pp. 1–23, January, 1952.
14. Pregnancy and Tooth Decay, editorial, *J.A.M.A.,* Vol. 141, p. 1060, Dec. 10, 1949.
15. CHISHOLM, RITA, Parents' Classes: A Fertile Field for Mental Health Concepts, *Pub. Health Nursing,* Vol. 44, pp. 273–275, May, 1952.
16. FITZGERALD, J. E., AUGUSTA WEBSTER, BRUCE P. ZUMMO, and P. C.

WILLIAMS, Evaluation of Adequate Antepartum Care for the Cardiac Patient, *J.A.M.A.*, Vol. 146, pp. 910–914, July 7, 1951.

17. BEILLY, JACOB S., MERVIN W. GREENBERG, JULES B. AARON, and SIDNEY J. PECK, Placenta Previa—An Eleven-year Review, *Am. J. Obst. & Gynec.*, Vol. 63, pp. 414–419, February, 1952.

18. WEINER, A. E., D. E. REID, and C. C. ROBY, Coagulation Defects Associated with Premature Separation of Normally Implanted Placenta, *Am. J. Obst. & Gynec.*, Vol. 60, pp. 379–386, August, 1950.

19. "Births by Person in Attendance: United States, Each Division and State, 1949," Vital Statistics—Special Reports, Vol. 36, No. 5, National Office of Vital Statistics, Washington, D.C., July 2, 1951.

20. GOLD, EDWIN M., JERE B. FAISON, HELEN M. WALLACE, and MARGARET A. LOSTY, Principles for Improving Patient Care in the Hospital Labor and Delivery Suite, *J.A.M.A.*, Vol. 146, pp. 1459–1461, Aug. 18, 1951.

21. "Standards and Recommendations for Hospital Care of Maternity Patients," Publication No. 314, Children's Bureau, Washington, D.C., undated.

22. KARTCHNER, FRED D., A Study of the Emotional Reactions during Labor, *Am. J. Obst. & Gynec.*, Vol. 60, pp. 19–29, July, 1950.

23. READ, GRANTLY DICK, "The Birth of a Child," Vanguard Press, Inc., New York, 1950.

24. (*a*) THOMS, HERBERT, "Training for Childbirth," McGraw-Hill Book Company, Inc., New York, 1950; (*b*) THOMS, HERBERT, and ROBERT H. WYATT, One Thousand Consecutive Deliveries under a Training for Childbirth Program, *Am. J. Obst. & Gynec.*, Vol. 61, pp. 205–209, January, 1951.

25. REID, DUNCAN E., and MANDEL E. COHEN, Evaluation of Present Day Trends in Obstetrics, *J.A.M.A.*, Vol. 142, pp. 615–622, Mar. 4, 1950.

26. MOORE, JOHN H., and FRANK A. HILL, The Postpartum Cervix, *J.A.M.A.*, Vol. 150, pp. 1187–1188, Nov. 22, 1952.

27. DAY, LOIS A., and PHILIP L. SMITH, The Reproductive Career of Women with Ovarian Dysfunction, *Am. J. Obst. & Gynec.*, Vol. 60, pp. 93–100, July, 1950.

28. JONES, G. E. SEEGAR, Some Newer Aspects of the Management of Infertility, *J.A.M.A.*, Vol. 141, pp. 1123–1128, Dec. 17, 1949.

29. SCHLESINGER, EDWARD R., Fetal and Neonatal Mortality: A Public Health Problem, *New York State J. Med.*, Vol. 52, pp. 1758–1763, July 15, 1952.

ADDITIONAL REFERENCES

1. BAIRD, DUGALD, Social and Economic Factors Affecting the Mother and Child, *Am. J. Pub. Health*, Vol. 42, pp. 516–520, May, 1952.

2. "Infant and Maternal Care in New York City: A Study of Hospital Facilities Sponsored by the Committee on Public Health Relations of

the New York Academy of Medicine," Columbia University Press, New York, 1952.

3. ADAIR, FRED L., editor, "Maternal Care and Some Complications: The Principles of Antepartum, Intrapartum, and Postpartum Care and of the Management of Some Serious Complications," University of Chicago Press, Chicago, 1939.

4. "Public Health Nursing in Obstetrics: Part IV, Mothers' and Fathers' Classes," Maternity Center Association, New York, 1948.

5. Selected Papers from the Public Health, Nursing and Hospital Administration Programs of the International and Fourth American Congress on Obstetrics and Gynecology, *Amer. Jour. Pub. Health,* Vol. 41, Part II, pp. 1–126, November, 1951.

6. "World Health Organization Expert Committee on Maternity Care, First Report: A Preliminary Survey," Technical Report Series No. 51, Geneva, Switzerland, June, 1952.

7. SIEGEL, IRVING, The Present Status of the Prenatal Record, *Am. J. Obst. & Gynec.,* Vol. 61, pp. 683–687, March, 1951.

8. BURKE, BERTHA S., and SAMUEL B. KIRKWOOD, Problems and Methods in Nutrition Services for Pregnant Women, *Am. J. Pub. Health,* Vol. 40, pp. 960–965, August, 1950.

9. ANDERSON, GEORGE W., Obstetrical Factors in Cerebral Palsy, *J. Pediat.,* Vol. 40, pp. 340–375, March, 1952.

10. POTTER, EDITH L., and WILLIAM JACK, The Responsibility of the Obstetrician in Perinatal Mortality, *Surg. Clinics No. Amer.,* Vol. 33, pp. 141–152, No. 1, 1953.

11. ENGLE, EARL T., editor, "Pregnancy Wastage," Charles C Thomas, Publisher, Springfield, Ill., 1953.

17 THE NEONATAL PERIOD

The neonatal period is a brief but highly important interval between the hazards of fetal life and the birth process on the one hand and the progressively safer periods of later infancy and childhood on the other. By giving separate consideration to this period, techniques for meeting the special needs of newborn infants can receive the emphasis due them. Although the neonatal period is defined for statistical purposes as the first twenty-eight days after birth, the early days are the critical ones for the welfare of the child. During these vital few days, hospital techniques are of the utmost importance, since the great majority of infants are cared for in groups in hospital nurseries.

Although the relative importance of the newborn period in the total picture of infant mortality had been pointed out before, it was only in the early 1940's, when the nation was immersed in a global war, that significant steps were taken in improving routine care of newborn infants. Since then, the strides made by hospitals, with the encouragement and assistance of community health agencies, have been so great that such procedures as individual nursing care, generally thought of previously as desirable but impractical, have become standard techniques in all well-run institutions.

HEALTH SUPERVISION

With the obvious exception of dental health services, the principles of health supervision are applicable to the newborn period, once the needs of the infant during and immediately after birth are met. Care in the delivery room provides for the major adjustments of the infant to an environment so different from his intrauterine existence. The infant's upper respiratory tract is cleared of mucus and other obstructing material. While respiration is being established, care is exercised to maintain the infant's body temperature. ·

1. *Health appraisal.* The first brief medical examination is made in the delivery room as soon as the adjustment of the infant permits, to be sure that no conditions of imminent jeopardy to the infant are present and to allow transfer of the infant to the newborn nursery with orders for his immediate care. The weight is also recorded, but other physical measurements are usually postponed for the less hurried atmosphere of the newborn nursery.

The first complete evaluation of the infant is performed as soon as possible after the infant reaches the nursery (1). A prompt physical examination, followed by close medical and nursing observation of the infant, is the surest way of discovering conditions, such as congenital malformations of the alimentary tract, for which early surgical intervention may be lifesaving. A careful, prompt examination is also of importance to reassure parents concerned about the condition of their infant, even though they may not have openly expressed their anxiety about the possibility of serious abnormalities. A final complete medical evaluation should be made before discharge of the infant from the hospital.

In the absence of medical attention in home deliveries, the public health nurse inspects the infant to be sure that no obvious abnormalities are present. This can be done readily during a demonstration bath without conveying the impression to the mother that a substitute for a medical examination has been provided. Even when the infant has been delivered in a hospital or has had medical attention at home delivery, an alert public health nurse may suspect abnormalities not evident at the time of the last medical evaluation. So long as the nurse first discusses her suspicions with the family physician, the three-way relationship of family, physician, and nurse will be strengthened and the infant's health will be safeguarded.

2. *Promotion of mental health.* The importance of the early neonatal period lies in its potentialities for building a firm foundation for favorable relationships between mother and infant; the period in the hospital is probably too short to exert influences on the emotional well-being of the infant that cannot be offset later at home. Maximum participation by the mother in the care of her infant, when the mother so desires, develops her confidence and helps prevent the difficulties commonly oc-

curring during the first days at home after discharge from the hospital. Maternal participation is practical today since the mother gets out of bed much earlier than formerly.

One measure hospitals can institute is to have mothers give all the artificial feedings, except the late night feeding, to their infants. Feeding by the mother also eliminates the temptation of nurses to prop bottles in the crib and helps ensure that infants on artificial feedings are held in the same position as for breast feeding. The mother can change the infant's diapers and participate in other ways at the time the infant is brought for feeding. When breast feeding is undertaken, the mother should be helped with the first few nursings. Attention to the rooting reflex, the turning of the infant's head in the direction of a tactile stimulus, will prevent the impasse following attempts by mother or nurse to push the infant's head toward the breast. Although rigid feeding schedules are considered undesirable, most hospitals must keep to some sort of schedule. The rigidity can be ameliorated somewhat by spreading out the feeding periods and taking infants to their mothers for feedings in the order of their apparent need.

Maternal participation reaches its peak in *rooming-in* arrangements during the postpartum period in the hospital. The infant may be kept with the mother at all times, or an adjacent nursery may be provided so that the infant may be wheeled out at night or at other times for the convenience of the mother. Rooming-in makes possible the nursing care of mother and infant as a unit. Whether or not it conserves nursing time has not been demonstrated conclusively; certainly it should not be introduced with this as a goal. Rooming-in requires careful planning of physical facilities and preparation of personnel if it is to be successful.

Rooming-in may be considered a return to universal practices which prevailed before hospital newborn nurseries were first established early in the twentieth century, with the major difference that it is accompanied by preparation of the nursing staff and by a planned program of parent education. The meaning of rooming-in

reaches beyond physical facilities and signifies an attitude in maternal and infant care and a general plan of supportive parental education which are based on the recognition and understanding of the needs of each mother, infant and family. It is a plan to maintain natural mother-infant relationships, to reinforce the potentialities of each mother and infant, and to encourage the family unit. (2)

In most hospitals in which rooming-in arrangements are available, the facilities are sufficient for only a small proportion of patients and the candidates for rooming-in are selected individually. Even when compulsory rooming-in is used, a significant proportion of infants must be separated from their mothers for maternal or infant causes (3). Under such circumstances, the harmful psychological effects of the exceptional separation upon the parents must be balanced against the favorable aspects of rooming-in for the majority.

Rooming-in is of public health interest for several reasons. It provides a method of parent education of a natural and practical character which fits into the over-all objectives of the maternal and child health program. The question of rooming-in frequently arises in consultative services of health departments to hospitals; flexibility is required to fit rooming-in arrangements into standards of care established for maternity and newborn services. Finally, a well-run rooming-in unit provides an outstanding facility for training of public health nurses in unit care of mother and infant, which corresponds closely to the type of service they render in the home.

3. *Prevention of infection.* Fortunately measures designed to foster good mother-child relationships are in no way incompatible with those aimed at the prevention of infection. Individual infant care and reduction in number of infants per nurse or attendant, often developed as barriers to spread of infection, make it possible to provide more adequately for the psychological needs of the infants as well.

The major hazard from communicable disease in the newborn nursery is the spread of infection through contact, with the possible exception of some respiratory illnesses. The frequent implication of air-borne infection in the past was due mainly to inadequate investigation of techniques in the newborn nursery which permitted transmission of infectious material by the hands of nursery personnel, through common equipment or common bathing and dressing facilities, or through artificial feedings or feeding equipment. Nursery procedures which cut the links in the passage of contaminated material from attendant to infant and from infant to infant help prevent infectious diarrhea of the newborn, impetigo neonatorum, thrush, umbilical infections, and other conditions which plague newborn nurseries in which poor techniques have been used.

The daily supply of diapers and linens for each infant may be stored on a rack or in a cabinet under the infant's bassinet. A simple rack attached to the crib holds thermometer, cotton, and other material. Bathing of infants during the newborn period has been eliminated entirely in many hospitals, reducing the danger of contact and releasing nurses for other functions; furthermore, infants not bathed before discharge from the newborn nursery are found to have healthier appearing skin with fewer impetigal infections. The most important single precaution on the part of all nursery personnel is careful washing, not scrubbing, of the hands before giving care to any infant. This cannot be done regularly unless sinks, operated by elbow, knee, or foot controls, are provided in each nursery.

Spread of infection through artificial feedings or fluids is prevented most readily by terminal heating of the bottled feeding, with the nipple and nipple cap on the bottle. Terminal heating may be done effectively with or without the use of pressure, provided the results are checked frequently by bacteriological examination of the product (4). The pressure method is preferable, using an autoclave in which the pressure and temperature can be properly controlled. Although preliminary sterilization of feeding equipment is not needed, careful cleaning with a detergent is still required for the sake of safety and appearance, and to minimize plugging of the nipples.

Limitation of the number of infants in a single nursery and the number cared for by a single nurse and provision of adequate space in the nursery are justified on the basis of reduction of spread of contact infection alone. When sufficient space cannot be provided, cubicles may be built as a barrier between cribs, not so much for the prevention of airborne infection as to prevent physical contact of the attendant with one crib while caring for an infant in an adjacent crib. A major disadvantage of cubicles is the additional housekeeping required to keep them clean.

Careful observation of infants for suspicious signs of infection is the final safeguard against outbreaks when infection finds its way into the newborn nursery, as it must inevitably do at times. A "suspect nursery" provides the means for caring for such infants without irrevocably removing them from the nursery. When an infant is found to have a diarrheal stool or some other suspicious sign, he may be rolled immediately into the suspect nursery in his crib with his own equipment. The same nurse may continue to provide care, using aseptic techniques. If suspicions of infectious illness are not confirmed after medical examination and further observation, the infant is returned to the regular nursery with little loss in nursing time and with no anxiety to the mother. If an infectious condition is found, the infant is transferred to an isolation unit or to the hospital pediatric service.

It is an almost universal legal requirement that a prophylactic against ophthalmia neonatorum be instilled in the eyes of infants soon after birth. The arguments relating to the use of silver nitrate or other prophylactics have been given in the discussion of ophthalmia neonatorum.

4. *Nutrition.* The shortness of the period in the hospital makes the dietary intake during the newborn period less important than the method of feeding. Less emphasis is placed at present on rapid recovery of the initial weight loss after birth since it has been found that supplementary feedings before the full milk flow is reached often result in failure of breast feeding. There is also no need of vitamin supplementation during the short stay in the newborn nursery. Terminal heating of the infant formula does not reduce significantly the level of even the heat-labile nutrients, so that possible loss of nutrients is no argument against terminal heating of the formula (5).

When artificial feedings of good nutritional and sanitary quality are provided, breast feeding no longer presents the clear advantage in promoting survival and health of infants that it possessed in former years (6). Breast-fed infants apparently have fewer respiratory infections in the second half year after birth than do artificially fed infants. Breast feeding is a definite protection against diarrheal diseases of infectious origin among groups living in poor socioeconomic conditions. However, under such circumstances, the nutritional needs of the lactating mother are often poorly met, so that breast feeding may become an added drain on her health.

The major argument in favor of breast feeding is of a psychological nature. When the mother has been physically and emotionally prepared during pregnancy, breast feeding favors the development of sound emotional relationships between mother and infant and of a feeling of security on the part of the infant. Close observation of mothers and infants has convinced many qualified observers of the validity of this statement, even though successful breast feeding cannot be readily separated from closely related factors making for sound emotional health. "One should enthusiastically favor giving the benefit of the doubt to breast feeding and advise earnest efforts toward establishment of it wherever possible." (7) These efforts should be tempered in the presence of certain psychological and physical contraindications. Some women have a deep-seated aversion to breast feeding, often a reflection of the attitudes of their social groups. Too vigorous urging of breast feeding in such instances may injure, rather than favor, a sound relationship between mother and infant.

The incidence of breast feeding varies widely in different parts of the country. The nationwide survey of 1946 showed that only 39 per cent of the infants in the Northeast were partially or wholly breast fed at the time of discharge from the newborn nursery; in the Southeast and Southwest, exclusive of the Pacific states, 82 per cent were still breast fed (8). How long the infants were breast fed at home is not known. There is a widespread impression that the incidence of breast feeding has declined markedly in the past two generations, especially in more economically favored population groups. However, it is in just these groups that interest in breast feeding for psychological reasons appears to be on the rise.

5. *Accident prevention.* During the newborn period and for some time thereafter, common-sense care is all that is needed to keep the infant safe from accidents. Even though the danger of suffocation has been exaggerated, it is desirable to have the infant sleep on a firm mattress without a pillow. Garments that may become entangled or constrict the neck should also be avoided. Bottle propping should be strictly prohibited.

Special hazards in the hospital nursery still cause occasional fatalities. Unless rigid care is exercised, there is always a chance that boric acid or other toxic agent may be used when parenteral fluids are administered. Aniline dyes and other benzol derivatives used in marking diapers and bedclothes of infants are readily absorbed through the skin to produce methemoglobinemia. This danger can be avoided if all marked materials are boiled before being stored for use in the newborn nursery.

Standards for Newborn Nurseries. Interest in improved care of newborn infants in hospital nurseries has resulted in the development of minimum or recommended standards by professional organizations and by official local, state, and Federal health agencies (9). These vary only in details; they cover the facilities and procedures already described in broad terms in this chapter. Regulations issued by state and local health departments as minimum requirements tend to emphasize measures specifically designed to prevent spread of infection. The development and maintenance of standards of newborn nursery care has been discussed in detail in Chapter 6 to illustrate principles relating to standards in general. Recommended standards prepared by other organizations suggest desirable medical procedures and hospital policies. Emphasis is placed, for example, upon having the physicians in the nursery part of the pediatric staff but working closely with the obstetric group; the importance of adequate round-the-clock nursing service is also stressed.

The program for the improvement and maintenance of adequate standards of care in newborn nurseries is similar to that for the maternity service as a whole. In many states, supervision of hospital maternity services included the newborn nursery from the start. In others, the program has been concerned only with the newborn nurseries. The techniques which have been described for consultation services to maternity services are even more readily applicable to newborn nurseries since there are more opportunities to suggest safer and more efficient procedures in the care of newborn infants. The elimination of bathing, having the mother give the infant his feedings, reduction in the frequency of weighing and temperature taking, use of a short-sleeved work gown rather than individual isolation gowns for work with normal newborn infants, and terminal heating of formulas without preliminary sterilization of equipment are examples of techniques by which hospitals can be helped to achieve higher standards of care without a prohibitive increase in nursing service.

Health departments may also be of assistance to hospitals in explaining new hospital policies to the public when an attempt by the hospitals to do so might be misinterpreted by the public. Restriction in the number of visitors and length of visits to the mother during the postpartum period, for example, is explained as a necessity to assure the mother enough rest to enable her to care for her own infant. When such a statement is issued by a health department, it tends to be accepted as an advance in hospital care; when issued by individual hospitals, unless done very skillfully, the public tends to feel that the hospital is simply trying to meet its own convenience.

SPECIAL PROBLEMS

PREMATURE BIRTH

The prematurely born infant suffers from many handicaps which constitute a serious threat to his survival and later well-being. The immature state of his respiratory system interferes with adequate oxygenation. The temperature-regulating mechanism is poorly developed, which, combined with the small amount of subcutaneous fat characteristic of the premature infant, results in rapid loss of body heat. The swallowing reflex is often absent or poorly developed, and the immature state of the digestive processes is one reason for the ease with which disturbances of the gastrointestinal tract develop. An ever-present threat to the premature infant is his susceptibility to infection from any source.

In spite of these handicaps, most premature infants can be saved. "Gestation can be curtailed at 75% of its normal span, and yet more than half the offspring can be made to live. And if 80% of the gestation period is accomplished, at least three out of four prematurely born fetuses can be adjusted to extrauterine existence." (10) Once the infant survives the hazardous neonatal period, his chances for normal physical and mental development are good, and even the small premature infant may be expected, by about five years of age, to attain the stage of development of a full-term infant born at the same time. Barring an unfortunate occurrence, such as an intracranial hemorrhage, during or shortly after birth, the fact of premature birth apparently does not adversely affect mental development (11). Unfortunately, the premature infant is highly susceptible to injury during and after birth, and the incidence of cerebral palsy and mental deficiency is therefore several times as great in premature infants as in full-term infants. A peculiar hazard to small premature infants is serious visual impairment from retrolental fibroplasia.

The severity of these handicaps is generally related to the size of the infant. The use of the birth weight of 2,500 gm., or $5\frac{1}{2}$ lb., or less as the criterion for the upper limit of prematurity, while necessary for statistical evaluation, cannot be used rigidly in the clinical care of premature infants. There is marked variation in the condition and prognosis of premature infants of the same weight (12). Infants born to mothers with complications of pregnancy have a case fatality rate several times higher than those in whom there was no apparent precipitating factor in the premature birth. Among premature infants of the same weight, those with longer gestation periods have a better chance of survival (13).

Causes and Prevention of Premature Birth. Among the conditions associated with premature birth are multiple births, premature separation of the placenta and other causes of maternal hemorrhage, toxemia of pregnancy, syphilis, and systemic conditions and abnormalities of the genital tract of the mother. In a high proportion of premature births, varying from one-third to two-thirds in different series, no specific complicating condition is found in the mother. Even when a complicating condition exists, however, it may have been merely coincidental, since pregnancy often goes to term in the presence of such conditions. Recent studies suggest that the nutritional status of the mother is closely related to the incidence of premature birth. In groups having adequate prenatal care, the incidence of premature birth is found to be much lower than in those lacking such care. The particular factors responsible cannot be isolated, however, since women lacking prenatal care also suffer from social and economic handicaps. It has been shown that the Negro and white mothers in more favored socioeconomic circumstances have fewer premature infants than less favored groups of women of corresponding racial stock (14).

The preventive approach to the problem of prematurity is simply the promotion and maintenance of a sound maternal health program, emphasizing certain of its aspects, such as the nutritional status of the pregnant woman. Measures to prolong gestation in pregnancies threatening to terminate early are the closest to a specific approach to this problem available. Expectant treatment for some complications of pregnancy, even though it may not be able to carry the pregnancy to term, can convert a small premature infant into one in a higher birth weight group with better chances for survival and ultimate health, and at less cost for his care. Admission of the mother to properly equipped and staffed hospitals gives the premature infant the benefit of more adequate care during delivery and immediately after birth.

Care of Premature Infants. Proper management of a premature delivery materially increases the infant's chances for survival and subsequent well-being. The following are among the more important measures recommended: use of conduction anesthesia or elimination of anesthesia entirely; routine use of vitamin K in mother and infant; routine episiotomy to prevent damage to the head against the perineum; and use of low forceps in case of delayed delivery, or possibly on a routine basis.

Care of the premature infant immediately after birth should be carried out by an adequately trained physician, whenever possible, especially when resuscitative procedures are needed. While the premature infant should be placed promptly in a previously heated incubator with an oxygen-rich atmosphere, sufficient time should first be taken to clear the infant's upper respiratory tract (10). The premature infant should be transported to the nursery in the heated incubator with oxygen provided. The importance of these and similar measures has been only recently appreciated so that their application is still rather limited. Interested physicians can do much in promoting broader application of these principles by studying and publicizing the management of premature deliveries and the early care of premature infants in their areas (15).

The premature infant continues to require highly individualized care after he leaves the delivery room. Special incubators are needed to provide proper humidity and to maintain his body temperature at an even level. Oxygen may have to be administered for a week or more. Extreme precautions must be taken against exposure to infection. Feedings must be carefully adjusted to his needs, starting not less than twelve to twenty-four hours after birth. For infants whose swallowing mechanism is poorly developed, feedings are given by gavage or stomach tube. The infant must be kept under close observation at all times since his condition may change suddenly for the worse. As the premature infant becomes more vigorous, the intensity of care diminishes progressively until he receives the care of a full-term infant in preparation for discharge.

To meet these complicated needs, skilled medical and nursing care should be provided in an adequately equipped special nursery (16). Many modern premature nurseries consist of several rooms, including an admission nursery, one or two rooms for intensive care, and a graduate nursery for infants being prepared for discharge. A demonstration nursery is desirable, so that mothers may have a chance to learn how to care for the infant under skilled nursing supervision. Piping oxygen into the nursery eliminates much traffic in the nursery and ultimately reduces the cost of providing oxygen. All premature infants, including those just under 2,500 gm., should ideally be placed in such a nursery, since the fatality rate among even the heavier premature infants is three to six times as high as among full-term infants. However, this can be done in comparatively few hospitals; in most hospitals, careful selection must be made of infants who most require the specialized care in the premature nursery.

Opinion generally favors locating the premature nursery in the maternity unit. The danger of infection is smaller, and there is less tendency to use nurses from the pediatric service to provide relief in the premature nursery. For similar reasons, it is preferable not to have isolation facilities for premature infants within the premature nursery unit. Nursing care of premature infants must be intensive around the clock. One adequately trained graduate nurse should not be required to provide care for more than four small or unstable premature infants. The nurse-infant ratio may be decreased in accordance with the size and condition of premature infants under care. When other than skilled nursing service is contemplated, it should be used in the normal newborn nursery or elsewhere in the hospital rather than in the premature nursery. The backing of the medical staff may be needed to ensure adequate nursing service in the premature nursery.

A hospital having less than a thousand births a year cannot be expected to provide the facilities and personnel for care of small premature infants. In hospitals of this size, there will be an average census of less than four premature infants throughout the year, the minimum that can be served at all efficiently by specially trained nurses on a full-time basis. It has, therefore, become increasingly common practice to transport premature infants born at home or in these smaller hospitals to special premature nurseries in centrally located hospitals having the necessary personnel and equipment. If this is done, infants should be transported as promptly as possible after birth under the care of skilled nursing personnel in special conveyances providing oxygen en route. The best results can be achieved if the infant is transported soon after birth, rather than after a period of waiting to see if the infant will do well in the hospital of birth. Physical separation of the infant at some distance from his parents is a serious objection to this type of care. The reasons for distant hospitalization must be fully explained to the parents, preferably supplemented by written explanation in pamphlet form for the parents to read at their leisure.

Aftercare. Premature infants face increased hazards even after the first month of life, since the fatality rate for premature infants from one month to one year of age is about three times as high as among full-term infants. Most premature infants are discharged home when they reach a weight of 2,500 gm., considerably less than the average weight of the full-term infant at birth, so that poor care after the infant is discharged from the hospital may negate all the expensive and time-consuming effort up to that point. Preparation of the home for reception of the infant can be achieved by exchange of information between the hospital and the public health nursing services; the public health nurse should be informed of the need for a home visit as soon as it becomes clear to the hospital staff that the baby will probably survive. Following the home visit, the nurse reports back to the hospital on the condition of the home which may influence the decision of the hospital staff about the proper time of discharge.

A well-equipped premature center should have facilities for demonstration of care for mothers prior to the infant's discharge. Several centers have established a graduate nursery in which the mother actually helps take care of the baby in the hospital for a period of time before discharge. The mother should be instructed by the public health nurse in the home in care of the infant, carrying out the family physician's recommendations and supplementing any training provided in the premature center. Medical social services should be called upon, at least in a consultant capacity, to help meet the social and emotional problems existing in the home, especially those which relate to the premature birth itself.

Community Programs. Programs for the care of premature infants are developing in many parts of the country (17). Through increased interest on the part of professional organizations of physicians, nurses, and hospital personnel, facilities for the care of premature infants are being expanded and improved at a rapid rate. This trend is encouraged by official health agencies in different ways. Recommended standards of premature infant care drawn up by voluntary and official groups are publicized, and hospitals assisted in meeting these standards through the provision of medical and nursing consultants. Modern incubators may be provided to hospitals as an incentive toward improved premature infant care. Financial aid may be offered for the construction of a modern premature nursery. In areas lacking hospital facilities, portable incubators may be provided for home care of the premature infant and the mother is instructed in his care by public health nurses.

More important than equipment and construction is assistance to hospitals in raising their level of medical and nursing care through graduate professional education. Hospitals are encouraged to take advantage of supplementary training offered at selected hospital centers in the country for which stipend and tuition are usually provided by the states with the aid of Federal funds. The training of hospital nurses through this mechanism has been provided widely since passage of the Social Security Act in 1936. More recently, emphasis has been placed on training of teams of physicians and nurses from hospital centers, since the joint postgraduate experience facilitates changes on return to the hospital. Institutes of one or two days duration may also be offered to hospital personnel on a local basis.

Primary emphasis in some areas has been placed on the development of special centers to which to transport premature infants born in the surrounding area. The premature center may provide supervised experience in nursing care of premature infants for other hospitals in the area. These educational functions are necessary even when a well-established program with a special center is in existence in the area, since the center cannot possibly take care of all premature infants born in the area, nor is it desirable to insist on this type of care for all premature infants.

The program of transportation and hospitalization of small premature infants has a dramatic and emotional quality which may be used to improve the care of all premature and even full-term infants in the area of the center. Judicious publicity of this program is generally well received and used by the local press, radio, and other mediums. The expense of such a program can therefore be justified by its wider ramifications in improving infant care. The method of financing hospitalization of premature infants at special centers varies under different programs. In some instances, the costs of hospital care are financed under the programs for all infants whose parents cannot meet all or part of the costs themselves, whether or not the infant is born in the hospital in which the special center is located. In others, financial assistance is granted to families only when the infant is brought into the special center from outside; with this approach financial assistance is used primarily as a means of promoting care of the infant at the special center.

Mother's Milk Banks. Human milk used to be considered so superior to other forms of feeding for premature infants that physicians went to extreme lengths to obtain it for infants under their care. Mother's milk banks were established in many cities, so that milk from human donors could be processed and stored until needed. However, there appears to be little point to expending the large amount of funds and effort needed for the establishment of a mother's milk bank. The higher content of protein, calcium, and phosphorus and lower percentage of fat in cow's milk, as compared with human milk, have been shown to approximate more closely the nutritional needs of premature infants. Infants fed a half-skimmed cow's milk formula have thrived as well as those on human milk; smaller premature infants actually gained weight more rapidly on the cow's milk formula (18).

What has been said about human versus cow's milk for the feeding of premature infants should not be interpreted as minimizing the psychological value of breast feeding to both mother and infant when the infant becomes vigorous enough to take the breast. Because of the particular need to establish a sound mother-infant relationship after a bad start because of the prematurity, the mother's milk supply should be maintained whenever possible, so that the infant might nurse when ready to do so.

Retrolental Fibroplasia. This ocular condition, peculiar to premature infants, has attracted widespread attention since 1941. Starting with tortuosity of the retinal arteries and veins some time after birth, it progresses through retinal detachment to ultimate internal destruction of the eyeball (19). Progress of the lesion may cease spontaneously, and it may even regress to some degree before the stage of severe retinal detachments. Although many leads about the etiology and treatment of retrolental fibroplasia have been reported, all have ended as false scents. Cooperative control studies involving a number of medical centers, in which such possible etiological factors as high oxygen concentrations are investigated, hold out hope of solution of this problem (20).

The reported incidence of retrolental fibroplasia has varied widely in different medical centers. A study of gross visual defect from retrolental fibroplasia covering a broad geographic area showed an incidence rate of 1.5 per cent in infants weighing less than 2,000 gm. at birth, with a rate of 15.9 per cent in infants under 1,000 gm., 4.3 per cent in those between 1,000 and 1,500 gm., and 0.7 per cent in those between 1,500 and 2,000 gm. (21). In infants in the same weight group, a higher incidence was found among those with a shorter period of gestation. Whether or not retrolental fibroplasia is increasing more rapidly than the improved survivorship of premature infants would lead one to expect is still a moot point.

ERYTHROBLASTOSIS FETALIS

Hemolytic disease of the newborn, or erythroblastosis fetalis, is, in about 95 per cent of all cases, the result of incompatibility of Rh antigens in the red blood cells of the parents, the mother being Rh negative and the father Rh positive (22). Although there are several antigens in the Rh group, most of the clinical cases are due to incompatibility with the Rh_0 antigen (the D antigen of the British or Race system of classification). For an Rh-positive infant to be affected, the Rh-negative mother must first have become sensitized to the antigen and the maternal antibodies must reach the fetal circulation. The danger of this occurring has been greatly exaggerated, especially in numerous articles in popular periodicals. Whereas incompatible matings constitute nearly 15 per cent of the total, erythroblastosis fetalis occurs in only about 0.5 per cent of all pregnancies. Even in the group of incompatible fertile matings, only one in twenty ever results in the birth of an affected offspring. The chance of having erythroblastosis fetalis develop increases with successive pregnancies.

Preventive Measures. Avoidance of sensitization of Rh-negative girls and women should be scrupulously observed. This requires Rh typing of all girls and of all women of childbearing age prior to transfusion, and the use of Rh-negative blood when indicated. The use of intramuscular blood for various purposes has fallen largely in the discard but, when it is used, the same precautions should be observed. Sensitization even many years prior to pregnancy in the absence of such precautions has been responsible for most cases of erythroblastosis fetalis occurring in the first pregnancy. It has also been found that the outcome in the offspring is much more serious when sensitization has been produced through administration of Rh-incompatible blood.

The same precautions should naturally also be observed when transfusions are given for hemorrhage occurring at any time during the maternity cycle. It is probable that many cases of erythroblastosis fetalis in second or subsequent pregnancies are the result of sensitization not directly related to a former pregnancy but rather to an incompatible transfusion at that time. Once sensitization has occurred in the mother, and the father is found to be homozygous for the Rh factor, avoidance of further pregnancies is the only method of preventing additional cases of erythroblastosis fetalis. Claims made about the specific preventive value of so-called Rh hapten have been disproved.

Management during Prenatal Period. When the pregnant woman is found to be Rh negative and her husband Rh positive, her blood should be tested periodically for the presence of different types of Rh antibodies (23). In nonsensitized women, these tests need be performed only two or three times during pregnancy, the last time a few weeks before expected term. In sensitized women, quantitative titrations should be done more frequently. Interruption of pregnancy before term has been advocated in instances in which the maternal antibodies are found to be rising. This procedure may be of value in a small group of carefully selected cases, but it has been found that the danger of premature birth has negated a great part of the value of avoiding the more severe manifestations of erythroblastosis fetalis. In addition, it is difficult to prognosticate the outcome of any pregnancy. A vital part of management during the prenatal period is suitable preparation for care of the infant after birth.

Care of Infants with Erythroblastosis Fetalis. These infants need good general care in the early neonatal period, with special attention to maintenance of body temperature and provision of oxygen, so that they must be handled almost like small premature infants. Specific treatment in all but the mild cases involves the administration of Rh-negative blood to the infant. Replacement transfusion is becoming generally accepted as the method of choice; multiple replacement transfusions in deeply jaundiced infants have been found to reduce sharply the danger of cerebral damage from the condition (24). In the absence of such skilled services locally, affected infants may be transported to a center where this procedure may be carried out, or they may be given repeated small transfusions locally.

Public Health Programs. The community approach to the problem of Rh incompatibility has been confined mainly to public and professional education and to the provision of laboratory services. The role of the Rh factor in the genesis of fetal and neonatal death needs to be sharply deemphasized in the public mind. This can best be done as part of routine health supervision of the pregnant woman confronted with the problem.

Public health laboratories are increasingly providing diagnostic procedures to assist the physician in his management of the problem (25). Simpler procedures like the initial Rh typing may be carried out in local laboratories; this can be done on the sample of blood submitted for a serological test for syphilis. Antibody titrations and other complicated procedures are best left for well-staffed and well-equipped central laboratories. Some states have a question on the birth certificate about the performance of Rh typing and the results of the examination during the prenatal period. Compulsory Rh typing is not indicated until there is assurance of quantitatively and qualitatively adequate facilities for such an extensive program.

CONGENITAL MALFORMATIONS

In addition to breeding strains of animals liable to develop defects, congenital malformations have been produced in the offspring of experimental animals by inducing deficiencies of vitamin A, riboflavin, and other nutrients in the pregnant animal's diet and by exposing the pregnant animal to a variety of traumatizing events or agents such as irradiation, trypan blue, cortisone, anoxia, and nitrogen mustard (26). The type of malformation in the offspring is related to the length of gestation at the time of the insult to the fetus rather than to the nature of the injurious agent. In human beings, some defects are genetically determined, and a small proportion have been shown to follow German measles or exposure to irradiation early in the mother's pregnancy, but the causation of the vast majority of congenital defects in man is still unknown.

Congenital malformations have been found in about 2.3 per cent of a large series of births at the Boston Lying-In Hospital (27). In infants surviving more than 10 days after birth, an incidence of 1.7 per cent was found. Musculoskeletal defects were the leading group in the surviving infants, whereas defects of the central nervous system were the leading group among the fetal deaths, and cardiovascular anomalies in the infants dying before ten days of age.

Until more is known about the causative factors in congenital malformations in man, there is little of a specific nature that can be done to prevent their occurrence. Even if a practical means should be developed to be sure women are immune to German measles before they become pregnant, the total incidence of congenital defects would be reduced only slightly. Genetic principles may be applied in the case of the more serious defects which are clearly of hereditary origin. While comparatively little of a preventive nature is possible at the present time, much can be accomplished in the treatment and habilitation of children with congenital defects. The contributions of a community approach to these problems will be discussed in Chapter 21 in relation to physically handicapping conditions of childhood.

CITED REFERENCES

1. DUNHAM, ETHEL C., "The Appraisal of the Newborn Infant," Children's Bureau Publication No. 242, Washington, D.C., 1947.
2. "Family Centered Maternity and Infant Care, Report of the Committee on Rooming-in of the Josiah Macy, Jr. Foundation Conference on Problems of Infancy and Early Childhood," Josiah Macy, Jr. Foundation, New York, 1950.
3. McBRYDE, ANGUS, Compulsory Rooming-in in the Ward and Private Newborn Service at Duke Hospital, *J.A.M.A.*, Vol. 145, pp. 625–627, Mar. 3, 1951.
4. WALLACE, HELEN M., HAROLD ABRAMSON, MARGARET A. LOSTY, MICHAEL BADE, and LEON BUCHBINDER, Formula Rooms for Newborn Infants in Lying-in Hospitals, *J. Pediat.*, Vol. 39, pp. 337–345, September, 1951.
5. HODSON, A. Z., Terminal Heating of Infant Formula: V. Retention of Nutritive Value of Milk Proteins, *J. Am. Dietet. A.*, Vol. 27, pp. 488–490, June, 1951.
6. NEWTON, NILES R., and MICHAEL NEWTON, Recent Trends in Breast Feeding: A Review, *Am. J. M. Sci.*, Vol. 221, pp. 691–698, June, 1951.
7. ALDRICH, C. ANDERSON, The Advisability of Breast Feeding: A Survey of the Subcommittee on Maternal and Child Feeding, National Research Council, *J.A.M.A.*, Vol. 135, pp. 915–916, Dec. 6, 1947.
8. BAIN, KATHERINE, The Incidence of Breast Feeding in Hospitals in the United States, *Pediatrics*, Vol. 2, pp. 313–320, September, 1948.
9. (*a*) "Standards and Recommendations for Hospital Care of Newborn Infants—Full-term and Premature," Committee on Fetus and Newborn, American Academy of Pediatrics, Evanston, Ill., 1949; (*b*) "Standards and Recommendations for the Hospital Care of Premature Infants," Children's Bureau Publication No. 292, Washington, D.C., 1943; (*c*)

Regulation 35, Chap. II, Sanitary Code, New York State Department of Health, Albany, N.Y., 1951.

10. SMITH, CLEMENT A., The Valley of the Shadow of Birth, *Am. J. Dis. Child.*, Vol. 82, pp. 171–201, August, 1951.

11. For summary of available data, see DUNHAM, ETHEL C., "Premature Infants: A Manual for Physicians," Children's Bureau Publication No. 325, Washington, D.C., 1948.

12. RUSSELL, G. R., and W. A. BETTS, Natal and Neonatal Factors in Premature Infant Mortality: Report of a Ten-year Study, *J. Pediat.*, Vol. 40, pp. 722–732, June, 1952.

13. STEINER, MORRIS, and WILLIAM POMERANCE, Studies on Prematurity: II. Influence of Fetal Maturity on Fatality Rate, *Pediatrics,* Vol. 6, pp. 872–877, December, 1950.

14. BLOCH, HARRY, HERBERT LIPPSETT, BERNARD REDNER, and DANIEL HIRSCHL, Reduction of Mortality in the Premature Nursery: II. Incidence and Causes of Prematurity: Ethnic, Socioeconomic and Obstetric Factors, *J. Pediat.*, Vol. 41, pp. 300–304, September, 1952.

15. WALLACE, HELEN M., HENRY RASCOFF, and HILDA KNOBLOCH, Pilot Study of Maternal and Neonatal Factors in Premature Infant Mortality, *J.A.M.A.*, Vol. 146, pp. 886–891, July 7, 1951.

16. WALLACE, HELEN M., MARGARET A. LOSTY, and LEONA BAUMGARTNER, Factors to Be Considered in Planning a Premature Center, *Am. J. Dis. Child.*, Vol. 83, pp. 54–64, January, 1952.

17. (*a*) Series of articles on the premature infant, *Child*, Vol. 14, pp. 146–163, April, 1950; (*b*) BAUMGARTNER, LEONA, Nation-wide Plan for Reduction of Premature Mortality, *J.A.M.A.*, Vol. 146, pp. 893–896, July 7, 1951.

18. GORDON, HARRY H., SAMUEL Z. LEVINE, and HELEN McNAMARA, Feeding of Premature Infants: A Comparison of Human and Cow's Milk, *Am. J. Dis. Child.*, Vol. 73, pp. 442–452, April, 1947.

19. LAUPUS, WILLIAM E., and FRANKLYN P. BOUSQUET, JR., Retrolental Fibroplasia: The Role of Hemorrhage in Its Pathogenesis, *Am. J. Dis. Child.*, Vol. 81, pp. 617–626, May, 1951.

20. KINSEY, V. EVERETT, Personal communication, February, 1953.

21. SCHLESINGER, EDWARD R., and ISABEL McCAFFREY, The Incidence of Gross Visual Defects from Retrolental Fibroplasia, *Pediatrics*, Vol. 11, pp. 238–245, March, 1953.

22. PIERCE, MILA, chairman, Round Table Discussion, Recent Advances in the Treatment of Blood Dyscrasias in Children, *Pediatrics,* Vol. 7, pp. 865–872, June, 1951.

23. WIENER, ALEXANDER, S., RAFFAELE NAPPI, and EVE B. GORDON, Studies in Rh Sensitization: V. Importance of the Titer of Rh Antibodies in the Sensitized Pregnant Rh-negative Woman for Prognosis, *Am. J. Obst. & Gynec.*, Vol. 63, pp. 6–15, January, 1952.

24. DIAMOND, LOUIS K., chairman, Round Table Discussion, Erythroblastosis Fetalis, *Pediatrics,* Vol. 10, pp. 337–347, September, 1952.
25. ARGALL, CLIFFORD I., A Public Health Rh Program on a State-wide Scale, *Am. J. Pub. Health*, Vol. 39, pp. 356–360, March, 1949.
26. FRASER, F. CLARKE, and T. D. FAINSTAT, Causes of Congenital Defects: A Review, *Am. J. Dis. Child.*, Vol. 82, pp. 593–603, November, 1951.
27. STEVENSON, STUART S., JANE WORCESTER, and ROBERT G. RICE, 677 Congenitally Malformed Infants and Associated Gestational Characteristics: I. General Characteristics, II. Parental Factors, *Pediatrics,* Vol. 6, pp. 37–50, 208–222, July and August, 1950.

ADDITIONAL REFERENCES

1. PARMELEE, A. H., The Newborn Infant: An Interpretive Review, *J. Pediat.*, Vol. 41, pp. 591–612, November, 1952.
2. SEELYE, WALTER B., chairman, Round Table Discussion on The Newborn, *Pediatrics*, Vol. 6, pp. 151–160, July, 1950.
3. BRUNS, PAUL D., and LLOYD V. SHIELDS, The Pathogenesis and Relationship of the Hyaline-like Pulmonary Membrane to Premature Neonatal Mortality, *Am. J. Obst. & Gynec.*, Vol. 61, pp. 953–965, May, 1951.
4. ROLF, BRUCE B., The Obstetrician's Responsibility to the Rh-negative Patient: The Management of the Rh-sensitized Obstetrical Patient, *Am. J. Obst. & Gynec.*, Vol. 61, pp. 139–146, January, 1951.
5. COURVILLE, CYRIL B., Ultimate Residual Lesions of Antenatal and Neonatal Asphyxia: Their Relation to Certain Degenerative Diseases of the Brain Appearing in Early Life, *Am. J. Dis. Child.*, Vol. 84, pp. 64–78, July, 1952.
6. BARNES, GEORGE R., JR., ANTON N. LETHIN, JR., EDITH B. JACKSON, and NILDA SHEA, Management of Breast Feeding, *J.A.M.A.*, Vol. 151, pp. 192–199, Jan. 17, 1953.

18 LATER INFANCY AND THE PRESCHOOL PERIOD

The early years of life, up to the time of entering school, constitute the most important single period after birth in the physical and psychological development of the individual. Growth and development proceed at such a rapid pace during these years that many deviations from good health, unless discovered early, progress more rapidly than at any later age. When discovered during the first few months of life, congenital dislocation of the hip, for example, may be corrected completely without surgical intervention, whereas even extensive surgery a few years later may not result in normal function (1). Emotional difficulties become established during this period and, since they are so often related to parental attitudes, tend to intensify unfavorable family situations unless they are given attention in their early stages.

Periodic medical examination of the presumably healthy infant, with advice on infant feeding, was probably the first general application of preventive medicine through personal hygiene. The past generation has seen widespread acceptance by the public of the importance of regular visits to physicians for "baby's checkups." Young parents expect guidance in matters relating to the infant's behavior, in addition to having the infant immunized and obtaining advice on feeding.

A gap has continued to exist in acceptance of comparable health services for children between the end of infancy and the beginning of the school years, even when such services have been readily available in the community. The country as a whole has progressed further toward the goal of adequate services during illness than it has in providing supervision for presumably healthy children during this period of life. The study of child health services in 1946 revealed that health supervisory visits by children in this age group were made at the rate of 5.5 per thousand children in the nation as a whole. This is only about one-third of the minimum number of visits required according to accepted schedules of visits for well-child care. Furthermore, although many of these visits were made mainly for changes in formula or for immunizations, they were counted as complete visits since the study made no attempt at qualitative evaluation. The difference between the actual amount of service given and the theoretically desirable amount therefore becomes even greater. This discrepancy in health supervisory services increases progressively as one proceeds from the metropolitan centers to the rural areas.

The principles of health supervision presented in Chapter 15 find their clearest expression during later infancy and the preschool years. Much of the illustrative material in the discussions of health appraisals, mental health and child safety, and nutrition services were drawn from the period of later infancy and the preschool years. To avoid needless repetition, the review of the elements of health supervision in this age period will therefore be fairly brief.

During infancy and the preschool years the possibility of providing the various elements of health supervision as integrated aspects of a single service reaches its peak. In no other age period do parents bear such direct responsibility for the child's entire day. At the start of this period, the infant has graduated from the newborn nursery, in which the infant's care is largely planned and administered by the hospital. At the end of the period, the child, who has passed through key stages on the road to emotional independence, enters school where a large part of his waking day is supervised by persons outside of his family. Patterns of regular medical care by the family, and of well-child care in particular, should therefore be promoted most intensively during these early years.

1. *Periodic health appraisal.* Various schedules of routine visits have been proposed, with frequent visits during the first year and lengthening intervals between visits as the child grows older. Starting with monthly visits during the first six to eight months of life, the visits may be planned every three months until two years of age, and every six months thereafter until the child's entrance into school. The medical history on the first visit includes the birth history and details of any illnesses or

symptoms, with attention to the child's behavior and to parental attitudes toward the child. A complete physical examination should be performed on the first visit, but it is not needed on each subsequent visit. The time that would be devoted to frequent physical examinations can be used to better advantage for discussion with the parents. Instead of a complete physical examination on each visit, the child may simply be observed for his general appearance, and examination of specific parts may be made in accordance with questions raised in discussion with the parents.

Physical measurements should be made even though a complete physical examination is not performed. These include routine recording of weight on each visit, with less frequent measurement of length. The circumference of the head is measured at intervals until about one year of age. The inclusion of other measurements is desirable for more complete appraisal, but these should not be done to the detriment of more important elements of the visit. Recording the weight and height as part of the health appraisal should also be used to discourage parents from making their own measurements. Parents tend to be too literal in their acceptance of average heights and weights for each age, so that minor deviations from the reputed norm may give rise to anxiety in the parents. Feeding problems may be aggravated when the parents urge food beyond the child's appetite or needs, in an attempt to get the child to reach the desired weight.

The developmental level of the child should be determined in broad terms as part of the health appraisal. Information on which such a determination is based is obtained in part from the parent's description of the child's behavior, supplemented by the physician's observations during the visit. Only a brief history can be obtained and a few observations made in the routine visit, but even such data on the speech and motor development of the child provide valuable clues to his developmental level.

Simple laboratory examinations should also be included in the health appraisal, whenever possible. For routine purposes only, analysis of the urine and a hemoglobin determination not oftener than every six months during the first year and every year thereafter are all that can reasonably be performed.

Screening tests for visual and auditory acuity are applicable only toward the end of the preschool period. When the child is three or four years of age his visual acuity for distance may be tested with the use of a Snellen chart in which "E" figures are used. The group phonograph audiometer is not reliable in the preschool period, and individual pure tone audiometers must be used for children under six years of age.

2. *Promotion of mental health.* The broadest opportunities exist in this period for contributing to improved mental health through health supervision, provided physicians and other professional personnel concerned are alert to the possibilities. Visits for well-child care should allow ample opportunity for discussion of the mental and emotional development of the child; the mother should be encouraged to ask questions that may be disturbing her in her relationships with the child or in other matters of concern about the child's health. Even routine visits for immunizations or adjustments of feedings provide additional opportunities to go over these matters with the mother. A physician can learn much about the attitude of the mother toward her child and its influence on the child's personality from observations during an ordinary visit. For example, "the mother's typical response, after praise of the baby, is to look at it . . . . The response to the compliment may be as tangible a bit of evidence as the response of a knee jerk to a tap on the patella." (2) A dependency relationship may be indicated when a child of four looks first at his mother for guidance before answering even a simple question. Anticipatory guidance attains its clearest expression during later infancy and the preschool years, and much can be accomplished through the early discovery and management of emotional difficulties during this period.

3. *Nutrition services.* The promotion of improved nutrition should cover not only the nutritional adequacy of the diet but also the emotional aspects of child feeding. If breast feeding has been established, it should be encouraged until the time for gradual weaning to bottle or cup has arrived. If artificial feeding is used, the mother should be instructed in safe and efficient methods of preparing the formula. Terminal heating of the formula in flowing steam has become the standard method of home formula preparation. Vitamin supplements are added to the diet starting during the second week of life and continued throughout the preschool period. Preparations with high concentration of vitamin D are supplanting cod-liver oil; preparations containing vitamin A are preferable to those with vitamin D alone. Natural fruit juices are preferred to synthetic ascorbic acid. Although the difference in cost between natural and synthetic vitamin C no longer exists, it is better

to have the infant develop a taste for natural foods, unless an allergy or some other contraindication exists.

Rigid feeding schedules have been falling into discard, but the self-demand schedule, by which infants are fed whenever they indicate the desire for food, has not been uniformly adopted in its stead. A middle course is recommended in educational materials distributed by most health agencies; a general feeding schedule, not stating specific hours for feedings as in former years, is suggested as a working guide to fit the individual needs of the infant. Even on self-demand, the infant generally works out his own schedule by two months of age, and this flexible schedule can be followed until he is on three regular meals a day.

Appraisal of the young child's nutritional status is carried out as part of the general health appraisal. Screening procedures, using physical measurements and laboratory tests apart from the medical examination, are not so helpful in the preschool period as they are during the school years. Children under six years cannot be assembled readily, so that a screening procedure alone is hardly justified in relation to the effort entailed. Even with the strides made in improving the nutritional status of young children in recent years, significant nutritional deficiencies are still found in this age group (3).

4. *Control of communicable diseases.* The program of immunization against diphtheria, whooping cough, tetanus, and smallpox can best be carried out during regular visits for well-child care. The desirability of completing the first series of injections by six to eight months of age has been enhanced by two factors recently emphasized: the increased incidence of paralytic poliomyelitis in infants over this age when they have been immunized within one month before onset of the disease, and the suggestion that infants are not as disturbed emotionally when the immunization is given before they are eight months of age (2). The mother should also be instructed in advance to bring her child to a physician for passive immunization or "booster" injections in the event of exposure to measles or whooping cough or following injuries which might lead to tetanus.

5. *Dental health services.* The physician is in an ideal position to promote regular dental supervision starting at two to three years of age. The physician should not wait until obvious caries is present. Examination of the teeth by a physician is not an adequate substitute for

examination by a dentist or dental hygienist using a dental explorer and mirror, since small cavities, which can be treated almost without discomfort to the child, can be found with any certainty only by the latter means. Topical sodium fluoride prophylaxis should be performed as soon after the third birthday as possible, to secure maximum benefits from this procedure. Dental correction programs using the principle of incremental care are possible only in selected situations, such as nursery school groups, in the preschool period.

6. *Promotion of child safety.* Serious illness and death from poisoning, falls about the home, and burns and scalds in the kitchen are most common during the preschool period. Characteristic of these accidents is the ease with which they could have been prevented, if elementary precautions had been taken in the home. It seems likely that promotion of child safety will become a prominent aspect of health supervision during the early years of life, along with the promotion of mental health. Indeed, the techniques of anticipatory guidance, described in Chapter 14, are equally applicable to these two types of services.

THE CHILD HEALTH CONFERENCE

The desired coverage for child health supervision is set forth in the following statement of the Committee for the Study of Child Health Services:

All children are entitled to preventive health services irrespective of the economic status of their parents. Opinion may vary about the extent which official health agencies should provide these services to certain economic groups. But there can be no difference of opinion about the right of every child to receive such service from either private practitioners or public health agencies. (4)

As pointed out earlier in this chapter, this need is being met only fractionally on a national scale. The same study showed further that preventive health services provided by health agencies, both public and private, were not adequately supplementing care by private physicians, since they provided less than 10 per cent of such services throughout the nation.

With such a wide discrepancy between services and needs, the community child health program must give high priority to the promotion of child health supervision, even before the promotion of many services relating to specific disease problems. Since many parents are not sufficiently aware of the value of these health services for their children, the community program must include the following closely related activities for the attainment of the goal of more adequate health supervision:

1. Bringing together all community services for educating parents in the prevention or solution of health problems in their children

2. Getting as many infants and preschool children as possible under the regular care of family physicians, in so far as physicians are willing and able to bear the load effectively

3. Providing similar services, under the auspices of governmental or voluntary health agencies, for children who are not or who cannot be brought under regular health supervision of family physicians; and

4. To supplement care by the private physician, with the physician's approval, with special services of public health personnel

The child health conference is the hub of these organized community health activities. Variously known as the well-baby or well-child conference or clinic, as the child health station, or even as the baby-keep-well station, the child health conference has become the accepted technique for providing health supervision to infants and preschool children not under the regular care of family physicians.

Promotion of Well-child Care. The primary function of the child health conference and its related activities at the present time is education of the community in the nature and value of well-child care. Lack of public demand for such care is probably the chief reason for the present inadequacy of these services in many areas. A child health conference is a tangible facility, one which the public can readily see and understand. By using the child health conference as a demonstration of the benefits of health supervision, it is easier to persuade parents to call upon their family physicians for this service. Needless to say, the service given must be of such quality as to serve as a real example for care.

Similarly, women's organizations, service groups, and other voluntary groups may be stimulated to support a child health conference, wholly or in part by financial aid or volunteer assistance. This may be done even when the conference is conducted by the health department, since the official health budget rarely includes items for toys and play equipment or for sufficient personnel as receptionists, clerks, and transportation aides. Through their personal or financial participation in a tangible service, they can be persuaded of the value of this care through private resources as well. Since these groups are generally influential in the community, their leadership is greatly to be desired in the promotion of regular health supervision. Furthermore, arousing their interest in well-child care tends to give more balance to the activities of these groups which are often concentrated on the support of services for children with specific types of handicapping conditions.

Professional Education. Physicians and other professional personnel benefit in several ways from a well-run child health conference program in the community. The most general benefit is the stimulation it provides to physicians to provide this type of service in their own practices. The stimulation may be direct if the physician participates in the work of the conference itself. This aspect appears to be increasing, since the tendency is to encourage more participation by local general practitioners rather than to bring in pediatricians from outside the community. Since many general practitioners have had little or no special undergraduate medical training in well-child care, as the nationwide study of 1946 demonstrated, some child health programs require preliminary participation of physicians in special child health conferences under the supervision of a well-trained pediatrician before they conduct conferences in their own areas. In a large community or at some selected point in a rural area, therefore, a special child health conference may be conducted as a training center in the techniques of child health supervision.

Other programs employ the services of pediatric consultants who visit child health conferences periodically to work with the general practitioners in charge. Another technique is the employment of physicians who have recently entered practice in the community. These younger physicians have the time to devote to public service and the experience gained under supervision in the child health conference carries over into their own practices, so that more service of a higher quality soon becomes available to the children of the area.

The opportunities for professional training and experience should be extended to others besides the practicing physician. Through arrangements with hospitals having approved internships and residencies, house officers can obtain experience in care of the presumably healthy child which may not be available in their own hospitals. Full use is not being made of the potentialities of this training facility. A survey in 1950 revealed that child health conferences conducted by only 28 out of 217 health departments replying to the questionnaire were being used for the training of house officers (5).

The experience in child health conferences is more valuable if the house officer conducts regularly scheduled conferences at intervals of two weeks to a month rather than having the experience concentrated in daily participation over a short period. An effective technique has been the assignment of several young infants to a house officer at the first session for him to follow for as long as his attendance at the child health conference permits. Longitudinal care of a small group of children resembles the type of care he will render later in his own practice.

Psychiatrists, particularly those training for a career in child psychiatry, may use the child health conference to gain experience in supervising emotional development in a normal setting and to see emotional problems in their incipiency. Nurses, nutritionists, and medical social workers should have similar opportunities. This is an essential part of the public health nurse's training since she will later bear the immediate responsibility for the management of child health conferences. The nutritionist finds an opportunity for practical experience in nutrition education in a setting in which the emotional aspects of infant and child feeding receive proper consideration.

Public Health Education. Education of parents in the community through the child health conference is greater than the actual number of children seen would lead one to expect. Education relating to the immediate health problems of their own children tends to be diffused to neighbors and other persons in the community. Methods of group instruction have been tried in different settings in connection with child health conferences. Some of these group sessions have been conducted by physicians, others by public health nurses, psychologists, or social workers. In some instances, they have been open to parents referred by their family physicians. Nevertheless, group instruction of parents of infants and preschool children is still experimental and has not approached the degree of standardization achieved in classes for expectant parents. The difficulties are greater because it is not possible to obtain the same community of interest as during the prenatal period.

Unless the person conducting the group sessions has had specific training and experience, the discussions should be kept generally within the sphere of anticipatory guidance. This is not a simple thing to do, even if parents of children of the same age are segregated in different sessions, since problems in child behavior and family relationships are bound to arise, and answers will be sought at the group discussions. The parents themselves may assume responsibility for organization and presentation of subject material in child study groups. These do not tend to go as deeply into problems of child rearing, but they should nevertheless have some degree of supervision and consultation from trained personnel.

Direct Services. While there is general agreement on the functions of health education and professional training served by a limited number of child health conferences in any community, the use of child health conferences for service to large segments of the population is being widely questioned in medical circles. There can be no question of the theoretical desirability of having the health promotional services of child health conferences incorporated in total medical care along with services for sick children. However, until the gap in health supervisory services for young children is at least partially closed, the child health conference remains the most convenient and inexpensive technique for providing the services to children who would otherwise have to do without them.

Even in communities with extensive child health conference programs, experience has shown that child health conferences have enhanced rather than reduced the opportunities of the physician in private practice. Many infants and children, who might otherwise have escaped attention, are referred for more definitive diagnosis and possible treatment. In addition, abnormalities coming to his attention at an earlier stage often permit the private physician to render effective treatment with the resources at his command, so that he is not faced with the need to refer the child elsewhere for specialized services.

Administration of Child Health Conferences. In practice, a great many child health conferences do not measure up to their theoretical advantages as presented. Physical facilities in the conferences are often inadequate, and emphasis is placed on the quantity rather than the quality of care rendered. Above all, the potentialities of the child health conference as a center for professional and parent education are infrequently realized.

The training and interest of the physician and other professional personnel are the most important single factor making for success or failure of the child health conference. Whenever possible, physicians with special training in well-child care should be chosen to man the conference, or an effort should be made to provide a minimum of such training through one or another of the techniques previously described. It is preferable not to have any one physician conduct too frequent conferences; it is difficult to maintain the needed degree of interest on an intensive basis, especially when the number of children seen in each conference is too large for adequate individual attention. In some smaller communities or rural areas, several local physicians may participate in a program in which only one session is held each month; when such is the case, it is advisable to have each physician conduct the conference for not less than six months at a time, to preserve a certain degree of continuity of care for the infants under supervision. In the large child health conferences held in densely populated areas, in which two or more physicians are present at each session, every effort should be made to have a given child followed by the same physician on successive visits.

Physical facilities for the child health conferences should be planned to make the best of what is available. The conferences are ideally held in a health center or a hospital in which the physical setup has been planned with the needs of the conference in mind. The efficient flow of movement can thus be assured from the reception room through the undressing room, the physician's examination and consultation room, the nurse's office, and back to a dressing room.

In rural areas, where the need for child health supervision is greatest, it is usually necessary to improvise less satisfactory arrangements in order to be reasonably close to the families served. The location of the less frequently held conference may be in a schoolhouse, a village hall, a church, or even a vacant store. Whatever the location, a separate room or at least an isolated screened-in corner is needed by the physician. Space must also be allowed for the receptionist, usually a volunteer who also supervises the children when the parents are otherwise occupied. Individual facilities, even though of a simple nature, should also be provided for undressing and dressing children, and a covered space should be available for the protection of baby carriages.

The number of children seen at any one conference should be limited, to allow a minimum of fifteen minutes for every newly admitted child and five to ten minutes for other children, depending upon the reason for return. An appointment system is desirable if overcrowding is to be avoided, and the staggering of appointments permits more efficient service. This may not be possible in rural areas when several women and children may be transported to the conference at one time by a volunteer. In some areas, also, in spite of all efforts to install an appointment system, the mothers insist on congregating at the start of the session and treat the conference as a social gathering. The waiting time of mothers has occasionally been used to advantage for group discussions of problems of interest at the time or for demonstration of methods of food preparation.

The public health nurse is generally responsible for immediate management of the child health conference, but the efficient nurse can delegate her routine duties to trained volunteers. This will permit the public health nurse to concentrate on her educational functions and to interpret and enlarge upon the recommendations of the physician. The nurse may also administer the immunizations. If this is done, it should be only with the clearly stated policy that she is acting as the agent and under the supervision of the physician.

Suspected deviations from good health discovered at the child health conference must be brought to the attention of the family physician or to the community agency concerned with providing medical service for the child. Adequate follow-up services must therefore be provided. Persons providing follow-up must not be content with a simple referral to the family physician; they must be sure that the physician is aware of community facilities which may help him provide specialized services beyond his own resources.

Auxiliary Services. Dental health services may be provided for children attending child health conferences. Those actually provided in the child health conference itself have been mainly of a prophylactic nature. Examination of the teeth starting between two and three years of age and cleaning of the teeth have been services given by dental hygienists for some time. More recently, topical application of fluoride solution has been introduced; while this procedure may be started on a routine visit of the child to the child health conference, additional visits will be needed to complete the series of applications. These additional visits may be scheduled apart from the child health conferences to avoid overcrowding and confusion.

Unless a sufficient number of children over two years of age are scheduled for the session which a dentist or dental hygienist attends, their services will not be used efficiently. It is usually preferable to provide dental prophylactic and treatment services in special clinics to which preschool children seen in child health conferences may be referred. Separate sessions also encourage broader use of the dental services, since children receiving well-child care from family physicians may also be referred for dental care when other dental services are inadequate in the community.

It it not advisable to have other professional personnel such as nutritionists provide direct services to parents and children in child health conferences, except for their own training. It is more satisfactory for the nutritionist to act in a consultant capacity to the public health nurse and to have advice on nutrition given by the physician and nurse. Apart from the possibility of conflicting advice by too many professional persons, the amount of information that can be absorbed and used efficiently by a mother is limited. The same reasoning applies to the use of psychologists in the conference, unless for purposes of research or training.

THE PRESCHOOL ROUNDUP

The preschool or summer roundup is a program promoted mainly by parent-teacher organizations in various parts of the country. It has as its objective a health appraisal for every child during the summer before he enters school, so that any remediable defects discovered may be corrected before school opening. Volunteers visit the homes of four- and five-year-old children in the community to urge the parents to have their children given a medical examination in preparation for school. If the parents cannot secure this examination from a family physician for any reason, they are invited to bring their children to a special clinic for the purpose. At this clinic, screening testing for visual and auditory acuity may be performed and immunizations administered.

The preschool roundup is a transitional service between preschool and school health services, and it may be approached from either direction. Public health nurses or specialized school nurses are usually brought into the activity to ensure proper follow-up services. The records of the roundup must be incorporated in the school health records if they are to have any lasting value. The preschool roundup serves a particularly useful function in areas lacking health supervisory services for infants and preschool children; the roundup and its related educational activities may serve as the first step in the development of health services for younger children.

SUPERVISION OF GROUP CARE

Although preschool children usually must be brought under supervision individually, they may be found in certain group situations outside institutions. The value of group activity under skilled supervision in nursery schools in furthering the social and emotional development of the young child is becoming more widely appreciated, so that the number of nursery schools under both private and public auspices is increasing. Supervised care of young children is also provided in day-care centers, mainly for children of working mothers. The demand for day care varies with the pressure of the economy for additions to the usual labor force. This reached its peak at the height of the Second World War, when liberal assistance was available to communities from Federal funds for the establishment and maintenance of day-care centers. The distinction between nursery schools and day-care centers is often not clear in practice. Many nursery schools, especially those located in public housing projects and in settlement houses, give preference to children of working mothers. The better day-care centers, on the other hand, incorporate accepted nursery school techniques in their programs (6).

Group care of children provides an opportunity for more adequate health supervision but at the same time requires additional safeguards against the hazards of close contact. All the services implicit in child health supervision may be planned for each child by the day-care center or nursery school, to be provided by the family physician, by a member of the staff of the center or school, or by a child health conference. Nursing and nutritionist services may be provided by persons employed as members of the staff of the school or center or be obtained either as a direct service or on a consultant basis from the local health agency. Daily observation for the presence of communicable disease is especially important in groups of highly susceptible preschool children; this function can be delegated to a specially prepared member of the child care staff if the services of a nurse cannot be obtained readily. Under careful health supervision, children attending nursery school have been found to have no more colds than other children (7).

Supervision of group care of young children, with or without formal licensure, is needed to safeguard the children against the special hazards to health inherent in the group situation. Minimum standards for the physical facilities, including protection against fire and accidents, must be established and enforced and adequate medical and nursing services assured. Diet practices, covering the nutritional value of the food and the sanitation of food services, must be supervised. Although total responsibility for such supervision and licensure is carried by the health agencies in a few places, the usual practice is to have the welfare and education authorities assume primary responsibility for supervision of the day-care centers and nursery schools, respectively, with health departments assisting with the aspects related more directly to health of the children.

ADOPTION PROCEDURES

Children who cannot be raised by their natural parents for any reason and who are legally free for adoption should be given the benefit of a properly supervised placement as soon as possible. Even children with a disability may be successfully placed with adoptive parents who understand the situation and who are willing to accept the responsibility involved. Children to be adopted "should have the protection of good laws that are effectively administered because they have the support of all who are interested in children, including professional groups such as the American Academy of Pediatrics." (8) The heavy demand for children to be adopted has led to many abuses harmful to both the adopted children and the adoptive parents, in spite of vigorous countermeasures (9).

State departments of social welfare usually supervise local agencies approved for arranging adoptions. These social agencies seek only the best interests of the children and adoptive parents and conduct careful investigations with this end in view. Physicians should encourage out-of-wedlock parents and couples wishing to adopt children to use only approved social agencies, rather than have them deal with individuals, no matter how well intentioned the latter may appear to be. The services of health agencies, through child health conferences or other means, are often used to obtain a health appraisal of the children prior to placement for adoption.

CITED REFERENCES

1. BOST, FREDERIC C., HELEN HAGEY, EDWIN R. SCHOTTSTAEDT, and LOREN J. LARSEN, The Results of Treatment of Congenital Dislocation

of the Hip in Infancy, *Am. J. Bone & Joint Surgery,* Vol. 30-A, pp. 454–468, April, 1948.

2. LEVY, DAVID M., Observations of Attitudes and Behavior in the Child Health Center, Sample Studies of Maternal Feelings, Dependency, Resistant Behavior, and Inoculation Fears, *Am. J. Pub. Health,* Vol. 41, pp. 182–190, February, 1951.

3. PRICE, JULIAN P., and WALTER M. HART, Malnutrition and Anemia in Young Children: Clinical Study of Fifty Cases, *J.A.M.A.,* Vol. 148, pp. 5–10, Jan. 5, 1952.

4. "Child Health Services and Pediatric Education, Report of the Committee for the Study of Child Health Services, American Academy of Pediatrics," Commonwealth Fund, Harvard University Press, Cambridge, Mass., 1949.

5. HARPER, PAUL, and SAMUEL M. WISHIK, The Use of Child Health Conferences for Training of House Officers and Medical Students, *Am. J. Pub. Health,* Vol. 41, pp. 312–318, March, 1951.

6. KEISTER, MARY E., Day-care Centers and Nursery Schools Have the Same Goals, *Child,* Vol. 15, pp. 159–162, May, 1951.

7. DIEHL, ISABELLE, The Prevalence of Colds in Nursery School Children and Non-nursery School Children, *J. Pediat.,* Vol. 34, pp. 52–61, January, 1949.

8. WEGMAN, MYRON E., Protecting the Child About to Be Adopted, *Pediatrics,* Vol. 5, pp. 903–906, May, 1950.

9. HUBBARD, JOHN P., Black Market in Babies, *Pediatrics,* Vol. 10, pp. 355–358, September, 1952.

ADDITIONAL REFERENCES

1. "The Child-Health Conference: Suggestions for Organization and Procedure," Children's Bureau Publication No. 261, Washington, D.C., 1941.

2. BLACK, IRMA S., Everyday Problems of the Preschool Child, *J. Pediat.,* Vol. 41, pp. 233–243, August, 1952.

3. WISHIK, SAMUEL M., Current Practices and Trends in the Child Health Conference, *Am. J. Pub. Health,* Vol. 41, pp. 57–65, January, 1951.

4. JEANS, PHILIP C., Nutrition in the Health Conference of the Preschool Child, *Pub. Health Rep.,* Vol. 66, pp. 834–836, June 29, 1951.

5. BAKWIN, RUTH M., and HARRY BAKWIN, Adoption, *J. Pediat.,* Vol. 40, pp. 130–134, January, 1952.

19 SCHOOL AGE AND ADOLESCENCE

Children of school age constitute about 20 per cent of the total population. The possibility of promoting the health of such a large group at an impressionable period of life is an opportunity that should not be lost, especially since health guidance and early detection of abnormalities can be provided fairly readily to the children attending school.

Although health services for school children had their beginnings before the turn of the century, there is general agreement that major deficiencies continue to exist in these services. One-half the counties in the United States, in which 22 per cent of all children of school age resided, had no organized system of medical examinations in relation to the schools in 1946 (1). The percentage of children lacking even a bare minimum of school health services is actually much greater than this since a county was considered to have school health services even if only one out of many schools in the county provided health examinations. Fully one-third of the counties had neither medical nor nursing services in any of the schools. The continued heated discussion of health services for the child of school age bears witness to the inadequacy of a large percentage of existing programs.

The school child is a member of the school group as well as the family. While the basic responsibility for his care must remain with his family, the educational authorities have immediate responsibilities for the child during the greater part of his waking day that he spends in school. In addition to doing what they can to promote good health in children under their charge as an end in itself, educational authorities are interested in good health as an essential factor which enables children to take advantage of their educational opportunities. Good health services also provide an educational experience, leading to desirable health habits in adult life, by serving as an example of the teaching set forth in courses in health education.

The physician and others in the health professions, while tending by tradition to make good health an end in itself, realize that, in the final analysis, good physical and emotional health is sterile to the degree that the individual lacks the social usefulness promoted by the educational process. Health services promoted or given in the schools may also help the practicing physician and the community health services outside the schools to provide better total care for children. There is more than enough common ground on which to establish an effective program of health services for the child of school age. Much of the difficulty that has existed in bringing together professional persons with differing backgrounds is the lack of a common language. Experience has shown that working together in a joint program, no matter how limited it may be at the start, produces mutual understanding and cooperation, even though previous prolonged discussions and attempts at planning have failed to bring this about.

Although mortality rates during the school years are lower than during any other period of life, the problems of rheumatic fever and its sequelae and of dental caries assume major importance at this time. Furthermore physical defects such as impaired vision and hearing can be readily discovered through available screening tests; these disabilities may not be severe enough to come to attention otherwise, but may nevertheless interfere with the child's emotional and social development and impede his educational progress.

Health services rendered in relation to the schools play their part within the broad community program. Health services as such during this age period include all the elements of adequate health supervision. In addition, efforts should be made to ensure a healthful school environment, to make provision for the child with special problems, and to take full advantage of the school curriculum to impart knowledge of sound health practices and to motivate the child to make these practices part of his daily living. Health education as part of the organized educational program is not considered the responsibility of the medical or related professions. While physicians should advise on the content of such instruction, the actual instruction is more effectively done by qualified teachers on the school staff, allowing physicians to function in fields for which they are specifically trained.

HEALTH SUPERVISION

1. *Health appraisal.* The health appraisal during the school years differs from that of younger age periods only in that correlation of information from more sources is needed. Medical findings and recommendations from the family physician, information from school health personnel and from community agencies, observations of teachers and guidance personnel in the schools, and the results of screening tests and measurements must be brought together by the school physician to decide about possible follow-up services or adjustments in school routine for each child. Health questionnaires for completion by parents have been used successfully as an additional source of information (2). While the recommendations of the family physician are carried out in so far as possible, the final responsibility for school adjustments for individual children must rest with the school administrator and, through him, with the health service personnel in the school.

The medical examination is an essential element in the total health appraisal. Family initiative should be encouraged to the greatest possible extent in having medical examinations performed by the family physician. "In view of the fact that the period of school life represents only about one-fifth of the individual's expected span of life, it would seem wise to provide for that school period a system of health service that will correlate with that received in the preschool period as well as with that to be received in later years." (3) When a child has been under the regular care of a physician prior to entering school, the health services in the school should certainly not supplant or duplicate this service. This is also highly desirable from the administrative viewpoint since it permits concentration of the school physician's time on the more urgent health problems among school children.

In geographic areas in which favorable socioeconomic conditions prevail, it has been found that a majority of the medical examinations are performed by family physicians, provided the program is interpreted properly to the practicing physicians of the community. A basis for such understanding can be reached through the local medical organizations. The school physician should further develop this relationship through individual contacts with family physicians, preferably by personal discussions over the telephone rather than by mail. In many areas, the initiative for promoting more active participation of the practicing physicians in the health programs of the schools has been taken by the local medical profession itself through the organization of school health committees of local medical societies (4).

The family physician must understand that the health appraisal is performed not only as a means of discovering conditions requiring medical attention but also as the basis for adjustments in the classroom and in physical education activities. The family physician must be furnished with adequately detailed, but not too long, forms explaining the type of information desired and allowing sufficient room for the physician's recommendations for medical care and for adjustments in the child's school program. He may provide the needed medical care himself, or he may request the aid of services provided through local health agencies. Space should be allowed on the form for the physician's recommendations about follow-up, with particular attention to his wishes about having the child brought back to him for further attention after a specified period of time.

When parents do not take their children to a family physician for medical examinations, the school must provide these examinations through its health services, if only to be sure that the child's health does not interfere with the educational services offered. Health examinations performed in the schools should be planned carefully as an educational experience for both parents and children. A well-performed medical examination is in itself a demonstration to the child which should teach him the value of continuing under medical care in adult life, especially if the school child can see benefits to his health as a result of the service. On the other hand, a poor examination is worse than useless in that it gives the child and his parents the wrong idea of what constitutes adequate care and, at the same time, leads to a false sense of confidence in the state of the child's health.

Parents should be present at the examinations, whenever possible. Discussion of the findings with the parents at the time of the examination not only saves considerable time and energy in follow-up, but it is effective in securing the desired action on the part of the parents. Health questionnaires may be sent home with the child for completion by the parents prior to the examination. These should not be used as a substitute for the parents' participation in the examination in the school; they should act rather as a stimulus to the parents' interest to provide additional leads for the school physician and nurse.

Arrangements for the examinations should provide privacy for the physician and child. A minimum of fifteen minutes should be allowed for each child so that there will be enough time to obtain a medical history and to allow discussion of the findings. How complete the examination in the school should be is a matter of some controversy. All such examinations are for purposes of screening, since they are not intended to lead to definitive diagnosis, and treatment is not instituted without further study by the physician to whom the child may be referred. Nevertheless, the more complete the screening is, the less likely significant abnormalities will be missed.

If privacy is assured and the child is draped, a complete rapid examination may be performed, including examination for possible hernia. By devoting less time to portions of the examination which are unproductive in children, more attention may be paid to the remainder of the examination, which is often neglected for lack of time. For example, careful auscultation of the lung fields is rarely indicated in the absence of positive leads in the history. On the other hand, examination for flat feet, aided by inspection of the shoes for evidence of wear on the inner aspects of the heels, is often neglected. Unnecessary disruption of the class may be avoided by having each child report on a prearranged schedule. The use of an appointment system, when possible, will also secure more complete parent participation in the program.

Teachers have an important part to play in the health-appraisal process (5). Since they are in close contact with children day after day, they can observe any changes in each child's appearance or behavior which may be the first evidence of many deviations from good health. Teachers have gained a basic understanding of child growth and development during their training. The school physician and nurse can build upon this foundation to make the teachers more aware of their potential contributions and instruct them in particular points to observe. Children with conditions that seem to merit prompt attention are referred to the school nurse, who may call upon the school physician to determine the seriousness of the condition and decide on the need for further care. Periodic conferences between the nurse and teacher, to review those observations of the teachers which did not appear to merit immediate referral, reinforce the need and value of this type of observation in the teacher's mind.

Medical examinations are of two general types. The first are the routine examinations, made at selected times during the child's school career. The other is the interval examination made for a variety of reasons. They may be made as a result of the teacher's observations, followed by preliminary screening by the school nurse. They may be used to check on the child's condition after a period of illness or an injury without adequate medical attention. Interval examinations are also helpful when assignment to a special class is under consideration or when special guidance work is to be undertaken.

Ideally, the routine periodic examination should be provided at short intervals, supplemented by special examinations as indicated. In practice, the frequency of the periodic examination must be determined on the basis of the returns to be expected from these examinations in relation to available medical manpower, school health budgets, and other administrative considerations. The old type of annual medical inspection, still performed in many places, has been found to be unproductive, both in terms of health benefits to children and in their educational value in inculcating sound health habits. Instead, less frequent but more complete examinations are recommended, with the examinations given at the time of school entrance, at the fourth or fifth grade, at the ninth grade, and prior to the time the pupil leaves school. Under such a program, it is possible to give adequate attention to interval examinations and other aspects of health services in the schools. Whatever the schedule of examinations adopted, reports on examinations performed by family physicians should follow the same pattern.

In some school systems, especially those in large cities, provision is made for the services of specialists in ophthalmology, otolaryngology, orthopedics, and cardiology. For the most part, these specialists perform a secondary screening, that is, they examine children suspected of some condition in their field of special competence prior to notification of the parents about the child's need for medical attention. This reduces the number of insignificant referrals to family physicians and tends to make the family physician treat referrals from the school with more attention.

a. Measurements and screening tests. Measurement and recording of the height and weight of children are all that are practicable in most school situations. These and such other measurements that may be selected are readily performed by the home class teacher at designated intervals and before periodic or special examinations by the school physician. The teacher may also maintain the growth chart which is made available to the nurse during the nurse-teacher conference and to the school physician when the child is referred to him for any reason.

Screening tests for visual and auditory acuity are performed in most schools as routine procedures. The simpler tests may be administered by teachers or volunteers after instruction. The more complicated tests should be given by trained technicians or by nurses, although generally this is a poor use of nursing time. These tests should be administered periodically to all children of school age since they may disclose visual or auditory disabilities in the absence of any suspicious symptoms. For children with presumably normal vision and hearing, every second year should be sufficient in view of the slow progression of most auditory and visual conditions in childhood.

The type of tests selected for testing of vision and hearing in a school must be determined by the circumstances in the community after consultation with any medical specialists practicing in these two fields. There is considerable difference of opinion among physicians as to what levels on the tests of vision and hearing constitute a significant impairment. In communities in which physicians are more conservative in their judgment of visual and auditory disabilities, irritation is created if many children with borderline conditions are referred for more definitive diagnosis and possible treatment. Whatever type of test is used, it is advisable to perform the routine tests of vision and hearing even if the child has been examined by his family physician, except when the physician indicates that he has conducted these tests himself.

b. Follow-up services. Disclosure of the same remediable defects in school children year after year without securing correction has been a major deficiency of many school health programs. Follow-up for the purpose of encouraging parents to secure more definitive diagnosis and indicated treatment for conditions discovered in the school health program is a more difficult task than comparable follow-up in the preschool period. The school health program must provide medical examinations for all children not examined by family physicians, whereas only a relatively small proportion are seen in child health conferences. Parents must be present with their preschool children, whereas a varying proportion are present at the time their school-age children are examined in the schools. Finally, more agencies are involved in the case of the child of school age, so that the role of the nurse in follow-up is more complex.

Effective follow-up services start with an adequate medical examination at which the parent is present. By explaining why additional medical care is needed, the school physician makes the referral an educational process. If the parent is not present at the examination, the public health nurse should try to have the parent come to school for an interview or she should visit the child's home, rather than simply send a note home with the child. Establishment of a priority order in follow-up by the school physician helps the public health nurse concentrate primary attention on the more urgent problems. Teachers can also be of help in working with individual children if the physician's records are interpreted for them, rather than simply passing the technical recommendations on to them.

2. *Promotion of mental health.* The discovery of children with emotional problems is part of the process of continuing health appraisal. The teacher is the central figure in this process within the school setting, more so than in the case of other health problems, since the teacher has the opportunity of observing the children a large part of each school day. The overly withdrawn, as well as the hostile child, can be brought to attention before possible serious mental illness develops, if the teacher has been prepared to understand the meaning of children's behavior. Specialized guidance personnel, such as psychiatrists, psychiatric social workers, clinical psychologists, or specially trained teachers, often devote a major segment of their time to promoting such understanding on the part of teachers, nurses, and other personnel in the schools (6). The school physician should enter into this program, by helping prepare the teachers, as well as by examining children before they are referred for special guidance services or psychiatric care.

The school physician should also work closely with personnel in the schools who evaluate children for special placements or school adjustments because of mental and emotional factors. School systems should provide psychological testing services for all children, with more complete evaluation of children who deviate markedly from the mid-range results in either direction, rather than call upon the limited facilities of child guidance clinics for this purpose.

The educational authorities have a responsibility to provide the best possible emotional climate in the school. The personality of the teachers is probably the most important single element in this. In this respect, care must be exercised in the selection of candidates for enrollment in colleges for teachers and services should be provided for guidance of students in these colleges. Within the schools, the impact of the school curriculum on the health and adjustment of the child must receive constant attention. The fostering of individual initiative must not be at the expense of undue pressures on the child. Sufficient time should be allowed for a leisurely lunch period and for changes in class-rooms. While these are activities directly related to the curriculum of the school, school physicians and other health personnel can often be helpful in offering suggestions for correcting unfavorable situations and for developing the desired emotional climate in the school.

3. *Nutrition services.* Special attention should be paid to the nutritional status of the child in the process of health appraisal. When a nutritional deficiency is suspected, the first effort should be to rule out any underlying condition responsible for it. At the same time, the food habits of the child and family should be investigated, either directly by the nurse employed in the school or by personnel of a community health agency to which the family may be referred for further investigation. Few nutritionists are employed by schools for work with individual children who present nutrition problems, or even for consultation to nurses working with school children; hence the need for a close working relationship between the school health service and community agencies having nutritionists on their staffs.

Apart from the health services for individual children, the schools promote improved nutrition by including instruction in nutrition in the regular curriculum. In the elementary school grades, this instruction is given as part of the teaching of other subjects, as opportunities for including the principles of sound nutrition present themselves. In the high schools, the instruction is usually included in courses in home economics or in special courses in health. The role of the school lunch program has been discussed in Chapter 13.

4. *Control of communicable diseases.* This still remains an important aspect of health services in the schools, in spite of the decreasing severity of most of the common communicable diseases of childhood. In instituting control procedures, school authorities generally follow the policies, regulations, and advice of the official health agency. State and local

departments of health generally make summary sheets or booklets available to the schools, giving brief descriptions of the common communicable diseases, along with required and suggested control measures for each disease. Legally, the school authorities must maintain the minimum requirements of the regulations on isolation and quarantine of cases and contacts of the reportable diseases. It should be understood that these regulations are intended only for the control of further spread of the disease in question and that a period of home care beyond the minimum isolation period is often needed to safeguard the health of the convalescent child. Imposition by the schools of additional requirements relating to the reportable diseases is undesirable, since the current trend is toward reducing the stringency of control measures in most communicable diseases of childhood. Special regulations may have to be developed by the schools for the so-called nuisance diseases because of their special significance in relation to school attendance, even though they are of minor importance from the standpoint of general health.

The policy of the educational authorities governing school attendance bears on the control of communicable diseases. Too frequently, perfect attendance is made a fetish, with commendation and special awards as inducements to the child. The most infectious period of the common cold and of most of the specific communicable diseases of childhood is at the time of onset of symptoms. Encouragement of perfect attendance tends to bring the child to school, in spite of symptoms, only to have him excluded after he has spread the infection. Financial aid from the state granted on the basis of average daily attendance rather than on the pupil enrollment encourages this practice. Physicians, as informed citizens, should try to have such outmoded practices changed, even if legislation is required.

The decision as to closure of a school in the presence of an outbreak is often a difficult one. Although the health department advises the school authorities and issues public statements on the situation, the final decision regarding closure must rest with the educational authorities, with the advice of the school physician. The nature of the epidemic disease and of conditions in the community influence whatever determination is made. Schools should certainly not be closed because of outbreaks of measles, whooping cough, German measles, mumps, or chickenpox. If adequate daily observation of children can be provided in the school, it is generally preferable to keep the school open in the presence of outbreaks of other diseases as well. It has been a frequent experience that closing of schools has resulted in increased exposure of children because of visiting in other homes and congregation of children in public places. The major exception to this policy is in central schools in rural areas in which the children gather from a wide area. Poliomyelitis is the disease which most frequently causes this question to be raised. In most instances, the outbreak is already on the wane before the start of the academic year and the further course of the outbreak is not demonstrably influenced by the opening of school.

Initial or stimulating immunizations against diphtheria, tetanus, and smallpox should be promoted through the health services in the schools. It is preferable to have the immunizations given by the family physician or the local health department, rather than for the schools to set up a duplicating service. The school authorities may make their facilities available to personnel of the official health agency to administer the immunizations within the school to those children not under the regular care of a family physician. They may usefully cooperate by obtaining the signed request slips for the procedures from the parents. An additional advantage in having health departments responsible for the actual immunizations, especially in rural areas, is that infants and preschool children may be given their immunizations at the same time as children attending school.

The close and prolonged association of school children with teachers, bus drivers, and other adults within the school environment requires that special precaution be taken that the adults have no infectious condition of hazard to the school children. Tuberculosis among school personnel constitutes the chief danger from this source. Preemployment x-rays of the chest should be mandatory, and periodic x-rays thereafter are desirable. A system of benefits should be arranged for school personnel found to have tuberculosis, to assure their full cooperation in the program.

5. *Dental health services.* Since dental caries is almost universal among children of school age residing in areas lacking fluoride in the drinking water, the school health services can make a valuable contribution to the dental health program even if they do not provide treatment services. Education in mouth hygiene has been traditionally carried out in the schools by both teachers and dental hygienists. With the demonstrated value of preventive measures in dental health, the dental hygienist has tended to concentrate on rapid cleansing of the teeth and the

topical application of sodium fluoride solution, rather than on relatively fruitless dental prophylaxes. Similarly, periodic dental examinations prior to referral for dental treatment is being replaced by a positive program encouraging regular care by the family dentist.

The school years are so vital for the retention of the permanent teeth that no community dental health program can hope to succeed without the active cooperation of the educational authorities, even though the corrective services are generally financed and administered by the health or welfare departments. Many school systems provide space for dental care within the schools for children who cannot be brought under the care of a family dentist. The provision of such facilities within the schools, helpful as it may be, is less important than the cooperation of the school in an organized program of case finding and follow-up. The key to success is a planned pattern of complete dental care of entering school children, with care of incremental defects in these children in succeeding years, and enrollment of new groups of entering school children each year. This program of care of incremental dental defects, described in more detail in Chapter 12, is most readily applicable to children of school age.

6. *Promotion of child safety.* During the school years, education begins to take precedence over passive protection of the child. Safety education within the schools is a valuable adjunct to a community program for the prevention of accidents. Check lists of accident hazards in the home may be profitably used with older school children to gain the interest of the entire family in the promotion of home safety. The high schools of the nation are rapidly providing instruction in driving motor vehicles. The common experience has been a sharp drop in the rate of automobile accidents in drivers under twenty-five years of age within a few years after the introduction of such courses.

The prevention of accidents on or near the school grounds is a responsibility of the school authorities. The school physician should see to it that periodic checks are made of the school and its immediate environs for the presence of accident hazards, and he should use his influence to have steps taken to correct them as soon as possible. Recreation on the school grounds should be supervised during and after school hours. Schools should work closely with the agencies responsible for elimination of traffic hazards near the school.

A planned program of first aid should be developed, setting forth the responsibilities of the teacher in case of specific types of accidents. It is desirable that one or two teachers, trained for the task, be made responsible for first aid in the school. When the nurse is called upon to render first aid, she should use the situation as an opportunity to instruct the teacher in the principles and procedures of first aid. This approach will release the nurse for more important functions such as home visiting. Standing orders for care of emergencies should be prepared under the direction of the school physician and posted in prominent places in the school.

OTHER ASPECTS OF SCHOOL HEALTH SERVICES

Health Services in Secondary Schools. Health service programs in the secondary schools are generally inferior in both extent and quality to those in the elementary grades. As a result, the special problems of the adolescent, from both the physical and emotional viewpoints, are frequently neglected in the later elementary school grades and in high school. Variation in individual growth and development presents acute problems to both the child and the teacher. A small amount of reassurance to an adolescent who is concerned about supposedly early or late sexual maturation or about social difficulties with persons of the opposite sex will go far in reducing anxiety which may seriously interfere with school work or social adjustment. Nutritional problems also come to the fore at this time. The individual needs of the secondary-school pupil reach a peak at a time when the school system uses a departmentalized approach, with no one teacher interested in the child as a person. It has been recommended that each secondary-school pupil have assigned to him "a single adult on the school staff to whom he can turn for all types of advice, including assistance on problems of physical, mental and emotional health . . . (and that) such a person should have available to him sound medical and public health advice and should know how to use it." (7)

Family physicians are called upon for advice in handling emotional problems in adolescents, as well as providing medical care for somatic illness.

The physician's understanding of the adolescent's and his parents' emotional needs and limitations may be of great help to the school counselor in formulating an appropriate academic or vocational training program for the individual child. In turn, the counselor by knowing of the child's limitations and potentialities can do a great deal to help the physician to relieve the tensions and anxieties by adjustment of the child's academic program. (8)

In other phases of the health program as well, every effort should be made to enlist the pupil's interest and to encourage him to carry through recommendations on his own behalf. Contrary to the situation in the lower and intermediate grades of elementary school, parents should not be present at the time of medical examinations in secondary schools. Particular emphasis should be placed on medical examinations of pupils who leave school prior to graduation, allowing sufficient time for follow-up to ensure correction of any remediable defects present. These examinations serve a dual purpose in that they can also be used as pre-employment examinations for pupils going to work. Vocational guidance also takes on great importance during the high-school years.

Physical Education and Athletics. Physical education and athletic competition with other schools require special health services to forestall any untoward happenings which may be laid at the door of the educational authorities. The frequent medical examination of athletes engaged in extramural sports often relegates other phases of the health service program to the background. Athletes are among the healthiest members of the student body. A medical examination at the beginning of the academic year should suffice for athletes, supplemented by careful observation during the athletic season on the part of the coach or physical training instructor. Of greater importance is supervision of regular physical education for the entire student body. It is desirable to exclude as few children as possible from the physical education program; the program should be adjusted to the child's needs, even if it is limited to very mild activities for some children.

Roles of School Physician and Nurse. Physicians may function either on a full-time or part-time basis in the schools. The most common pattern in the larger school systems is probably the employment of a physician part-time for morning hours during the academic year. The physician should be accepted as a member of the school staff who takes part in "planning all parts of the school program affecting the physical, emotional and social health of children and staff." (9) His primary function is "to give medical guidance in the development of a school environment and an experience which will contribute to the healthy development of children, and to give specific help to children with health problems." (9) This is in contrast to the older limited concept of his functions in assisting in the control of communicable diseases and the identification of children with physical defects. To fulfill his wider functions, the techniques for selecting children for health appraisal and for carrying out the examinations discussed earlier in this chapter must be employed. Of the utmost importance is the school physician's role in follow-up procedures in which his medical background and prestige will help gain the understanding and support of private physicians and community health agencies in the health program for school-age children.

Nursing services may be provided by a generalized public health nurse spending part of her time in the schools in her area or by a specialized nurse devoting full-time to school nursing. The nurse acts as liaison between the physician and school personnel, assisting with the arrangements for the medical examinations and with the medical histories and, above all, in carrying out the follow-up services needed to implement the physician's recommendations. The nurse serves an educational function as well in her conferences with teachers to review the health status of children in each class. The school physician should use his influence to keep the nurse from being assigned nonnursing duties such as investigation of all absences and immediate provision of first aid, apart from the aspects of these activities which are productive in health benefits for school children.

School Health Councils and Coordinators. Because every activity in the school has some bearing on the health of children, it is highly desirable in all but the small schools to bring together representative personnel from the various types of activities for better understanding and planning of the health program. Health councils within the schools should include not only the school physician and nurse and other persons in health services but also the school administrator and representatives of the fields of health education and physical education. One or more persons from this intramural school health council should serve on community health councils, when these exist, to promote more effective working arrangements in community health services for children of school age.

The work of the school health council is greatly enhanced by a health coordinator in the school, who may also act as chairman of the council. The health teacher, when one is employed, is generally designated health coordinator, or some other teacher may be selected and allowed to devote a major segment of time to this function. The coordinator has no specific administrative or teaching responsibilities apart from regular teaching assignments. He is encouraged to be alert to the health implications of all aspects of school activities, in interpreting the school health services to the teachers and to parents' groups, and in encouraging parents to assume their general responsibilities for securing health services for their children.

Sanitation of the School Environment. Municipal school systems usually employ or have technical consultation available on problems of ventilation and lighting. Water supply and sewage disposal in schools in large cities present no problems, except in antiquated school plants. In the smaller rural schools, the responsibility for periodic sanitary inspection of the school and grounds often falls upon the school physician or school nurse. Such inspection is obviously inadequate in determining the safety of the water supply or of sewage disposal. It is very unusual for school systems to hire technically qualified environmental sanitarians for this purpose. Cooperative arrangements have therefore been worked out in a number of places to have the sanitary engineers or sanitary inspectors on the staff of the health department check the sanitary conditions in the schools and submit reports to the school authorities. Carrying out the recommendations of the sanitary engineer is the responsibility of the school authorities.

Administration of Health Programs in the Schools. The legal responsibility for the administration of health services in the schools varies widely in different states. Of the 34 states having specific legislation covering such services, responsibility is vested in the state education department in 13 and in the state health department in 8; in the remaining 13, authority under the law is shared by the two agencies (10). Health education as part of the program of organized instruction is conceded to be the responsibility of the educational authorities. Conversely, the schools have almost universally refrained from providing treatment services.

An equal amount of variability in the administrative pattern exists locally. As a general rule, health services in the schools are provided through the education authorities in large cities and through health departments in rural areas. No blanket recommendation can be made as to which agency should administer school health services. Where full-time local health departments exist under progressive leadership, it is probable that at least the medical aspects of school health services can be provided more efficiently under their administration. Where adequate local health services do not exist, and this is the case in large areas of the country, school authorities must provide the health services themselves if the job is to be done at all.

Much of the discussion about the administration of school health services has arisen in those areas of the country in which school health services have been administered by the school authorities for several decades, long before the development of a modern health department, and in which adequate full-time local health services developed subsequently. In such situations, the jurisdictional dispute engendered has often retarded the development of an effective health program for children of school age.

Evaluation of Services. The effectiveness of health services for children of school age can be judged ideally by the actual benefits in health accruing to the children. This can be done periodically or at the end of the child's elementary- or high-school career. No reliance can be placed on routine reports on the number of "defects" found and corrected; the wide variation in interpretation of what constitutes a defect and of the adequacy of follow-up makes such reports almost meaningless. For a more adequate evaluation, independent health appraisals of a selected group of children should be performed by qualified examiners employed by the schools or by an outside agency (11).

This type of careful evaluation is applicable to only limited portions of the program and even then only infrequently. For evaluation of the adequacy of the total health program, as in meeting the needs of children with specific handicapping conditions, a step-by-step review of the program itself is the obvious alternative approach. Such an evaluation may be made in relation to the stated objectives and procedures of the local program, or reliance may be placed on statements by recognized leaders of what constitutes an adequate program. Appraisal forms have been developed in which the elements of a well-rounded program are set forth in some detail (12). Use of such appraisal forms is also helpful in promoting a more complete program.

CITED REFERENCES

1. HUBBARD, JOHN P., KATHERINE BAIN, and MARYLAND Y. PENNELL, School Health Services: A Report from the American Academy of Pediatrics Study of Child Health Services, *Am. J. Pub. Health,* Vol. 39, pp. 781–786, June, 1949.
2. SINGER-BROOKS, CHARLOTTE, Of What Value Are Health Inventories

Filled Out by Parents? *Am. J. Pub. Health,* Vol. 42, pp. 661–664, June, 1952.

3. SMILEY, DEAN F., and FRED V. HEIN, editors, "Health Appraisal of School Children: Standards for Determining the Health Status of School Children—Through the Cooperation of Parents, Teachers, Physicians, Dentists, Nurses and Others," A Report of the Joint Committee on Health Problems in Education of the National Education Association and the American Medical Association, Chicago, 1948.

4. HEIN, FRED V., and DONALD A. DUKELOW, "Physician Participation in School Health Services: A Report of the Analysis of the Questionnaire to Medical Societies on Physicians and Schools," American Medical Association, Chicago, 1950.

5. WHEATLEY, GEORGE M., and GRACE T. HALLOCK, "Health Observation of School Children," McGraw-Hill Book Company, Inc., New York, 1951.

6. SPOCK, BENJAMIN M., Schools Are a Fertile Field for Mental-health Efforts, *Child,* Vol. 15, pp. 10–11, August–September, 1950.

7. Suggested Standards for Health Services in Secondary Schools: Report of the Committee on Health Service Programs for Secondary Schools, School Health Section, *Am. J. Pub. Health,* Vol. 42, Part II, pp. 139–147, May, 1952.

8. SCHONFELD, WILLIAM A., General Practitioner's Role in Management of Personality Problems of Adolescents, *J.A.M.A.,* Vol. 147, pp. 1424–1428, Dec. 8, 1951.

9. BIERMAN, JESSIE M., and DOROTHY B. NYSWANDER, Letter, *Pediatrics,* Vol. 3, pp. 357–359, March, 1949.

10. STAFFORD, FRANK S., "State Administration of School Health, Physical Education and Recreation: A Status Study," Bulletin 1947, No. 13, Office of Education, Washington, D.C., 1947.

11. (*a*) YANKAUER, ALFRED, Designs for Evaluation Needed in the School Health Services Field, *Am. J. Pub. Health,* Vol. 42, pp. 655–660, June, 1952; (*b*) Evaluation Studies Which Have Contributed to School Health Services and Education: Report of the Chairman of the Committee on Evaluation to the School Health Section, *Am. J. Pub. Health,* Vol. 42, Part II, pp. 125–129, May, 1952.

12. Appraisal Form for Evaluating School Health Services, Prepared by the Michigan School Health Association in Cooperation with the American School Health Association, Approved by the Governing Council of the American School Health Association, *J. School Health,* Vol. 18, pp. 1–12, January, 1948.

ADDITIONAL REFERENCES

1. "Suggested School Health Policies: A Charter for School Health," Health Education Council, New York, 1946.

2. NYSWANDER, DOROTHY B., "Solving School Health Problems: The Astoria Demonstration Study," Commonwealth Fund, Harvard University Press, Cambridge, Mass., 1942.

3. Special issue devoted to health services for the child of school age, *Child,* Vol. 15, pp. 2–39, August–September, 1950.

4. Report of the Committee on School Health, American Academy of Pediatrics, *Pediatrics,* Vol. 7, pp. 826–830, June, 1951.

5. "An Eye Health Program for Schools," Publication No. 141, National Society for the Prevention of Blindness, New York, 1951.

6. GALAGAN, DONALD J., Progress in School Dental Programs, *Am. J. Pub. Health,* Vol. 42, pp. 834–839, July, 1952.

7. STIX, REGINE K., and ARTHUR LENZ, For the Health of Working Boys and Girls, *Child,* Vol. 16, pp. 118–122, April, 1952.

8. SELLERY, C. MORLEY, Role of the School Physician in Today's Schools, *Am. J. Pub. Health,* Vol. 42, pp. 813–817, July, 1952.

9. CREE, MARGARET A., Present-day Views on School Nursing, *Am. J. Pub. Health,* Vol. 42, pp. 818–824, July, 1952.

10. WISHIK, SAMUEL M., Administrative Jurisdiction of the School Health Service, *Am. J. Pub. Health,* Vol. 41, pp. 819–823, July, 1951.

11. YANKAUER, ALFRED, Use and Abuse of Newer Knowledge of Growth and Development in Schools, *Pediatrics,* Vol. 10, pp. 627–633, November, 1952.

Part IV

SPECIAL PROBLEMS

20 SERVICES COMMON TO CHILDREN WITH SPECIAL PROBLEMS

Up to this point, emphasis has been on community health services for the entire child population and the application of these services to children at successive periods of development. Incidental to these discussions, certain special problems have been presented as a matter of convenience. The subjects of premature birth and erythroblastosis fetalis, for example, were included in the discussions of the maternity cycle and the newborn period, since these conditions occur at no other time. The remainder of a large group of children with special problems also need the help of the community health services, and these children deserve separate consideration.

The health problems presented by these children are of all degrees of severity. Some are so mild as to be detectable only by careful health appraisal including screening tests for specific conditions. Others are evident to the casual observer, but appear to be causing no difficulty for the child at the moment. At the other end of the scale are the children with extreme single or multiple disabilities which prevent them from taking care of even their own daily needs. In recent years, children with the more severe disabilities have received a major share of attention. Children with subclinical or clinically mild conditions, though not considered handicapped in the usual sense of the word, deserve their share of attention in an effort to avoid potentially serious disabilities.

In educational circles, the term *exceptional children* is applied to "those who deviate from what is supposed to be average in physical, mental, emotional, or social characteristics to such an extent that they require special educational services in order to develop to their maximum capacity." (1) This definition includes groups such as gifted children who require special educational attention to encourage full development of their potentialities and, indeed, to prevent maladjustment from sheer boredom with the usual curriculum. It has been estimated that 12.4 per cent of all children of school age are exceptional in this sense (2). In considering children with handicapping or potentially handicapping conditions in the discussion that follows, whether the manifestations appear to be primarily of a physical, emotional, or social nature, only those children will be included for whom health services should be provided.

Health Supervision. Children with special problems have the same basic needs as other children. Their total adjustment should not be lost from view because of concentration on a weak limb or poor eyesight. "If the ultimate goal for the child who is handicapped is participation with nonhandicapped children in normal life situations, the total needs of the child, as well as those for his specific handicap, must be considered." (3) The child with cerebral palsy or epilepsy goes through the same stages of emotional development as a presumably healthy child. His emotional needs, fundamentally the same as other children, are exaggerated or distorted by his special problem. When the disability is an obvious one, this in itself creates disturbances in the child's relationships with other persons. Long periods when the child is homebound or institutionalized deprive him of some of the basic experiences needed for the development of a healthy personality. A child who might otherwise have been well adjusted may withdraw into himself or become overly aggressive and self-assertive. Parental attitudes of overprotection or rejection, partially stemming from the child's condition, may aggravate the emotional difficulties of the child.

Children with many special problems may need to have nutrition services more than other children. Their disabilities may introduce difficulties in ingesting or absorbing food, and periods of acute illness may further increase the possibility of nutritional deficiencies. Dental health services, even when not a specific element in the child's rehabilitation program, should be provided routinely. The handicapped child may need special protection against accident hazards in the environment, but every effort should be made to emphasize the educational, as opposed to the protective, phase in promoting his safety, so that the child might develop confidence in his ability to protect himself.

The child with a special problem, therefore, needs regular health supervision, just as any other child, in addition to, or as part of, health services connected with his specific condition. For children with minor disabilities, this presents no greater problem than for presumably healthy children. Such children usually require relatively simple special services which can be provided by occasional visits to a clinic or treatment center, if a family physician cannot provide these services, while regular health supervision is continued through ordinary channels.

More difficulty is encountered in the provision of general health supervision to children with severe disabilities because they may be separated from their families for special care or because attention is riveted on the specific condition present. This difficulty is overcome in the comparatively few centers providing well-rounded services through a team approach of personnel from several professional disciplines. In such teams, a physician specially trained in the care of children, aided by other health personnel, supervises the over-all care of the child. When a functioning team approach does not prevail, it may be necessary to bring in a physician periodically for general health appraisal or use an outside community resource for the purpose, if the child is not otherwise under the care of a family physician.

Prevention of Disabilities. The two phases of prevention, the avoidance of all conditions which are potentially disabling and the early care of children with potential or actual handicaps, must proceed at the same time. The individual child cannot be neglected while research is seeking out the causative factors involved, nor can the development of basic health programs be overlooked because of exclusive concern for care of handicapped children.

There are many examples of identical causes resulting in different types of disabilities. Perinatal factors may be the immediate or remote cause of orthopedic impairments, cerebral palsy, mental deficiency, and possibly, epilepsy. It is fortuitous what type of injury an accident may produce, with residual disability affecting almost any organ or system, manifested as mental deficiency, blindness, epilepsy, or orthopedic handicap. Nutritional disorders have been responsible for orthopedic and cardiac disabilities, as well as mental deficiency. Recurrent infections of the upper respiratory tract due to the hemolytic streptococcus may lead to rheumatic fever and cardiac disease or to impaired hearing. Other communicable diseases, such as encephalitis, may result in mental deficiency, intractable behavior disorders, or paralytic conditions with subsequent orthopedic problems.

These examples of identical causes leading to many different types of disabilities indicate that the prevention of factors ultimately responsible must be accomplished through the general community health program, in so far as this is possible in the light of present knowledge. Health services during the maternity cycle and during the newborn period are of particular importance in this regard. The promotion of child safety also requires greater emphasis from the viewpoint of the extent of serious disability resulting from accidents.

Early Discovery. The prevention of serious or permanent disabilities after the occurrence of the primary factor is most completely accomplished through early discovery and care. Neglect to provide early care and follow-up for children with apparently nonparalytic poliomyelitis, for example, may result in deformities of the spine. Similarly, disregarding a discharging ear may lead to irreversible hearing impairment; or waiting for a child to "outgrow" strabismus may result in loss of vision in one eye because of lack of use following suppression of the double image.

Equally as important as the permanent physical disabilities as a result of neglect to discover and treat special problems in their early stages are the emotional problems that may develop. The younger the child at the onset of the neglected problem, the more important in general are the emotional complications. Preschool children suffering from marked but undiscovered hearing loss are often found in groups of children coming to attention because of behavior difficulties. Deliberate concealment by their parents of children with conditions thought to carry a social stigma accentuate the emotional handicaps associated with the condition by superimposing a forced isolation. This is too often the case among children with epilepsy or mental deficiency; the social stigma attached to cerebral palsy appears to be declining as a result of the widespread attention this condition has received.

Lack of early discovery and care may result in other serious after-effects in the young child. The abnormality distorts the normal patterns of growth and development in addition to causing damage to existing structures and patterns. For example, a postpoliomyelitic paralysis of one lower extremity in a young child may inhibit growth of the extremity and result in a marked waddle gait which would not develop in an adolescent child or an adult similarly affected; early care, including artificial inhibition of growth of the opposite extremity, prevents the disproportion. When a disability occurs in a young child, it is more serious also because the child has not had a chance to learn normal patterns. Once abnormal patterns are acquired, retraining is a costly, time-consuming, and often ineffectual process. This is evident in the case of speech disabilities resulting from impaired hearing, cleft palate, or cerebral palsy.

Early discovery of most special problems is achieved with the greatest economy of effort through the over-all child health program. It would be automatically attained if all children were under adequate health supervision, whether by a family physician, a child health conference, or the health services in the schools, including the use of mass screening techniques. Since regular health supervision is far from universal, other techniques must be used to make up for the deficiency. When supplementary information on the condition of the offspring is given on the birth certificate, the case should be followed up to be sure the infant is under care. Children reported to have certain communicable diseases, such as poliomyelitis, meningitis, and possibly hemolytic streptococcal infection, should be followed for possible sequelae. In areas in which a census of children of preschool and entering-school age is taken in connection with enrollment in school, emphasis should be placed on the discovery of handicapped children. Finally, the public health nurse often learns of neglected or concealed children with special problems.

Early discovery of special problems is fostered by a campaign of public education and by efforts to increase the understanding of physicians and other professional persons in the nature of these problems. This is needed because of a still common fatalistic attitude toward some of these children and a belief that nothing can be accomplished in any case before the child is of school age.

Diagnostic Services. Every child suspected of a handicapping or potentially handicapping condition should be given an adequate evaluation as early as possible, including a complete medical examination as well as a careful appraisal of the special problem. This will ensure discovery of conditions which may be unrelated or contributory to the special problem, and which may interfere with any specific plan of management outlined. Arriving at a medical diagnosis is only the first step in a complete evaluation. The evaluation should also include an individual plan for medical treatment, rehabilitation, and special education as well as an estimate of the extent of return to normal function if the complete plan is carried out. Knowledge of what can be expected is particularly important as an incentive to the child and his parents, while it does not give rise to false hopes which may lead to frustration.

For less complicated conditions, the family physician need not call upon community facilities if the family's resources can cover the costs of consultation services. In the case of more complicated conditions, the family may not be able to afford the series of consultation visits needed, even if they can readily manage their usual medical expenses. Referral to a community facility may be requested by the family physician, with the understanding that a full statement of the diagnosis, the outlook as to function, and a suggested plan of management will be returned to him for his decision as to further care of the child. In many instances, the community resources may be the only means of obtaining needed services, and the family may pay for this care.

The three steps—diagnosis, prognosis, and plan of management—can be provided ideally through the team approach of a group of specialized workers from related fields for those conditions in which different types of services are needed. This may appear unnecessarily expensive; in the long run, however, it will save unnecessary procedures and help ensure greater earning capacity and social adjustment of the handicapped child. A team approach implies more than a series of examinations by a group of specialists, each making his own recommendations for further care. The group must discuss the findings and reach a common understanding of the child's status and needs, in which the relative importance and the timing of the various components of care are weighed. For example, a child with a cleft palate is more than simply a subject for oral surgery. He may be in poor nutritional state because of difficulties with chewing and swallowing, and the actual and potential speech disability and the orthodontic deformity may be severe, to mention some of the usual problems presented by the child with a cleft palate. The team must weigh all these factors to secure the best possible total functional result for the child. Surgical repair with less than complete anatomical closure of the cleft may be selected for the sake of better speech development. It may be necessary to delay certain aspects of care until the child's nutritional state has been improved.

Medical Treatment and Rehabilitation. The methods of obtaining medical treatment and hospital and convalescent care have been discussed at some length under the services of professional personnel and of hospitalization and related services in Chapters 7 and 8. Adequate rehabilitative services should be provided for children whose condition can be functionally improved even though the underlying condition may not be changed. Rehabilitation has been defined as the "restoration of the handicapped to the fullest physical, mental, social, vocational and economic usefulness of which they are capable," or from the medical viewpoint, as "the third phase of medical care." (4) The same concept and terminology is used in the case of children with congenital defects or conditions acquired early in life even though, strictly speaking, these children are not being rehabilitated to a former state of health, but are being "habilitated" or aided in the fullest use of their potential capacities.

Medical rehabilitation first of all employs all physical means of reducing the extent of a disability—surgical procedures, the modalities of physical and occupational therapy, and mechanical aids such as prosthetic devices. To accomplish even the first step in rehabilitation requires the active participation of the individual patient. When adverse emotional factors are present in the child or the parents, the child may resist the rehabilitative plan. The child may have become discouraged as a result of repeated falls or failures, and he may not wish to face the risk of repetition of unpleasant experiences. Special methods may have to be used in motivating children to participate actively in the attainment of improved function (5). To discover and overcome the emotional factors impeding care may require a detailed investigation of the social situation or interpersonal relationships of the child by a medical social worker (6).

Modern rehabilitative techniques are keyed to daily living (7). In neuromuscular disorders, for example, muscle retraining is not an end in itself; muscle training is taught in relation to everyday activities, such as getting in and out of bed and wheelchair without support or, when the individual has progressed further, in crossing streets within the time a traffic light would ordinarily take to change. In speech training, instruction goes along with the material being taught in the regular school grade of the child.

In the course of rehabilitation, the child's progress must be evaluated periodically. This is necessary as a guide to further care and, in some instances, to avoid waste motion by determining whether or not maximum restoration of function has been achieved. Evaluation of progress in children is more difficult than in adults, in that development of the child may account for the so-called progress, independent of any treatment given. This is especially important in conditions such as cerebral palsy in which muscular coordination is a major factor. Methods of evaluation must therefore be used which take normal development into consideration (8).

A team approach is as necessary in carrying out the medical rehabilitation program as it is in achieving a diagnosis and outlining a plan of care. Therapists of various backgrounds are essential members of any team carrying out a plan of treatment and rehabilitation of the handicapped child (9). The three major fields in which this important group of ancillary health personnel functions are in physical therapy, speech therapy, and vocational therapy; of these, the field of physical therapy is the oldest and most firmly established. Physical and occupational therapists function legally under the specific direction of physicians; when this has not actually been the case in practice, it has rendered the work of the therapist more difficult and has often resulted in wasted effort on the part of the therapist.

Most physical and occupational therapists are employed in hospitals, convalescent institutions or clinics, or in other types of circumscribed situations such as rehabilitation centers or special schools. With the increasing trend toward a more complete type of home care, physical therapists are being employed more frequently by official and voluntary agencies for services in the home. In general, two types of children are given care. The first group consists of children whose stay in a hospital or convalescent institution can be shortened if a small but essential amount of physical therapy can be continued in the home or community in which the child resides. The other group consists of children with lesser degrees of handicap who were never hospitalized, but who will benefit from exercises or some other type of physical therapy that can be performed or supervised by the parents with proper instruction. The physical therapist may provide the service herself or assist the public health nurse in doing so, depending on the type of problem presented by the child. To a lesser extent, occupational therapists are also employed to provide service to homebound parents. The occupational therapist likewise serves as a supervisor of volunteers who visit homebound children to give a simple form of recreational or play therapy.

The position of the speech therapist is not clearly defined in relation to that of the speech teacher. Theoretically, the speech teacher is able to handle speech problems of any nature. Actually, the training of most speech teachers has been in the teaching of clear speech and the correction of the more common speech defects found in the school setting. The more specialized services needed in auditory and speech training of children with severe handicaps, such as deafness, cerebral palsy, and cleft palate, are often not adequately covered in her training, nor is adequate time allowed in her teaching program to give the individual attention needed by these children. Until such time as these services are provided in the schools, auditory and speech training must be provided by speech therapists in relation to health services for handicapped children, whenever there is a physical handicap requiring highly specialized care.

The various activities described are integral parts of a minimum program of medical rehabilitation, to achieve functional restoration. Medical rehabilitation is only one aspect of care needed to achieve total rehabilitation; the latter requires the joint efforts of educational, vocational rehabilitation, and other personnel in a broad community program.

Rehabilitation Centers. The complicated nature of rehabilitation services makes it difficult for any one institution or agency, established primarily for another purpose, to provide the full range of services needed. Rehabilitation centers are community facilities designed to fill the gaps in existing services, supplementing, not replacing, the services of the private physician, the general hospital, the social agency, and the school. Rehabilitation centers have started from widely different points of origin and have developed to meet varying community needs. For the most part, they have no inpatient facilities; patients coming from a distance are boarded in nearby homes or rooming houses and are transported to and from the center. At a typical well-established center, the following are among the services provided: medical examinations by specialists in various fields; physical, occupational, and speech therapy; braces and other prosthetic appliances; nursery school for young children with severe disabilities; vocational testing, counseling, and training and actual work experience; and services for the homebound (10). In such a center, each department and each worker considers its responsibilities toward total care of each patient.

An outpatient rehabilitation center can serve the needs of a sizable community through referrals from the general practitioners of the area. . . . The members of the medical profession are beginning to understand that the center is built to serve the needs of the doctors, the patients and the public and that professional support by the physicians is essential to successful rehabilitation. (11)

When services for children are provided in the rehabilitation center, these are usually brought into close relation with other community facilities for children with special problems. Arrangements must be made with the schools so that services for handicapped children of school age may be provided with minimum disruption of their class schedule. Services for specific children at the center may be financed through the official agency administering the program for handicapped children.

Education of Children. General educational opportunities should be available to the handicapped child to the extent he can benefit from them. In certain respects, these opportunities must be greater for the handicapped child than for other children because his selection of a vocation is more limited. The provision of such opportunities is naturally the responsibility of the educational authorities, but the manner in which they are provided is influenced by the nature and adequacy of health services in the schools and in the community at large.

Since the goal of all services for children with special problems is their participation in normal life situations to the greatest possible extent, placement in the school is guided by the same principle. When the child can be kept in the regular class with suitable adjustments to meet his special needs, this is the method of choice. The adjustment may be a simple one, such as seating a child with a moderate hearing loss at the front of the classroom. In the case of a child with epilepsy, instruction of the classroom teacher and careful but casual preparation of the class may spell the difference between successful and unsuccessful school adjustment for the affected child. A handicapped child should never be placed in a regular class as a matter of convenience to the school administration; when the class cannot meet his needs, the experience will be frustrating to the child and will only handicap him further by increasing his fear of new situations.

Special classes must be provided for children whose needs cannot be met in a regular class. In the special class, the method of instruction is adjusted to the specific handicaps of the children. The grouping of children in special classes makes it efficient to provide special services such as speech or physical therapy in this setting, rather than to remove the children from school individually at frequent intervals to be given these services elsewhere. In the larger cities, a special school may be maintained for children with special problems, particularly those of an orthopedic nature. Some of these schools are well equipped with modern forms of physical therapy. The tendency is to make the facilities of the special classes and schools more widely available by providing bus transportation even to children living at some distance; when handicapped children live outside the boundaries of the school district in which the special facility is located, financial arrangements are usually made between the two school districts concerned.

The importance of continued instruction of children in hospitals or convalescent institutions for long periods of time has been stressed. Special visiting teachers should be provided for such children, as well as those who are homebound. In a few places, homebound children are able to participate in classroom activities through the use of a two-way telephone connection between the home and school.

Some children with severe handicaps such as blindness, deafness, or mental deficiency may have to spend all or part of their school career in special residential schools. Although prolonged separation from the home is undesirable for these children, whose emotional needs are often greater than those of other children, facilities similar to those available in residential schools are rarely available near home.

The needs of preschool children with special problems are becoming more generally appreciated. In widely separated parts of the country there are a few special nursery schools for young children with severe handicaps. They are maintained in an effort to provide the stimulation of relationships with other children often not otherwise available to these children. Elsewhere, regular nursery schools have been opened to children with special problems for the same reason.

The health services in the schools must provide close supervision over children with special problems. The school physician should review the health status of each child recommended for placement in a special class or school, or for whom any significant adjustment in the classroom situation or curriculum is being considered for reasons of health. The status of these children should also be reviewed at periodic intervals to be sure that the special placements are still suitable for the child. The school nurse interprets these recommendations to the classroom teachers and checks to see if they are being carried out.

Some school systems provide additional medical consultation and even treatment services for certain types of problems. Most common among these are ophthalmological consultation and fitting of glasses for children with eye defects, for whom private medical care or even clinic care cannot be arranged. The services of otologists and cardiologists are also used in the schools, although not so frequently as in the case of eye conditions. When they are, it is usually to assist in proper placement of the child concerned, rather than to recommend treatment.

Vocational Rehabilitation and Guidance Services. Vocational rehabilitation is the process of preparing handicapped persons to be self-supporting and finding suitable employment for them. The vocational rehabilitation program seeks maximum medical rehabilitation as the necessary first step, since it is an axiom in vocational rehabilitation never to train around a disability that can be corrected or reduced. Federal grants-in-aid administered by the states cover the costs of medical and surgical care and rehabilitation. These services have limited applicability to children since the minimum eligible age is fourteen years and few persons under eighteen years of age are given care under the program.

The child with a disability severe enough to limit his choice of future occupations should have the help of a vocational guidance counselor early in his school career. Using the results of the child's health appraisal and of psychological testing, the counselor evaluates the child's potentialities for employment in terms of his abilities rather than simply ruling out certain types of work because of his disabilities. Vocational rehabilitation workers should have an opportunity to see handicapped children at an earlier age to obtain a better picture of the children's problems. Working with the guidance counselors and others in the schools, these specialists can point out methods for preparing the child for training prior to employment.

Parent Education. In all types of handicapping conditions, work with parents, individually and in groups, helps ensure a successful effort in rehabilitating the child to the greatest possible extent (12). The parents' handling of the child may greatly facilitate or hamper the rehabilitative process. In congenital deafness, for example, the parents are instructed to talk and sing to the infant and young child as much as possible, as a stimulus to later acquisition of lip reading. In other instances, parents may carry out recommended exercises or other activities in the home, to supplement outside rehabilitative services. Whatever the special problem, parents need encouragement to give their children sufficient rein to develop as individuals.

A striking development of recent years has been the development of groups of parents of children having certain special problems, such as cerebral palsy or mental deficiency, organized by the parents themselves. As local groups have formed, they have tended to coalesce to form state and national groups, which have exerted a strong influence in broadening governmental and voluntary activities in the specific field. Local parents' groups in association with clinics or institutions have been helpful to the agency in interpreting its policies to the parents and in bringing the needs of the parents to the attention of the agency. It has been suggested that a parent of an affected child be on the board of every institution and community agency providing services to handicapped children.

Community Education. Along with health and educational services, an active program of public education is needed in every community to promote acceptance of the handicapped individual as a person who has positive contributions to make to the life of the community, if his special needs are met. Prevailing attitudes toward the handicapped vary from one of pity, to indifference or a feeling of defeatism, and even to one of fear or horror, depending on the particular handicap and the traditions of the community.

In some instances, handicapped children find their way barred to education because of the attitudes of school authorities. This is particularly the case with respect to children with epilepsy. Possibly more serious is the attitude of employers, as well as employees with whom the handicapped person would work. Demonstrating the potentialities of the handicapped to both employers and employees is a function, strictly speaking, outside the realm of health services for children. It is so important, however, that physicians and others interested in rehabilitation of the handicapped child should lend their influence to any efforts in that direction.

Coordination and Follow-up Services. In many of the special problems of childhood, long-term care is needed and the child is shuttled back and forth among various agencies, which may not know of services he has received or may still be receiving. Ideally, one agency, most logically the local health department, should maintain a register of children with selected types of problems, to be sure that each child has been brought under care and that recommendations made for care are being carried out, in so far as possible. Although mandatory reporting is rarely desirable or effective, the cooperation of professional groups and voluntary agencies should be sought to make the registration more complete. Even without a case register, the use of an interagency referral system will eliminate much duplication in service and provide more efficient service for the child.

CITED REFERENCES

1. "The Education of Exceptional Children, Part II of the Forty-ninth Yearbook of the National Society for the Study of Education," University of Chicago Press, Chicago, 1950.
2. MARTENS, ELISE H., "Needs of Exceptional Children," Leaflet No. 74, U.S. Office of Education, Washington, D.C., 1944; cited in reference 1.
3. WILSON, EUNICE W., The Handicapped Child, *Pediatrics,* Vol. 5, pp. 569–573, March, 1950.
4. RUSK, HOWARD A., Rehabilitation, *J.A.M.A.,* Vol. 140, pp. 286–292, May 21, 1949.
5. SCHWARTZ, R. PLATO, FREDERICK N. ZUCK, FRANCES H. PARSONS, KATHLEEN WINGATE, THOMAS LACEY, II, and MOULTON K. JOHNSON, Motivation of Children with Multiple Functional Disabilities: Hartwell Method, *J.A.M.A.,* Vol. 145, pp. 951–955, Mar. 31, 1951.
6. SENSENICH, HELENE, Team Work in Rehabilitation, *Am. J. Pub. Health,* Vol. 40, pp. 969–972, August, 1950.
7. BUCHWALD, EDITH, "Physical Rehabilitation for Daily Living," McGraw-Hill Book Company, Inc., New York, 1952.
8. (a) BLUM, LUCILLE H., and NINA D. FIELDSTEEL, Method for Objective Measure of Developmental Progress, *Am. J. Dis. Child.,* Vol. 83, pp. 306–308, March, 1952; (b) "Blum-Fieldsteel Development Charts," World Book Company, Yonkers, New York, 1953.
9. SANGER, WILLIAM T., Careers in Rehabilitation: A Place on the Team, *The Crippled Child,* Vol. 30, pp. 18–20, December, 1950.

10. GREVE, BELL, The Cleveland Rehabilitation Center, in "Rehabilitation of the Handicapped: A Survey of Means and Methods," William H. Soden, editor, The Ronald Press Company, New York, 1949.
11. JONES, ARTHUR C., The Community Rehabilitation Center and the General Practitioner, *J.A.M.A.*, Vol. 144, pp. 994–995, Nov. 18, 1950.
12. MILMAN, DORIS H., Group Therapy with Parents: An Approach to the Rehabilitation of Physically Disabled Children, *J. Pediat.*, Vol. 41, pp. 113–116, July, 1952.

ADDITIONAL REFERENCES

1. WENKERT, WALTER, Community Planning for Rehabilitation, *Am. J. Pub. Health,* Vol. 42, pp. 779–783, July, 1952.
2. CHAPMAN, A. L., and J. H. GERBER, Rehabilitation: The Role of the Health Department, *Pub. Health Rep.,* Vol. 66, pp. 529–534, Apr. 27, 1951.
3. KRUSEN, FRANK H., The Scope and Future of Physical Medicine and Rehabilitation, *J.A.M.A.*, Vol. 144, pp. 727–730, Oct. 28, 1950.
4. "One in Three Hundred: Children Served by the Crippled Children's Program in 1948," Statistical Series No. 10, Children's Bureau, Washington, D.C., 1951.
5. "Emotional Problems Associated with Handicapping Conditions in Children," Publication No. 336, Children's Bureau, Washington, D.C., 1952.
6. BAHLKE, ANNE M., Rehabilitation of the Handicapped: The Place of the Official Agency, Medical Clinics of North America, Vol. 37, pp. 933–941, May, 1953.
7. RUSK, HOWARD A., Rehabilitation Pays Dividends, *J.A.M.A.,* Vol. 150, pp. 837–840, Nov. 1, 1952.
8. "The Job of the Physical Therapist," The American Physical Therapy Association, New York, 1951.
9. HAWK, SARA S., "Speech Therapy for the Physically Handicapped," Stanford University Press, Palo Alto, Calif., 1950.
10. DUNTON, WILLIAM R., JR., and SIDNEY LICHT, editors, "Occupational Therapy: Principles and Practise," Charles C Thomas, Publisher, Springfield, Ill. 1950.
11. SHANDS, A. R., The Care and Treatment of Crippled Children in the United States, *J. Bone & Joint Surg.,* Vol. 35-A, pp. 237–244, January, 1953.

21 CHILDREN WITH PHYSICAL HANDICAPS

Although the general approach to special health problems of childhood has been discussed at some length, specific aspects of some of these problems deserve brief consideration. The conditions selected for discussion by no means include all that deserve emphasis. Their selection has been based on the size and urgency of the particular problem, on the amount of professional and public interest shown in it, and upon the possibilities of accomplishing worth-while results through community effort.

The separation of these problems into physical and mental, emotional and social handicaps is somewhat arbitrary. The grouping of any condition has been based upon the relative importance of the usual responsibilities of health agencies in meeting the needs of affected children. Physical handicaps have emotional and social components, as has been repeatedly pointed out. Many cases of mental deficiency, and some of behavior disorders, on the other hand, are the result of physical damage to the brain. The grouping is, nevertheless, necessary from the practical viewpoint.

AUDITORY PROBLEMS

Surveys of the results of screening tests of hearing among children of school age indicate that about 4 per cent of the children have a significant impairment of hearing (1). While all these children with impaired hearing should be followed for complete diagnosis and possible treatment, less than one-quarter, or somewhat under 1 per cent of all children of school age, are actually handicapped to any degree by virtue of their hearing loss. About 0.3 per cent of children of school age are deaf, *i.e.*, whose hearing loss is so severe that the child cannot communicate because he has never heard speech.

With the rapid strides in electronics during and since the Second World War, many children with severe degrees of hearing loss are able to hear through amplification of the spoken voice, so that the practical distinction between hard of hearing and deaf children varies with the facilities available for testing and specific training. The degree of hearing loss for conversational speech, as measured by speech audiometry, is a determining factor for medical and educational services. From this viewpoint, a mild hearing loss is considered as one in which the spoken voice cannot be detected at a threshold of 30 to 40 decibels; the threshold for the spoken voice is 40 to 70 decibels in a moderate loss, and more than 70 decibels in a profound loss (2).

A moderate decline may be occurring in the prevalence of mild to moderate hearing impairment in children. In a nationwide survey of the results of hearing tests in the late 1930's the prevalence of significant hearing loss was found to vary between 4.9 and 6.1 per cent, as compared with 4.0 per cent in the 1947–1948 school year (1). This reported decline occurred during a period when more sensitive types of testing equipment were introduced and widely used. On the other hand, there is no reason to believe that there has been any decrease in the prevalence of severe auditory handicaps in children; the lives of some children with formerly fatal infections are being saved as a result of newer developments in therapy, only to have the children left with marked hearing loss.

The two main types of hearing loss are impairment in conduction of sound from the outer to the inner ear and disturbance in sound perception in the inner ear or the auditory nerve. Conduction disorders prior to adolescence are usually due to infections of the middle ear or to a reduction in air pressure in the inner ear as a result of obstruction of the orifice of the eustachian tube by lymphoid tissue, or to a combination of the two factors. It has been estimated that early and adequate treatment of these forms of potential or actual conduction loss would prevent one-half to two-thirds of the cases of profound hearing impairment otherwise occurring in adults under forty years of age. In adolescent children, progressive hearing loss may be due to otosclerosis, a familial condition of unknown origin characterized by hardening of the structures about the inner ear.

In younger children, most cases of profound hearing loss are examples of disturbances of sound perception either in the inner ear or in the auditory nerve. In the first year or two of life, hereditary and congenital deafness comprise most of this group; with advancing age, deafness complicating infectious diseases forms an increasing proportion of the total. Multiple factors may be present in any child with an acoustic handicap.

Early Detection and Diagnosis. During infancy and the early pre-school years, only fairly severe hearing loss comes to light, and then often after some delay. This is unfortunate since auditory and speech training should be started as early as possible. "New methods of testing should be instituted so that the deafened children are detected and evaluated at the earliest possible age. If this is not accomplished, too many hard of hearing children will eventually be sent to schools for the deaf without having had the chance to overcome their handicap in a normal environment." (3)

No screening methods exist for the detection of hearing impairments in children under three to five years of age. In children who are under regular health supervision or in nursery schools, hearing impairment may be suspected when speech is unduly retarded or when children, having progressed normally through the babbling stage, stop making an effort to talk. Finding cases of severe hearing defects in the early years may be expedited by concentrating upon vulnerable groups, for example, children with one or both parents who were deaf from childhood, children who have recovered from serious infections such as meningitis, and children whose mother had German measles during the first trimester of pregnancy. Clinical history and examination may heighten the suspicion of hearing loss, but determination of the severity of the condition depends upon the availability of objective audiometry. In trained hands, this procedure, based on the use of conditioned reflexes, is reliable in children well under one year of age. Free field sound tests provide another useful tool, especially when there may be disturbances of intersensory perception which may be confused with deafness (4). Bells and other sound makers of known frequency and intensity range are used at a given distance from the child's ear when the child is engaged in some activity. Presence of hearing is indicated by temporary cessation of the activity.

In the school years, screening audiometric tests are widely available.

Screening tests for hearing are only one facet of a broader program of case finding; teachers should be encouraged to report children to the school health services who appear inattentive or who ask to have questions repeated. Children with frequent colds and ear infections also require interim follow-up.

Since the concepts of modern audiology, the name applied to the diagnosis and management of disorders of communication from hearing loss, are not widely known and practiced, the school physician should be sure of his ground before instituting follow-up for children with suspected hearing impairment. Abnormal screening tests should be repeated; if a child has had a recent infection which may be the cause of a transient hearing loss, follow-up should be postponed until a retest is performed after one or two months. To increase the value of follow-up, otologists may be employed to perform a screening clinical examination in the school; the results of these examinations may be forwarded to the family physician for whatever use the latter wishes to make of them. An adequate audiological appraisal is needed by every child with hearing loss, as a basis for treatment and rehabilitation services and for special placement in school. This may be provided by a local otologist interested in audiology or in a community facility. Mobile units equipped with pitch range and speech audiometers may be used for the purpose in smaller population centers and rural areas.

Treatment and Rehabilitaton Services. For children with severe perceptive hearing loss, medical treatment has little to offer, although treatment of any concomitant conductive disturbance is essential to retain any residual hearing. Training is centered around any degree of serviceable hearing present. When hearing aids are used, they should be selected after adequate appraisal of the hearing loss, using a speech audiometer; the child and his parents should be trained in its use, and the child should be followed up to be sure its use is continued. Auditory training units have been developed to make amplification as pleasant as possible for the child. Simple purchase of hearing aids without these precautions results in rapid discarding of instruments in a high proportion of cases. Audiological training may be needed to teach the child the meaning of what he hears, and the child must be taught intelligible speech through speech training. Speech reading (or lip reading) is a useful supplement, since the child may not hear all sounds clearly even with the use of a hearing aid. The child with no serviceable hearing can still be taught through special techniques to speak intelligibly and to read the speech of others.

Additional treatment procedures are vital in the case of conductive disorders. These consist of adequate treatment of any local infections, removal of impacted wax in the ear canal, and removal or shrinkage of hypertrophied lymphoid tissue obstructing the eustachian tube. There is general agreement that any large adenoid masses should be removed surgically. The role of irradiation of the nasopharynx for any remaining lymphoid tissue is still unsettled, although it is probable that this procedure, either by x-ray or radium, is of value in arresting or reversing the course of many cases of conductive hearing impairment, provided adequate precautions are observed in its use (5). Surgery is effective in many cases of otosclerosis.

A community conservation of hearing program may center its attention on case finding and medical rehabilitation (6). A recent development has been the emergence of speech and hearing centers, in which rehabilitative services are provided for all types of speech difficulties, in addition to audiological appraisal and training for children with hearing impairment. Most of these centers are affiliated with universities and are used for training of specialized personnel (7). Community rehabilitation centers are also tending to broaden their services to include care for the acoustically handicapped.

VISUAL PROBLEMS

Disturbances of vision are probably the most common of all special health problems of a chronic nature in childhood. Fully one-quarter of the children attending school have eye problems requiring further medical attention (8). The majority of these children have some impairment of visual acuity, usually of a degree that does not necessitate any significant adjustment in school or in the community. It is generally estimated that seriously handicapping visual impairment is found in 1 out of every 500 to 1,000 children of school age. Most of these partially sighted children can receive instruction through the sense of sight with the benefit of special visual devices and techniques. For educational purposes, the partially sighted group includes children whose visual acuity is found to lie between 20/70 and 20/200 in the better eye after corrective measures have been completed, when tested with the Snellen chart. With few exceptions, use of the eyes for educational purposes does not affect the underlying ocular condition. From the viewpoint of health services, greater emphasis is placed upon those children in whom the underlying condition is not static or irreversible.

About 1 in 5,000 children of school age is so severely affected as to be considered blind. For purposes of classification and education, children are defined as blind if their visual acuity is 20/200 or less in the better eye after corrective procedures have been completed, or if they suffer from other handicaps affecting the usefulness of vision to a similar degree.

Factors responsible for the development of the common ocular conditions are poorly understood. Significant inroads can probably not be made in their numbers through preventive techniques available at present. Certain of these conditions tend to be familial, especially myopia and strabismus and other imbalances of the external ocular muscles. Strabismus is also known to occur more frequently in premature infants than in full-term infants. Disturbances during early fetal life may produce congenital cataracts and other types of ocular abnormalities.

In contrast to the common ocular disturbances, many of the causative factors in serious visual handicaps are known, and several of these causes are clearly preventable (9). Infectious diseases such as ophthalmia neonatorum and syphilis, formerly among the leading causes of blindness, have decreased markedly in importance, and new cases should virtually cease to appear in the near future if the present trend continues. The incidence of blindness due to accidents and other traumatic causes has also shown a moderate decrease. On the other hand, blindness of prenatal origin or following retrolental fibroplasia in premature infants appears to be increasing. Among blind children of school age, the onset of blindness was found to be before birth in 54 per cent; in an additional 26 per cent, the age at the time of onset was between birth and five years.

Detection and Diagnosis. The major specific measure applicable during early infancy is the periodic ophthalmoscopic examination of premature infants for evidences of retrolental fibroplasia. Without such examinations, serious impairment of vision may not be suspected by parents until the infant is four to six months of age. Less severe types of visual disturbances cannot be easily detected during the first year of life. Coordination of the eye muscles is usually not established before the age of four months so that a diagnosis of muscular imbalance may not be made definitely until several months later. When strabismus or definite imbalance is suspected or diagnosed, the parent should be encouraged to keep the child under competent ophthalmological care, rather than to delay such care with the hope that the condition will be outgrown.

The selection of a screening test for use in a health program for children of preschool or school age should be made in the light of local conditions. The difficulty in selection is increased by the fact that the additional information disclosed by the more complicated screening tests has not been definitely shown to be worth the effort involved. More highly trained personnel is needed for the complicated tests, and more conditions of questionable significance are found, resulting in unnecessary referrals. Community facilities for the diagnosis and treatment of visual defects must approach adequacy if the more complicated testing program is not to defeat itself. In most situations, the Snellen test, used by properly instructed personnel under carefully controlled conditions, is the screening test of choice.

As with hearing problems, periodic screening tests are only one aspect of case finding in the conservation of vision program. The teacher is in a strong position to suspect the presence of visual disturbances because she observes the child in both close and distant use of his eyes over long periods of time. She also should observe the presence of inflammatory conditions of the eyes, such as conjunctivitis or styes, and of symptoms such as headaches which may suggest visual disturbances.

Suspicion of some ocular abnormality by the school health services should lead to referral to the family physician, with the decision as to further care up to him. Very often, however, parents by-pass the family physician and take their children directly to an ophthalmologist or an optometrist. The optometrist may prescribe glasses, but not being a physician, he is not permitted to treat eye conditions with drugs or by surgery, nor is he equipped to make a complete medical diagnosis of any ocular abnormalities. Since optometrists often provide the bulk of services for children with impaired visual acuity, even when there are practicing ophthalmologists in the community, they should be brought into the program for the conservation of vision early in the planning stage along with local medical specialists. In some programs, this has resulted in an agreement between the two groups which ensured better service for children. The optometrists may agree to refer to ophthalmologists those children whose visual acuity is not normal after fitting of glasses or who show an abnormality of the eye which is not within the province of the optometrist to treat; the ophthalmologists, on their part, agree to return the child to the referring optometrists for optometric services.

An adequate vision-testing program in the schools should include testing of children already wearing glasses. These children may have neglected to return to their physician or optometrist as requested, or some change may have occurred since their last visit. When their visual acuity is found to be abnormal with their glasses on, it is preferable to communicate directly with the ophthalmologist or optometrist about further follow-up, rather than institute routine follow-up through the parents.

Treatment and Rehabilitation. Apart from a few programs in municipal school systems in which ophthalmologists employed by the schools provide definitive examinations and prescribe glasses, health agencies rarely offer organized treatment services for children with eye defects, either through clinics or hospital care. Reliance is generally placed upon available private or clinic resources. Financial aid is provided in only a few health programs for medical or surgical correction of strabismus or similar services of a sight-saving nature. For children whose families cannot afford private care but who are not eligible for public welfare, service clubs and similar organizations are often of the greatest assistance in obtaining needed services.

Rehabilitation of children in the partially sighted or blind groups is almost entirely an educational process, with medical services playing a relatively small role. Orthoptic training is useful in the management of conditions characterized by disturbed coordination of the external ocular muscles, when it is performed under ophthalmological direction as part of a program in which adequate use is made of surgery. Children in sight-saving classes in the regular schools and those in residential schools or other institutions for the blind should have continued medical supervision and adequate care for any local or systemic conditions which may be even partially remediable. Vocational guidance and rehabilitation is particularly needed by the visually handicapped.

RHEUMATIC FEVER AND RHEUMATIC HEART DISEASE

Rheumatic fever, the term which will be used for convenience in this discussion to encompass acute rheumatic fever and Sydenham's chorea and acute and chronic rheumatic heart disease, is responsible for almost all the heart disease developing during the school years. It is a chronic, recurring disease of childhood and early adult life and a leading cause of death during this age period. There is almost universal agreement that rheumatic fever follows clinical or subclinical infections with the group A streptococcus, usually within a period of one to three weeks. In outbreaks of hemolytic streptococcal infections which have been studied carefully, 2 to 5 per cent of those infected subsequently developed acute rheumatic fever.

The first attack of rheumatic fever occurs most frequently in children between six and eight years of age, and recurrences are most likely to occur before puberty. The chance of further attacks diminishes progressively as the child grows older and as the interval following the previous attack lengthens. While susceptibility to rheumatic fever is a familial characteristic, its prevalence is increased under overcrowded housing conditions, and the disease and its aftereffects are found more often in urban areas than in suburban and rural districts. Rheumatic fever is most prevalent in the northern and central states along the Atlantic Coast and in some of the Rocky Mountain states, although it occurs with sufficient frequency in the South to merit attention there as well.

The trend in mortality from rheumatic fever and heart disease in children has been steadily downward since the first statistics of any reliability became available about 1920 (10). The mortality rate among children from five through nineteen years of age decreased to half its former level in the two decades following that date. The rate of decline accelerated after 1940, with another 50 per cent decrease occurring during the following decade alone. There is no indication that the saving of lives has resulted merely in a shift of the problem to one of increased prevalence of heart disease among the survivors. On the contrary, a number of recent surveys have shown a relatively low prevalence of rheumatic heart disease and acute rheumatic fever. Whereas most surveys in areas of medium to high mortality have previously shown a prevalence of rheumatic heart disease of 1 to 2 per cent among school children in the higher grades, some of the more recent surveys have disclosed less than 0.5 per cent in these groups (11).

The factors responsible for the sharp decline in rheumatic fever mortality and the probable decline in rheumatic fever incidence can only be surmised. The intimate association between rheumatic fever and hemolytic streptococcal infections suggests that whatever factors were responsible for the decline in the severity, and possibly the incidence of, the latter may have played a similar role in relation to rheumatic fever. The general rise in living standards, including improved nutrition and housing, is probably concerned in this. The accelerated rate of decline since 1940 is probably due in part to the development and application of improved methods of prevention and treatment of hemolytic streptococcal infections and of rheumatic fever itself.

Many nonspecific measures, such as maintenance of an adequate diet and others of a general hygienic nature, contribute to the prevention of the initial attack of rheumatic fever, emphasizing the importance of adequate health supervision of children in families having a history of rheumatic fever. In such families, special efforts should also be made to reduce the amount of exposure to hemolytic streptococcal infections. Such measures are admittedly applicable to only a limited extent even in rheumatic families. Specific prophylaxis against hemolytic streptococcal infection in the population at large is not justified. Sulfa drugs cannot be used for the purpose because of the development of sulfa-resistant strains of streptococci, and penicillin is ruled out because of its expense. The prevention of rheumatic fever through intensive treatment of streptococcal infections with penicillin immediately after their onset has been advocated for this purpose (12). The availability of long-acting penicillin preparations makes this a practical procedure.

Although rheumatic fever has been characterized as an obsolescent disease, community efforts based on recent developments can greatly accelerate the rate of its decline and prevent much disability that would otherwise carry over into adult life for some time to come. A community approach to the problem of rheumatic fever in childhood is needed because of the inherent difficulties in its diagnosis, in the prolonged care needed, and in the number of individuals and community agencies involved in follow-up. The changing nature of the disease in recent years also necessitates continued professional and public health education. Furthermore, rheumatic fever tends to be concentrated in those segments of the population least able to bear the burden of the medical and social care required.

Detection and Diagnosis. Early discovery of children with rheumatic fever permits prompt treatment which may minimize or prevent permanent cardiac damage. This requires the prompt examination of all children who do not appear well, even though their symptoms may not be characteristic of rheumatic fever. Medical screening of these children in the schools, as well as children who return to school after illnesses of an indefinite nature, is an effective method of early case finding. This can be facilitated by careful teacher and nurse observation of children who do not appear well.

Although major attention should be paid to the discovery of children with active rheumatic fever, the child with a heart murmur often receives greater attention in many localities. The overwhelming majority of heart murmurs in childhood are of no significance to the health of the child. Careful examination of groups of children has shown that more than 50 per cent have so-called functional murmurs or other innocent cardiac sounds (13). When heart murmurs of doubtful significance are discovered on routine examination, every effort should be made to determine their nature without arousing apprehension in the parents. Indiscriminate follow-up of children with heart murmurs of doubtful significance, for fear that an occasional child may have progressive cardiac disease, will do relatively greater damage to the much larger number of children with insignificant murmurs. Removal of the false label of organic heart disease in children assumes great importance in any community program. It is often hard to persuade parents to a contrary opinion when they are convinced that their children have heart disease, but neglect to do so may result in a fixed anxiety more disabling to the individual than even a fairly severe organic heart disease.

Even after a careful medical appraisal by a well-trained physician, with full use of the erythrocyte sedimentation rate determinations and other laboratory studies, and of electrocardiography and fluoroscopy, a child may have to be seen several times before a definite diagnosis can be reached. Similarly, it is often difficult to be sure when the active rheumatic fever has subsided. For these reasons, diagnostic and consultation services are a prominent part of any community rheumatic fever program. By itself, however, a children's rheumatic fever or heart clinic should not be thought of as a community program. "An irreducible minimum for a new program must include adequate follow-up services to insure that a diagnosis is made insofar as possible, that recommendations for the care of patients are carried out, and that patients are not lost after diagnosis." (14)

Treatment and Aftercare. The basis for the treatment of a child with active rheumatic fever is bed rest; this may be provided in the child's home, in a general hospital, in a special hospital or convalescent institution, or in a foster home, depending on the patient's medical and social condition and upon available facilities in the community. Wherever care is provided, special precautions must be taken to protect the patient against exposure to fresh hemolytic streptococcal infections, which may light up the rheumatic fever, and to the prompt and energetic treatment of such streptococcal infections when they occur. The value of ACTH and cortisone, in relation to salicylates or to bed rest alone, in suppressing the active rheumatic process, and in preventing residual cardiac damage, is still a controversial question.

At the end of the convalescent period, careful follow-up must be instituted to protect the child against recurrences of the disease and to restore him to the maximum physical activities permitted by his condition. Many community programs provide periodic health appraisal in special clinics for children who have no family physicians or for whom the latter requests such service. Facilities may also be provided in the program for administration of a sulfa drug or antibiotic throughout the year or during the winter and spring months as prophylaxis against hemolytic streptococcal infections. Sulfadiazine has the advantages of low cost and ease of administration (12). When sufficient funds are available, some prefer to use oral penicillin because of its low toxicity. The antibiotic may be provided free or at reduced cost through community programs to children who remain under the supervision of family physicians (15). The availability of a long-acting repository penicillin preparation which gives detectable blood levels a month after a single injection may combine the advantages of low toxicity and low cost, and injections at monthly intervals may not prove to be a significant objection (16).

Once all evidence of rheumatic activity is over, a medical determination must be made of the amount of physical activity permitted the child. When the child is allowed full activity or when only competitive sports are prohibited, both parents and child should be encouraged to take this recommendation at face value rather than continuing limited activities "to be on the safe side." Delay in returning to normal activities may result in permanent fear and invalidism on the child's part. Health services in the schools can play a particularly important role in this aspect of aftercare.

CONGENITAL CARDIOVASCULAR DISEASE

The outlook for a normal life for children with several types of serious congenital anomalies of the heart and great vessels has improved markedly as a result of rapid advances in diagnostic methods and surgical treatment. Cardiac surgery has progressed to the point of relieving pulmonary stenosis by intracardiac attack upon the stenotic area (17). While the prevalence of these conditions has probably not changed, a community approach to the problem is now possible which has resulted in a heightened demand for services. A special grant of Children's Bureau funds finances care for a limited number of children in selected centers in different parts of the country, when these children cannot obtain the services through other means.

In many children with anomalies that do not cause cyanosis, the condition is suspected only on medical examination. In some cases the child may present no symptoms until irreversible damage has occurred; yet the condition could have been readily detected by simple means. The finding of diminished pulsation on palpation of the femoral artery raises a strong suspicion of the presence of coarctation of the aorta. Similarly, cardiac murmurs due to congenital lesions are usually easy to differentiate from innocent murmurs and sounds.

The major diagnostic problems are the differentiation of congenital lesions from rheumatic heart disease and the determination of the type of congenital lesion present. Diagnostic and consultation clinics and other services, set up initially as part of a rheumatic fever program, have proved very helpful in overcoming these difficulties. Such clinics are especially useful in separating out children whose condition definitely cannot be ameliorated by surgery from those who may benefit from such treatment. With the passage of time, the proportion of children with congenital cardiovascular anomalies seen in these clinics has tended to increase, with children with congenital lesions constituting more than 50 per cent of the total number with organic lesions in many areas (11).

This is due to the probable decline in the occurrence of rheumatic fever and the simultaneous increase in interest in congenital heart disease.

The definitive diagnosis of the nature of the congenital heart lesion often requires complicated procedures such as cardiac catheterization and angiocardiography. As a result, the complete evaluation of a child with congenital heart disease is available in comparatively few medical centers, generally those in which surgical treatment is also provided. Since these centers can handle only a limited number of children, it is the responsibility of local services to eliminate those children with clearly nonoperable conditions.

SUBACUTE BACTERIAL ENDOCARDITIS

Subacute bacterial endocarditis in children, usually due to *Streptococcus viridans,* is almost always superimposed on preexisting rheumatic or congenital lesions. Until the advent of the era of sulfonamides and antibiotics, a fatal outcome was the rule. Since then, well over 90 per cent of those affected recover from the infection, but many succumb later or are severely handicapped from the scars of the bacterial infection, especially when the condition is not discovered early and treated promptly (18).

The child health program can help overcome this problem by promoting adequate preventive measures. *Streptococcus viridans* is frequently found in the blood stream after surgical procedures, especially tooth extractions and operations on the nose or throat. In children known to have rheumatic heart disease or congenital cardiovascular anomalies, an antibiotic should be used before and for a few days after surgical procedures to minimize the possibility of the subsequent development of bacterial endocarditis. Since it is not practical to require a general health appraisal before every minor surgical procedure, parents may be given cards to present to their children's dentists or to physicians not aware of their medical background, prior to such procedures. On these cards, a statement signed by the physician knowing the cardiac status of the child recommends the prophylactic use of the antibiotic.

ORTHOPEDIC PROBLEMS

Orthopedic problems of childhood, originally the only conditions covered under "crippled children's" programs, consist of a varied group of neuromuscular conditions. Of the milder conditions in this group, flat feet and simple postural defects are the most common. Poliomyelitis and cerebral palsy are responsible for the majority of the more severe handicaps. Serious disabilities from rickets and from tuberculous and suppurative infections of the bones and joints, which filled children's orthopedic hospital services in former years, have become of minor importance. On the other hand, outbreaks of poliomyelitis have tended to increase in frequency and severity.

The general discussion of the needs and services common to children with special problems is most specifically and completely applicable to the children with conditions of an orthopedic nature. The causes of orthopedic conditions run the gamut of genetic, congenital, infectious, nutritional, and traumatic factors. Similarly, elimination of these causative factors, in so far as this is possible, requires few measures which have not been brought out in other phases of the total health program for children.

The early discovery and treatment of orthopedic conditions deserve further emphasis as a means of preventing the development of more severe and possibly irreversible handicaps. Congenital club foot and dislocation of the hip have been cited as examples of conditions in which early nonsurgical treatment is of the utmost value. The same concept applies to less serious but far more frequent conditions. Too often, search for these conditions is postponed until school age when they have progressed and are much less amenable to treatment. If the significance of pronated feet and the resultant wearing down of the inner portion of the heels of the shoes is appreciated, simple measures such as wedging of the shoes can help prevent progression by making the child use his feet in the correct position.

Children of school age with functional postural problems are in particular need of an adequate health appraisal prior to measures directed specifically at the posture. Poor posture is frequently only one feature in a child of low vitality, in whom malnutrition, emotional problems, and poor general health habits all play a part. Rarely is specific orthopedic consultation needed for these children; if so-called posture clinics are held in the schools, the children to be seen should be selected only after screening by the school physician. Progressively poor posture due to spinal curvature in preadolescent and adolescent children, on the other hand, is of great significance and warrants intensive follow-up and possible surgical treatment.

Postpoliomyelitic Handicaps. The epidemic nature of poliomyelitis sets it apart from other causes of orthopedic problems. Whereas congenital and traumatic factors tend to operate fairly uniformly in different localities over a period of time, the impact of poliomyelitis in a given locality and year is unpredictable. In the presence of an outbreak, available facilities are likely to be severely overtaxed; conversely, in a long period between epidemic years, hospitals and convalescent institutions specializing in the care of children with postpoliomyelitic handicaps may function inefficiently because of a low census, especially if they serve a limited geographic area. For a full decade starting in the late 1930's, poliomyelitis and its aftereffects stood out sharply from other special health problems in childhood in another respect; the heavy financial aid for poliomyelitis patients given by governmental health services and by the National Foundation for Infantile Paralysis and other voluntary health agencies was not duplicated until much later for children with other conditions.

The erratic epidemic character of poliomyelitis requires a high degree of community planning to be prepared for any sudden need. A representative committee, in which practicing physicians take an active part, can accomplish more than isolated agencies. It can more easily influence general hospitals to admit patients with poliomyelitis in the acute stage, if these hospitals have followed a contrary policy. It can maintain a registry of inactive nurses and physical therapists who are willing to serve in an emergency. By developing temporary foster placement for children with less urgent chronic conditions in special institutions, additional facilities can be provided for children convalescing from poliomyelitis.

Since even the best prepared community cannot cope with an outbreak of major proportions, planning should also proceed on a regional or state basis (19). Broad geographical planning helps prevent wasteful expenditures for local facilities which may be used rarely. For example, depots of respirators may be maintained for shipment on a moment's notice, perhaps even accompanied by a skilled operator. Respirator centers have been developed in which groups of patients with respiratory difficulties may be given efficient care with greater chances of being rehabilitated after being weaned from the respirator.

The outlook for recovery from poliomyelitis varies with the care rendered. Local studies have shown that about 55 per cent of those recovering from clinically diagnosable poliomyelitis have no residual involvement, slight residual paralysis is found in about 25 per cent, and moderate to marked involvement in the remainder (20). The case fatality rates in various epidemics have varied from 3 to 10 per cent. The importance of bed rest in the early convalescent stages has been stressed as a means of preventing muscle weakness and pathological gaits (21). Under adequate care from the start of the illness, it is probable that only about 15 per cent of all patients have any permanent disability.

Recent trends have altered the approach to children with poliomyelitis. Hot packs are used over the affected muscles in the acute phase of the disease, and manipulation is resorted to at an earlier stage. An increasing proportion of children with nonparalytic disease or minor involvement is being cared for at home by choice during the acute stage, with hospital care available if needed (22). The family physician may be relieved of the need to suggest hospitalization for diagnostic purposes if the local health department makes the services of consultants available for those to whom such services are not otherwise readily available. The provision of nursing and physical therapy services in the home during the acute stage of the disease and of the latter on an outpatient basis during the convalescent and chronic stages further reduces the need for hospitalization in selected cases. The formerly widely accepted view that a period of one to two years must elapse before any surgical treatment is attempted is giving way to early surgery in selected cases. Prolonged stay in hospitals or special institutions followed by occasional medical checkups thereafter is also a questionable procedure. "It is better to hospitalize the child for a shorter period initially and to readmit him at regular intervals for short periods of evaluation, specific treatment, fitting and instruction in use of apparatus and reinstruction of parents. It is only when faulty or inadequate care is given (at home) that long periods of hospitalization are necessary." (23)

A major function of a community program is the long-term follow-up of children who have had poliomyelitis until their full growth has been reached. Assistance may be offered to practicing physicians by having physical therapists perform muscle testing at their request. Long after the condition of the child has apparently been stabilized, his functioning ability may become worse as a result of muscular incoordination. A severe spinal curvature may develop in a child who had what was considered to be nonparalytic poliomyelitis.

Cerebral Palsy. In the group of orthopedic conditions when broadly defined, the subgroup included under cerebral palsy warrants separate consideration because of the size of the problem and because of the prolonged and complicated services needed in most cases. The term pertains to all varieties of motor disabilities due to disturbances in the motor centers of the brain; as commonly used, it refers to conditions which had their onset during infancy and childhood. Although any of the causative factors previously discussed may produce cerebral palsy, those operating immediately before and during birth are probably the most important. Spasticity, muscular rigidity and tremors, athetoid movements, and ataxia are the clinical manifestations predominant in affected children; birth trauma or postnatal infections of the central nervous system have been found in association with almost one-third of a series of asymmetric spastic cases, whereas these factors were not implicated in the other types studied (24).

The prevalence of cerebral palsy, according to data obtained from a survey in a single county in New York State, has been found to be 5.8 per 1,000 children in the age group five through fourteen years (25). A lower prevalence rate was found in younger children, presumably because of underdiagnosis or concealment. Of those under twenty years of age, it was found that about 10 per cent would probably benefit from a period of hospital care, about 17 per cent needed chronic institutional care with little hope of improvement, an additional 67 per cent could be served through outpatient facilities; the remainder had such mild cases as to require no special medical or habilitative services. Other surveys have disclosed somewhat lower prevalence rates than the one found in New York State.

Children with cerebral palsy present a diversity of problems. In addition to disabilities of speech, a severe acoustic or visual impairment may be present. In a recent study, 50 per cent of the children with cerebral palsy were found to be mentally deficient and nearly three-fourths were of below-average intelligence (26). Convulsive seizures are found more often in children who are not considered educable. The motor difficulties may conceal a low-grade intelligence or, conversely, they may discourage efforts to assist children who are falsely considered to be mentally defective.

Cerebral palsy can be suspected and diagnosed in most cases before the infant reaches his first birthday. "If the condition is treated from infancy much of the deformity associated with spastic forms of the disease can be prevented." (27) Since there is no screening test available, early case finding is dependent upon the alertness of the physician in health supervision of the presumably normal infant. "Ordinarily the physician in general practice, because of his early contact with these infants, will first be in position to suspect the diagnosis. The general practitioner should assume a leading role in diagnosing cerebral palsy and in the all-important job of parent counseling." (28)

Adequate evaluation and effective treatment can scarcely be provided for most children with cerebral palsy without a multidisciplinary approach of a number of medical specialists with particular interest and training in cerebral palsy. Similarly, physical, occupational, and speech therapists, under medical direction, have important contributions to make as members of the team in habilitation of these children. The voluntary health agencies interested in cerebral palsy have promoted or financed special diagnostic and treatment centers and classes for cerebral palsied children alone. While this has resulted in more extensive services for these children, it has also tended to keep them isolated from activities in regular schools and even from other groups of handicapped children.

Muscular Dystrophy. This is a group of chronic familial conditions of unknown etiology usually having their onset in early childhood, characterized by progressive muscular weakness with a fatal termination from intercurrent infection due to respiratory embarassment, sometimes two or more decades after the onset (29). Prevention of contractures and maximal physical activity help retard the rate of development of disability. Increasing public interest and financial support raise the hope that methods of treating and rehabilitating affected children will become available.

EPILEPSY

Epilepsy is a health problem deserving a high priority in the community attack upon handicapping conditions of childhood. The problem is vast; the condition is present in about 1 in every 200 young adults, according to minimal selective service figures from two world wars. Effective methods of diagnosis and treatment are available (30), and there are no insuperable barriers to their broadest application. Without care, the child, and later the adult, becomes a serious burden to his family and community. With adequate care, including attention to the serious emotional problems involved in the adjustment of the children with epilepsy, 70 to 85 per cent of epileptic persons can be as useful as if their condition did not exist. The chief obstacle to normal adjustment of the epileptic patient is the mistaken attitude of the public which sharply impedes integration of the epileptic child in the school and community and which later prevents him from obtaining employment, often even of a type far below his capabilities. This public attitude can be overcome through community health education. Finally, the cost of providing care for children with epilepsy is very small in relation to the returns involved, especially in comparison with some other special problems of childhood. In spite of these compelling reasons, interest in the problem of epilepsy has been slow in developing (31).

Epilepsy is predominantly a childhood problem; of a group of children fifteen years of age or over with epilepsy, 60 per cent have their first seizure before four years of age (32). The two main types of seizures in childhood are *grand mal* and *petit mal,* the former being the popularly known episode of convulsions with loss of consciousness, and the latter a brief interruption of consciousness without convulsions. Only a small proportion of epileptic children are mentally defective, and it is estimated that less than 5 per cent of all epileptic persons need chronic institutional care. The relative importance of hereditary factors and brain injury in the causation of epilepsy is not well understood; the genetic factor is probably operative in only a small minority of affected children.

Diagnosis and Treatment. Since no screening device exists for the discovery of epilepsy applicable on a mass scale, early discovery depends upon the alertness to episodes suggestive of epilepsy on the part of the family physician, aided by parents, teachers, and others in close association with children. Electroencephalography, which records the electrical patterns of the brain, is particularly helpful in the diagnosis of petit mal episodes, but it cannot be used for mass screening because of its expense and because many individuals without seizures of any kind show abnormal electroencephalographic patterns.

Examination of the child should include psychometric testing and evaluation of his emotional adjustment. Management of any emotional disturbances will be dependent upon whether they are due to an organic lesion, possibly the same one underlying the seizures, or whether they represent an emotional reaction to the epilepsy and to parental handling of the child (33).

For those children whose condition cannot readily be diagnosed and brought under control through measures available to the family physician, central clinics have been established in some areas to provide adequate diagnostic studies including electroencephalography. In these clinics, various types and dosages of drugs to control the seizures are tried until the most suitable treatment for the individual child is found. A complete report of the diagnostic and therapeutic studies is sent to the family physician who continues regular supervision of the child, aided by the public health nurse in the area. Since the condition of the child may change and the maintenance dosage of the drugs may have to be modified accordingly, these clinics usually make themselves freely available to physicians for further consultation either by mail or telephone. This type of consultation may be sufficient for further care of the child in many instances. If more detailed reevaluation is needed, the child may be returned to the clinic for the purpose.

Most diagnostic and treatment services for epileptic children can be provided on an ambulatory basis, and an adequately staffed and functioning clinic service conserves funds that would otherwise have to be spent for hospitalization for diagnostic studies. Surgical removal of a localized, irritative focus responsible for the epilepsy should be considered for the small proportion of children who fail to respond to anticonvulsant medication (34). Financing of this type of surgical care and needed follow-up services may be provided through a community program.

Rehabilitation of epileptic children must include measures for overcoming the social and emotional handicaps associated with the condition. Exaggerated parental concerns and the withdrawal of the affected child may otherwise nullify the benefits of successful control of seizures. Where epilepsy clinic centers exist, they are convenient places in which to evaluate the social and emotional difficulties of the epileptic child and to institute measures which will alleviate parental concern and pave the way for acceptance of the child in the school and community.

CLEFT PALATE AND LIP

Congenital clefts of the palate and lip are found in about 1 out of every 800 live births. The condition ranges in severity from an insignificant cleft of the soft palate to a serious deformity involving both sides of the entire upper jaw with marked facial disfigurement and dental distortion. Various degrees of feeding and speech difficulties are present in all but the mildest types of malformation, and hearing impairment is a frequent complication.

The outlook for complete rehabilitation of the child with a cleft palate is excellent when he has the advantages of the well-developed clinical and rehabilitative techniques in this field. This is in sharp contrast to the situation formerly prevailing, when attention was focused on correction of the anatomical defect in the palate, without proper consideration of speech development or dental alignment (35). The needed services are complicated, calling upon the contributions of a diversified group of specialists, and must be spread over a period from the early days of life through adolescence (36). Even when families can afford the expense involved, they may not know what is needed and in only a few communities can they find the needed services available. Having these services available at the time the child needs them, and follow-up to ensure their use, must be a community responsibility.

All children with cleft palate, except those whose cleft is covered with mucous membrane, may be located during the newborn period through even a cursory health appraisal. Whenever possible, the clinical condition of the child should be evaluated by a team of specialists soon after discovery and a plan of management developed; the child with a cleft palate has already been cited as exemplifying the needs of all handicapped children in this respect. The cleft in the lip, when present, is usually repaired by plastic surgery during the first few months of life. Surgical closure of the palatal defect is generally deferred until late in the preschool period; in some instances, surgery may be rejected in favor of continued use of a prosthetic appliance to close the gap without interfering with speech development or with growth of the oral structures. Orthodontic treatment is often needed during the school years.

In addition to specific medical and dental care, the child with cleft palate needs rehabilitative services to help him overcome the social and emotional handicaps resulting from peculiarities in speech and cosmetic effects when the deformity is visible. Speech training should be started soon after surgical treatment. When care has been adequate in the preschool and early school years, there will be little need for vocational guidance and rehabilitation services later on. When difficulties in speech or social adjustment persist in adolescence, vocational services are of the utmost importance.

MALIGNANT DISEASE

The problem of cancer in childhood has come to the fore with the decline in other causes of disease and death. As with other disease problems affecting the population as a whole, this interest has been developing simultaneously among those whose primary concern has been with children and those leading the attack on cancer as a disease problem. The joint concern of the two groups has been expressed in the Children's Tumor Registry, sponsored by the American Academy of Pediatrics, which is maintained at the Memorial Hospital, a specialized institution located in New York City for the study and treatment of cancer patients of all ages (37). The Registry serves the threefold purpose of providing consultant services for physicians from all parts of the country, accumulating information on cancer in childhood, and conducting professional and public education on the problem.

Cancer may develop at any time of life; the death rate from cancer is higher before five years of age than during the later periods of childhood. Although all parts of the body may be affected, cancer originates in childhood mainly in the reticuloendothelial system, the central nervous system, the kidney, the eye, and the bones. In the leukemias and other malignant conditions of the reticuloendothelial system, only palliative measures are available, although there is hope that early detection may permit of cure with the newer agents already shown to be of great palliative value (38). In other forms of cancer, early discovery, followed by prompt treatment by surgery and radiotherapy, results in a high proportion of recoveries.

The causes and methods of prevention of childhood cancer are largely matters for future research. The major contribution to be made by the child health program is the early discovery of suspected cases of those types of malignant disease for which effective treatment is already available. In mixed or Wilms' tumor of the kidney, the outlook for cure is found to be far better in infants under one year of age than in older children, even though no difference can be shown in the grade of malignancy in tumors occurring in various age groups. "It is quite possible that the better outlook for babies is related to the fact that infants are examined more often by physicians and that they are handled more frequently by the mother who bathes, changes, and otherwise cares for them; it is quite probable that these lead to earlier detection of intra-abdominal masses." (39) Continuation of adequate health supervision beyond the first birthday would probably improve the outlook in older children as well.

For definitive diagnosis and treatment of suspected malignancy in children, reliance must be placed on facilities which are beyond the scope of the child health program as such. Special units are being developed for children in cancer hospitals, aided by funds from national voluntary health agencies. When the malignant condition itself or necessary treatment results in some permanent handicap, such as amputation of an extremity, the usual rehabilitative services in the community are called into play.

DIABETES MELLITUS

Although diabetes mellitus is mainly a problem of the older age group, it is not infrequent in childhood and has been reported in infants. About 8 per cent in one series of diabetic patients of all ages had their onset before twenty years of age (40). The National Health Survey of 1936 revealed a prevalence of diabetes of 1 in 2,500 children under fifteen years of age; a higher prevalence rate in childhood probably would be found today as a result of improved diagnosis and longer survival of children with the disease.

Juvenile diabetes usually presents a clinical picture and course markedly different from the disease in adult life. The onset tends to be sudden, often precipitated by an infection, and the progression of symptoms tends to be more rapid. The severity of the disease, the need to obtain the cooperation of the child in maintaining the prescribed diet and in administering insulin, and the varying need for insulin as a result of intermittent physical activity are factors making the disease more difficult to control in childhood. Yet the disease must be kept under control to reduce the chances of coma and to postpone the development of vascular changes and of loss of vision (41).

As in the case of rheumatic fever, juvenile diabetes is most readily found by the prompt examination of children who show deviations from good health, especially when the change has been noted to follow an infection. Routine screening tests of blood or urine are far less productive in children than in adults, mainly because the disease does not usually remain asymptomatic for long after its onset. Even so, one mass survey of school children uncovered 18 previously unknown diabetic children among 38,500 children tested (42).

The health services in the schools should pay special attention to diabetic children, requiring instructions from the family physician about handling of any emergencies. Effort is needed to help the child participate in all activities to prevent him from feeling different from other children. Apart from the school health program, the public health nurse may be helpful in applying the physician's recommendations in the home. A consultant nutritionist is usually needed to assist the public health nurse in implementing the details of dietary management recommended by the physician.

CITED REFERENCES

1. GARDNER, WARREN H., chairman, Committee on Hard of Hearing Children, Reprint No. 227, American Hearing Society, from *Hearing News*, February–May, 1950.
2. LESSER, ARTHUR J., "Services for the Child Who Is Hard of Hearing; A Guide for the Development of Programs," Publication No. 334, Children's Bureau, Washington, D.C., 1950.
3. HUIZING, HENK C., and DOREEN POLLACK, Effects of Limited Hearing on the Development of Speech in Children under Three Years of Age, *Pediatrics*, Vol. 8, pp. 53–58, July, 1951.
4. MYKLEBUST, HELMER R., Differential Diagnosis of Deafness in Young Children, *J. Exceptional Children*, Vol. 17, pp. 97–101, January, 1951.
5. GARLAND, L. H., H. A. HILL, M. E. MOTTRAM, and M. A. SISSON, Nasopharyngeal Irradiation: Relative Merits of Roentgen and Radium Therapy for Benign Conditions, *J.A.M.A.*, Vol. 146, pp. 454–460, June 2, 1951.
6. HAYMAN, CHARLES R., BENJAMIN S. RICH, and ELEANOR STARK, A Conservation of Hearing Program for School Children: Review of Three Year Experience in Harford County, Maryland, *Am. J. Pub. Health*, Vol. 41, pp. 1509–1520, December, 1951.
7. FORTUNE, GEORGE J., A Community Welfare Agency and a University Coöperating in a Speech and Hearing Program, *Am. J. Pub. Health*, Vol. 41, pp. 1390–1394, November, 1951.
8. CRANE, MARIAN M., RICHARD G. SCOBEE, FRANKLIN M. FOOTE, and EARL L. GREEN, Study of Procedures Used for Screening Elementary School Children for Visual Defects: Referrals by Screening Procedures versus Ophthalmological Findings, *Am. J. Pub. Health*, Vol. 42, pp. 1430–1439, November, 1952.
9. KERBY, C. EDITH, Causes and Prevention of Blindness in Children, Publication No. 110, National Society for the Prevention of Blindness, Reprint from *The Sight-saving Rev.*, Vol. 20, pp. 67–80, Summer, 1950.

10. WOLFF, GEORGE, Death Toll from Rheumatic Fever in Childhood, *J.A.M.A.,* Vol. 145, pp. 719–724, Mar. 10, 1951.

11. GARDINER, J. H., and JOHN D. KEITH, Prevalence of Heart Disease in Toronto Children: 1948–1949 Cardiac Registry, *Pediatrics,* Vol. 7, pp. 713–721, May, 1951.

12. The Prevention of Rheumatic Fever, Statement of the Committee on Prevention of Rheumatic Fever of the Council on Rheumatic Fever and Congenital Heart Disease of the American Heart Association, *Pub. Health Rep.,* Vol. 68, pp. 12–15, January, 1953.

13. FRIEDMAN, SIDNEY, WILLIAM A. ROBIE, and T. N. HARRIS, Occurrence of Innocent Adventitious Cardiac Sounds in Childhood, *Pediatrics,* Vol. 4, pp. 782–789, December, 1949.

14. "Guide for Local Rheumatic Fever Programs," New York State Department of Health, Albany, N.Y., 1949.

15. SMITH, MARY A., A Community Program for the Prevention of Rheumatic Fever Recurrence, *Pub. Health Rep.,* Vol. 68, pp. 16–19, January, 1953.

16. STOLLERMAN, GENE H., and JEROME H. RUSOFF, Prophylaxis against Group A Streptococcal Infections in Rheumatic Fever Patients: Use of New Repository Penicillin Preparation, *J.A.M.A.,* Vol. 150, pp. 1571–1575, Dec. 20, 1952.

17. DRY, THOMAS J., Present Status of Surgical Treatment for Cardiac Diseases, *J.A.M.A.,* Vol. 150, pp. 19–24, Sept. 6, 1952.

18. Treatment of Subacute Bacterial Endocarditis, editorial, *J.A.M.A.,* Vol. 145, pp. 734–735, Mar. 10, 1951.

19. Coordinated State Planning to Combat Poliomyelitis: A Suggested Guide for Use by State Poliomyelitis Planning Committees, *Child,* Vol. 14, pp. 41–42, September, 1949.

20. LENHARD RAYMOND E., Prognosis in Poliomyelitis, *J. Bone & Joint Surgery,* Vol. 32, pp. 71–79, January, 1950.

21. GREEN, WALLACE, Importance of Rest in the Treatment of Early Convalescent Poliomyelitis, *Am. J. Dis. Child.,* Vol. 33, pp. 4–7, January, 1952.

22. STIMSON, PHILIP M., Home Care of Patients with Acute Poliomyelitis, *J.A.M.A.,* Vol. 149, pp. 719–721, June 21, 1952.

23. BENNETT, ROBERT L., Care of Children Convalescing from Poliomyelitis: Discussion of Several Points of Controversy, *J.A.M.A.,* Vol. 144, pp. 377–379, Sept. 30, 1950.

24. YANNET, HERMAN, Infantile Cerebral Palsy Cases with Severe Mental Deficiency: Relationship of Etiology to Type of Neurological Syndrome, *Pediatrics,* Vol. 3, pp. 820–823, June, 1949.

25. "Report of the New York State Joint Legislative Committee to Study the Problem of Cerebral Palsy," Legislative Document No. 55, Albany, N.Y., 1949.

26. MILLER, ELSA, and GEORGE B. ROSENFELD, The Psychological Evaluation of Children with Cerebral Palsy and Its Implications in Treatment: Preliminary Report. *J. Pediat.*, Vol. 41, pp. 613–621, November, 1952.

27. PERLSTEIN, MEYER A., and HARRY E. BARNETT, Nature and Recognition of Cerebral Palsy in Infancy, *J.A.M.A.*, Vol. 148, pp. 1389–1397, Apr. 19, 1952.

28. FULDNER, RUSSELL V., Physical Examination of the Cerebral Palsied Child, *J. A. M.A.*, Vol. 148, pp. 34–41, Jan. 5, 1952.

29. RAMSEY, ROBERT H., and H. R. McCARROLL, Problem of Muscular Dystrophies, *J.A.M.A.*, Vol. 150, pp. 659–662, Oct. 18, 1952.

30. YAHR, MELVIN D., DANIEL SCIARRA, SIDNEY CARTER, and H. HOUSTON MERRITT, Evaluation of Standard Anticonvulsant Therapy in Three Hundred Nineteen Patients, *J.A.M.A.*, Vol. 150, pp. 663–667, Oct. 18, 1952.

31. BALDWIN, RUTH, EDWARD DAVENS, and VIRGINIA G. HARRIS, The Epilepsy Program in Public Health, *Am. J. Pub. Health*, Vol. 43, pp. 452–459, April, 1953.

32. BRIDGE, EDWARD M., "Epilepsy and Convulsive Disorders in Children," McGraw-Hill Book Company, Inc., New York, 1949.

33. BRADLEY, CHARLES, Behavior Disturbances in Epileptic Children, *J.A.M.A.*, Vol. 146, pp. 436–441, June 2, 1951.

34. Surgical Treatment of Focal Epilepsy, editorial, *J.A.M.A.*, Vol. 146, p. 820, June 30, 1951.

35. GRABER, T. M., Changing Philosophies in Cleft Palate Management, *J. Pediat.*, Vol. 37, pp. 400–415, September, 1950.

36. COURSIN, DAVID B., Treatment of the Patient with Cleft Palate: Present Day Concepts of a Pediatric Responsibility, *Am. J. Dis. Child.*, Vol. 80, pp. 442–453, September, 1950.

37. Children's Tumor Registry, *J. Pediat.*, Vol. 21, p. 703, November, 1942.

38. CRAVER, LLOYD F., "Value of Early Diagnosis of Malignant Lymphomas and Leukemias: A Monograph for the Physician," American Cancer Society, New York, 1952.

39. GROSS, ROBERT E., and EDWARD B. D. NEUHAUSER, Treatment of Mixed Tumors of the Kidney in Childhood, *Pediatrics*, Vol. 6, pp. 843–852, December, 1950.

40. JOHN, HENRY J., Diabetes Mellitus in Children: Review of 500 Cases, *J. Pediat.*, Vol. 35, pp. 723–744, December, 1949.

41. GRAYZEL, HAROLD G., and HYMAN B. WARSHALL, Clinical Survey of Vascular Complications in "Juvenile Diabetes Mellitus," *Pediatrics*, Vol. 8, pp. 506–512, October, 1951.

42. SHARKEY, THOMAS P., PAUL TROUP, RICHARD MILLER, H. C. VAN KIRK, ROBERT FREEMAN, and H. H. WILLIAMS, Diabetes Detection Drive in Dayton, Ohio, *J.A.M.A.*, Vol. 144, pp. 914–919, Nov. 11, 1950.

ADDITIONAL REFERENCES

1. HARDY, WILLIAM G., "Children with Impaired Hearing: An Audiologic Perspective," Publication No. 326, Children's Bureau, Washington, D.C., 1952.
2. FOOTE, ROBERT M., Public Health Aspects of a Speech and Hearing Program, *J.A.M.A.*, Vol. 150, pp. 1390–1392, Dec. 6, 1952.
3. WOHLMAN, REGINE F., The Integrated Treatment of a Young Child with a Speech Disorder, *J. Pediat.*, Vol. 40, pp. 525–529, April, 1952.
4. LANCASTER, WALTER B., and FRANKLIN M. FOOTE, The Battle against Blindness, *J. A. M.A.*, Vol. 145, pp. 26–29, Jan. 6, 1951.
5. LOWENFELD, BERTHOLD, Meeting the Needs of Visually Handicapped Preschool Children, Publication No. 144, National Society for the Prevention of Blindness, Reprint from *The Sight-Saving Rev.*, Vol. 20, pp. 145–150, Fall, 1950.
6. "Program Guide for Heart Associations," American Heart Association, New York, 1952.
7. BLAND, EDWARD F., and T. DUCKETT JONES, Rheumatic Fever and Rheumatic Heart Disease: A Twenty Year Report on 1000 Patients Followed since Childhood, *Circulation*, Vol. 4, pp. 836–843, December, 1951.
8. THOMAS, LEWIS, "Rheumatic Fever: A Symposium," University of Minnesota Press, Minneapolis, Minn., 1952.
9. The General Hospital in the Poliomyelitis Program, series of articles in *Hospitals*, Vol. 25, pp. 37–60, March, 1951.
10. ABBOTT, LeROY C., The Orthopedic Care in Anterior Poliomyelitis, *J. Pediat.*, Vol. 39, pp. 663–671, December, 1951.
11. Symposium on Cerebral Palsy, *J. Pediat.*, Vol. 40, pp. 403–404, 489–524, 606–633, March, April, May, 1952.
12. DENHOFF, ERIC, and RAYMOND H. HOLDEN, Pediatric Aspects of Cerebral Palsy, *J. Pediat.*, Vol. 39, pp. 363–373, September, 1951.
13. MEERLOO, LUCY, and JOOST A. M. MEERLOO, Some Psychological Problems in Cerebral Palsy Children, *Quart. J. Child Behavior*, Vol. 2, pp. 381–389, October, 1950.
14. WISHIK, SAMUEL M., To Restore the Child with Cleft Palate: Professional and Community Teamwork Will Bring Success, *Child*, Vol. 15, pp. 141–143, April, 1951.
15. "Diagnosis of Congenital Cardiac Defects in General Practice," booklet, American Heart Association, New York, February, 1953.
16. BUFKIN, JESSIE H., and WILBURT C. DAVISON, Childhood Cancer (Tumors, Leukemia, and Hodgkin's Disease): A Review, *J. Pediat.*, Vol. 42, pp. 612–632, May, 1953.

22 CHILDREN WITH INTELLECTUAL, EMOTIONAL, AND SOCIAL HANDICAPS

The heterogeneous group of children with handicaps primarily of an intellectual, emotional, or social nature deserves consideration together because of the difficulty and undesirability of setting up fixed diagnostic categories to differentiate them from one another. There is no single tool, for example, for determining mental retardation. The widely used criterion of an IQ of 70 on the Stanford-Binet scale as the upper limit of feeble-mindedness has led, in years past, to the institutionalization of many children who could have been helped to a satisfactory adjustment in the home and community. A child who may be properly motivated toward the psychometric tests in the presence of emotional disturbances may be intellectually adequate. One child's emotional difficulties may come to attention in antisocial behavior under the heading of juvenile delinquency when he comes into conflict with the law. In another child, marked personality changes may occur, with withdrawal of the child into a world of his own, necessitating psychiatric hospitalization. It should be understood, therefore, that the headings used in this chapter, as in the previous separation of physical from other handicaps, are purely for convenience in presentation.

INTELLECTUAL HANDICAPS

The physician is confronted with children having all grades and types of intellectual handicaps in the course of his regular care of children.

Understanding the possible causes of such handicaps helps him gain parental acceptance of the potentialities and needs of these children. A certain proportion of the children with borderline intellectual capacity represent the lower end of the scale of normal variations in human intelligence on a hereditary basis (1). An additional number of children in this borderline or slightly lower group have suffered a relatively slight cerebral damage from the same types of causes responsible for the more severe degrees of handicaps. Marked mental retardation is probably always due to extensive organic damage or interference with the metabolism of the brain. Infections before or after birth, birth trauma in its broad sense, and erythroblastosis fetalis are examples of such causative factors.

The figure of 1 per cent has been commonly cited as the prevalence rate of intellectual handicap in the population as a whole, but this figure is meaningless unless the criteria on which it is based are known. Grouping by intelligence quotient has little bearing on the ultimate social outcome of children with intellectual impairment when they are given ample opportunities for development and proper vocational training. Trainable mental defective children can make as satisfactory an adjustment in adult life as other individuals (2). In certain clinical syndromes in which mental deficiency is present, more reliable quantitative data are available. The incidence of mongolism, for example, has been found to be 1.2 per 1,000 live births, with a rate of 2.9 per thousand children among premature infants as compared with 0.9 per thousand in infants born at term (3).

Early Discovery and Diagnosis. Early discovery of children with intellectual handicaps is important in helping the parents develop a plan of management for the child and in encouraging them to provide as much social stimulation for the mentally retarded child as possible. Early discovery is dependent to a large extent upon regular health supervision. Selected children, such as those who have a history of difficulty delivery or erythroblastosis fetalis, deserve more careful follow-up.

The more severe the handicap, the earlier will deviations from expected growth and development become manifest and the sooner will an adequate total evaluation of the child become possible. An adequate evaluation must take into consideration the possibilities of social adjustment and training of the child as well as his physical and intellectual status. Care must be taken to rule out hearing impairment and other communicative disorders and possible emotional factors. In some areas, facilities of child guidance clinics are made available to assist physicians in this evaluation, especially for infants and preschool children. For children of school age, an evaluation is generally done in the schools, with emphasis on the type of school placement needed by the child. Special diagnostic clinics with pediatricians, social workers, and psychologists with knowledge of intellectually handicapped children are being developed on an experimental basis in a few communities (4). Where these exist, they can be of the greatest help to family physicians and physicians in community clinics in arriving at an early evaluation of the child and in providing guidance for the parents of the affected child.

Treatment and Habilitative Services. Specific treatment of the condition underlying mental deficiency is rarely possible once the intellectual handicap has developed. The use of glutamic acid in bringing about a slight to moderate increase in the intellectual capacity of mentally defective children is still a highly controversial question (5). Medical care is needed to be sure that any associated conditions which may interfere with full use of the child's limited capacity are corrected to the greatest possible extent.

Children whose intellectual impairment is so severe as to preclude a reasonable adjustment with proper training are usually placed in special institutions under medical direction. A fair proportion even of these children can be trained to care for their own immediate wants. This is a worth-while objective, especially since the life span of so many of these individuals has been greatly increased as a result of effective treatment of infections formerly causing early death. Unfortunately, many institutions for mental defectives are crowded with untrainable adults, so that the staffs are unable to provide the attention needed by the children and there are long waiting lists for admission. Special institutions are also used for children with intermediate degrees of intellectual handicap, preliminary to placing them in occupations suitable to their mental level and general capabilities.

For children with lesser degrees of mental handicap, special classes are usually provided in the regular schools or adjustments may be made in regular classes. There has recently been increased pressure from groups of parents of intellectually handicapped children to provide special classes in regular schools for so-called uneducable children previously excluded from school.

EMOTIONALLY DISTURBED CHILDREN

In discussing the promotion of mental health in Chapter 9, it was pointed out that the less severe emotional problems in children and, indeed, many of the more pronounced problems would have to be handled without benefit of specialized psychiatric advice, if they were to receive any help at all. A shortage of psychiatrists trained to meet the emotional needs and problems of children exists throughout the country, and their services are lacking entirely in broad areas of many states. Nevertheless, significant progress is being made through demonstration programs and public education, to bring the needs before the public and in establishing community facilities for helping emotionally disturbed children. Expansion of facilities, limited mainly by shortages in professional personnel, has been greatly accelerated since passage of the National Mental Health Act in 1946.

The size of the problem of behavior disorders and other overt emotional disturbances of childhood is vast. Estimates of well over a million, or about 4 per cent, of children in the country being in this category (6) have been projections of local studies. Criteria for diagnosis vary widely, so that any such estimates must be accepted with strong reservations. To a large extent, it is also an academic question, since a much greater proportion of all children and their parents could benefit from the services of skilled professional personnel oriented in the dynamics of children's emotional needs and development, if such services could be provided.

Child Guidance Clinics. The children's mental health clinic, or child guidance clinic, is a widely accepted mechanism for the provision of specialized diagnostic and therapeutic services for emotionally disturbed children (7). It has also been used in many places to provide services for mentally deficient children and in the appraisal of children being placed out for adoption. The modern child guidance clinic has grown from a varied background. While the majority of new child guidance clinics are being developed as separate community entities, possibly as part of a mental health clinic serving all age groups, many are conducted in association with hospitals, juvenile courts, teacher-training institutions, and school systems. Their sponsorship and financial support are equally varied, with voluntary health agencies playing an important part in supplementing and promoting use of funds from official sources.

The child guidance clinic really treats the parent-child relationship, rather than the child himself. Apart from the ill-defined influence of heredity on personality make-up, and the direct causative relationship between brain damage and behavior disorders in certain instances, the child's personality develops largely as a result of his life experiences. His relationships with other persons, and mainly with his parents, form the matrix of these experiences. Contrary to the original concepts in the older child guidance clinics, the child participates actively in the therapeutic process. The child guidance clinic centers about the child's problem and does not aim at a basic change in the personality structure of either child or parent, although this may occur to some extent as a result of the clinic's services. It is probably true that treatment of the parents of young children with emotional disturbances would help clear up most of the problems of the children. This approach faces two major obstacles, namely, the unwillingness of many such parents to accept psychiatric care and the impossibility of providing the intensive treatment needed.

It is generally stated that a community of 100,000 or more population can support a child guidance clinic, even though this would be insufficient to meet even the more urgent demands for service. The pattern of organization of service in clinics established in regular quarters in the larger communities is fairly well standardized (8). The clinic team consists of at least three professional persons, the psychiatrist, the psychiatric social worker, and the psychologist, perhaps with a pediatrician, a public health nurse, or an additional social worker.

The psychiatrist acts as the clinic director and provides technical supervision over the other members of the clinic staff. He is ultimately responsible for the total diagnostic evaluation and plan of treatment, although these are usually evolved as a joint process of all team members. He usually provides the direct treatment services for the child. It has been found undesirable for the psychiatrist to perform the general medical examination of the child. This may be required before referral to the clinic or be performed by a pediatrician in the clinic.

The psychiatric social worker generally handles the intake procedures in the clinic, works with the mother in gaining her understanding and cooperation and in maintaining relationships with community agencies. She often assists in actual therapy under the immediate supervision of the psychiatrist. The clinical psychologist usually works only in the clinic, assisting in the total evaluation of the child by the use and interpretation of psychometric and projective tests and by diagnostic interviews; in some places, the psychologist may provide educational and vocational guidance and handle relationships with the schools as well. Where mental health nurses have been employed, she "chiefly has served in a liaison capacity for the clinic in its relationship with the existing community nursing groups in health activities." (9)

In several states, child guidance clinics are conducted in smaller communities on an itinerant basis, returning at intervals of one week to one month or even longer. Some of these provide only diagnostic services. Others attempt to provide whatever brief therapeutic experience is possible during the occasional visits (10). The full team of the community type of clinic may provide the itinerant services, or the team may consist of a psychiatrist and psychologist only, depending upon a local child welfare worker or public health nurse to prepare patients for admission and to follow up on the understandings reached at the clinic. Whatever success such itinerant clinics can achieve depends upon how deeply rooted and well accepted they are in the communities they serve.

The relationship of any child guidance clinic to the practicing physicians and other professional persons and agencies is a key to the clinic's effectiveness in a community. The most progressive clinics invite the referring physician to attend case conferences, or the psychiatrist discusses cases individually with the physician concerned. Some clinics provide consultation services for children under the care of practicing physicians. The physician in turn can help interpret to his own patients that the child guidance clinic must exercise selectivity in the acceptance of its case load, since its limited facilities cannot accommodate all children in the community in need of some type of care. He can help prepare the child and his parents for referral to the clinic, and he can explain to parents that specific treatment for such symptoms as bed-wetting and stuttering, which are only manifestations of a broader problem, should not be expected. The physician can carry through on the relationship with the parents during and after the time the child is seen in the clinic, provided the clinic offers and the physician takes advantage of detailed discussion of the problems involved.

Other Community Services. Many school systems offer services for emotionally disturbed children. In a few of the large metropolitan centers, these may be developed to the extent of a full child guidance setup with related services. In others, a psychiatrist may be employed full-time or part-time to provide psychotherapy to selected school children for whom this service cannot be obtained through other channels.

In most schools in which any special services for emotionally disturbed children are available, these are provided by a social worker, often designated as a visiting teacher, who is called in to help evaluate the problem in the school and in the home, seeking to obtain indicated adjustments to help the disturbed child through the school and with the help of community agencies. Clinical psychologists employed by some schools perform similar functions, in addition to being able to do a more inclusive evaluation of the child. Since supervisory and consultant services of a psychiatrist are not available in the vast majority of schools, it is desirable to have such specialized school personnel work closely with the school physician as a link between the health services and the instructional program in these special problems.

A variety of other community agencies may provide treatment or guidance services for emotionally disturbed children, usually only for children in families receiving other services from the particular agency. Most often, this consists of services by social workers under the guidance of part-time psychiatrists on the staffs of the agencies. The family physician should be aware of the services available through the agencies in his community, so that he can make use of them for his own patients as the need arises.

Institutional Care. Various types of institutional care are needed by more severely emotionally disturbed children, but facilities for this type of care are grossly inadequate in most areas. For psychotic children, special psychiatric hospitals or segregated portions of psychiatric hospitals for all age groups should be available. Too often, when the children's service is part of a psychiatric hospital caring for adults as well, it tends to be subordinated to the acute needs of the remainder of the institution, so that the children's special needs may not receive the consideration they deserve.

In a certain group of emotionally disturbed children who are not psychotic, there is little hope of helping the child as long as he remains in the home or other situation which is largely responsible for his condition. Removal of such a child from the aggravating situation for a period of time may help break the vicious circle. Special boarding homes or residential institutions are ideal for these children. The child can be helped in a permissive atmosphere while work proceeds simultaneously with the parent or guardian who, for possibly the first time, can view the problem with some objectivity in the absence of the child. Unfortunately, these residential institutions are under considerable pressure to accept many children causing trouble in the community who may not benefit from the special type of care provided, and it is often hard for the institutions to withstand such pressure without losing the support of the community.

SOCIALLY HANDICAPPED CHILDREN

Socially handicapped children are those who lack physical or emotional security as a result of conditions within their own family, their social group, or their community. Children born out of wedlock or coming from broken homes, children from minority groups, and children in the families of migrant workers often face special obstacles to their full development.

The proper care of children deprived of a normal home life can now be seen to be not merely an act of common humanity, but to be essential for the mental and social welfare of a community. For, when their care is neglected, as happens in every country of the Western world today, they grow up to reproduce themselves. Deprived children, whether in their own homes or out of them, are a source of social infection as real and serious as are carriers of diphtheria and typhoid. (11)

The social agencies of the community bear the primary responsibility for meeting many of the needs of these children, but those responsible for health services must make a special effort to have these services available for the children and to motivate the parents to use the services offered. This aspect of health services has been touched upon in relation to some of the specific health services, especially in discussing the role of the public health nurse in reaching community groups out of the main stream of community life. Families in isolated rural areas are in a sense also socially handicapped, since it is usually much more difficult for them to obtain needed health services.

Two groups of children with special problems of a social nature, the juvenile delinquent and the narcotic addict, deserve brief consideration. In both of these, the presenting symptoms are socially unacceptable and social handicaps of various sorts are generally found in the young person's background.

Juvenile Delinquency. Juvenile delinquency is, by definition, a legal concept. It implies that children under a specific age, usually sixteen years, have committed an act which contravenes the law; since the law varies in time and place, the reported incidence of juvenile delinquency likewise varies. Juvenile delinquency is far more common in areas with unfavorable social and economic conditions. Reduction of juvenile delinquency in these areas is ultimately dependent upon amelioration of these conditions. However, even full correction of adverse factors outside the home would not prevent the development of the overt hostile acts, characterized as juvenile delinquency when detected by the legal authorities, which presumably result from emotional factors within the home. Programs for the prevention of juvenile delinquency must be as inclusive as a broad program for the promotion of mental health, since juvenile delinquency is only one of many possible outcomes of emotional disturbances.

Juvenile delinquency, as an insistent community problem, was one of the earliest mental health problems in children to receive attention. Child guidance clinics in relation to children's courts were a major impetus to the development of similar services for other children as well. Special clinics are conducted in many of the larger cities for children coming to attention as a result of delinquent behavior, or the services of other child guidance clinics may be called upon for the same purpose.

A number of studies have indicated that juvenile delinquents have more health problems of a physical nature than other children in the same community. These probably bear no causal relationship in most cases to the delinquency, except when a physical handicap underlies the need for the child to gain recognition through antisocial behavior. Even so, the general health of the delinquent child should be promoted as part of the management of the child. The health appraisal should also attempt to determine whether an organic condition, such as brain trauma or previous encephalitis, might not be the basic cause of the child's aberrant behavior.

"The delinquent child has, on the one hand, the same needs as all children and, on the other, special needs. Just like other children who require attention from public or private social agencies, the delinquent child may need casework treatment, psychiatric treatment, or foster care —singly or in combination." (12)

Narcotic Addiction. The problem of narcotic addiction among adolescents has received widespread publicity in the lay press, although there is no evidence that the problem exists outside a few areas within the major metropolitan centers in the country. Drug addiction develops when the drugs are available to, and are tried by, persons whose emotional needs are temporarily, if destructively, satisfied by use of the drugs. The reasons for the emotional susceptibility to drug addiction by certain individuals in a given environment are incompletely understood. The major preventive measure must consist of police action in cutting off the supply of the drugs.

The youthful narcotic addict generally starts with the smoking of marihuana cigarettes, progressing through the stage of ingestion of heroin or other truly narcotic drug, finally administering the drug intravenously to get the maximum satisfaction from the drug as tolerance develops. The scars from infected lesions at the sites of the injections are a major diagnostic sign of drug addiction. Rehabilitation of the drug addict, even when the drug addict is an adolescent, is a difficult matter. Getting youths to stop taking the drug is relatively simple, but the experience at the Federal hospitals treating drug addicts has been that the majority relapse into their old habits on return to their old environment. Social rehabilitation must be continued in follow-up clinics, with emphasis upon occupational training, guidance, and placement services. Counseling clinics which would provide the necessary psychiatric and other services have been proposed (13).

When there is a suspicion of narcotic use among school children, the same general policies in screening should be used as for other conditions coming to the attention of health services in the schools. Undue publicity and heightened suspicion on the part of schoolteachers, with direct referral to a police or treatment agency, have been found to result in false stigmatization of many school children thought to be drug users on the basis of nonspecific symptoms (14).

A GLIMPSE INTO THE FUTURE

The future of health services for the children of the United States is bright. Barring a major cataclysm, there is no reason to believe that the spectacular progress of the past several decades will not continue through the remainder of the twentieth century.

Much of what remains to be done is clearly apparent, and advances are being steadily recorded. Additional gains may be made by the broader application of what is already known. Adverse social attitudes which increase the burden of those already handicapped must be overcome more fully, so that children and adults may have adequate training centered about their abilities and full opportunities to function within their capacities as members of the community.

For those problems which are still beyond reach of solution, there is strong hope that research of a fundamental or applied nature will shortly yield more effective methods of attack. Significant progress may be made, for example, in the prevention of premature birth, congenital malformations, cerebral palsy, and mental deficiency by a clearer understanding of maternal factors to the extent that the latter bear responsibility in their causation.

For more rapid progress in maternal and child health, there must be an ever closer working partnership in broad community efforts between the practicing physician and his counterpart in other professional disciplines and the health workers in official and voluntary health agencies. If this book has made any contribution toward that end, it will have achieved its purpose.

CITED REFERENCES

1. BENDA, CLEMENS E., MALCOLM J. FARRELL, and CATHERINE E. CHIPMAN, The Inadequacy of Present-day Concepts of Mental Deficiency and Mental Illness in Child Psychiatry, *Am. J. Psychiat.,* Vol. 107, pp. 721–729, April, 1951.
2. YANNET, HERMAN, Trainable Mental Defectives, A Comment on Prognosis, *J. Pediat.,* Vol. 37, pp. 816–818, November, 1950.
3. PARKER, GEORGE F., The Incidence of Mongoloid Imbecility in the Newborn Infant: A Ten-year Study Covering 27,931 Live Births, *J. Pediat.,* Vol. 36, pp. 493–494, April, 1950.
4. BUCK, ELIZABETH W., Developing the Community's Responsibility for the Adjustment of the Mentally Retarded, *Am. J. Ment. Deficiency,* Vol. 55, pp. 407–414, January, 1951.
5. GADSON, EUGENE J., Glutamic Acid and Mental Deficiency—A Review, *Am. J. Ment. Deficiency,* Vol. 55, pp. 521–528, April, 1951.
6. "Statistics Pertinent to Psychiatry in the United States," Report No. 7, Group for the Advancement of Psychiatry, Topeka, Kans., March, 1949.
7. PENNELL, MARYLAND Y., DALE C. CAMERON, and MORTON KRAMER, Mental Health Clinic Services for Children in the United States, 1950, *Pub. Health Rep.,* Vol. 66, pp. 1559–1572, Nov. 30, 1951.
8. REYMERT, MARTIN L., The Organization and Administration of a Child Guidance Clinic, in "Handbook of Child Guidance," edited by Ernest Harms, Child Care Publications, New York, 1947.
9. HENDERSON, ADELE L., Activities of a Mental Health Nurse, *Pub. Health Rep.,* Vol. 65, pp. 331–336, Mar. 10, 1950.
10. COLEMAN, JULES V., and ROBERT E. SWITZER, Dynamic Factors in

Psychosocial Treatment in Traveling Child-guidance Clinics, *Ment. Hyg.,* Vol. 35, pp. 386–409, July, 1951.

11. BOWLBY, JOHN, Maternal Care and Mental Health, *Bull. World Health Organ.,* Vol. 3, pp. 355–533, special number, 1951.

12. BECK, BERTRAM M., Focus on Delinquency, *Child,* Vol. 4, pp. 59–62, December, 1952; special issue of *The Child* devoted to juvenile delinquency.

13. BERRY, LEONIDAS H., Medical Counseling Clinics for Young Narcotic Addicts, *J.A.M.A.,* Vol. 147, pp. 1129–1132, Nov. 17, 1951.

14. JACOBZINER, HAROLD, Epidemic of Narcotic Use among School Children in New York City, *J. Pediat.,* Vol. 42, pp. 65–74, January, 1953.

ADDITIONAL REFERENCES

1. MULLEN, FRANCES A., and MARY M. NEE, Distribution of Mental Retardation in an Urban School Population, *Am. J. Ment. Deficiency,* Vol. 56, pp. 777–790, April, 1952.

2. DIMICHAEL, SALVATORE G., "Vocational Rehabilitation of the Mentally Retarded," Rehabilitation Service Series No. 123, Office of Vocational Rehabilitation, Washington, D.C., 1950.

3. YANNET, HERMAN, chairman, Round Table Discussion, The Problem of Mental Deficiency in Children, *Pediatrics,* Vol. 10, pp. 223–230, August, 1952.

4. NEWELL, H. W., Principles and Practices Used in Child Psychiatric Clinics, *Ment. Hyg.,* Vol. 35, pp. 571–580, October, 1951.

5. ROONEY, HERBERT L., Cultivating Community Relationships in a Mental Health Program, *Pub. Health Rep.,* Vol. 66, pp. 637–643, May 18, 1951.

6. LEMKAU, PAUL V., Public Health Administration in Mental Hygiene, *Am. J. Pub. Health,* Vol. 41, pp. 1382–1387, November, 1951.

7. LURIE, LOUIS A., and MAX L. LURIE, Psychoses in Children—A Review, *J. Pediat.,* Vol. 36, pp. 801–809, June, 1950.

8. ALLEN, FREDERICK H., Developments in Child Psychiatry in the United States, *Am. J. Pub. Health,* Vol. 38, pp. 1201–1209, September, 1948.

9. REID, JOSEPH H., and HELEN R. HAGAN, "Residential Treatment Centers for Emotionally Disturbed Children," Child Welfare League of America, New York, 1952.

10. "Directory of Psychiatric Clinics and Other Resources in the United States," The National Association for Mental Health, Inc., New York, 1952.

11. "Residential Treatment Centers for Emotionally Disturbed Children: A Listing," Children's Bureau, Washington, D. C., 1952.

12. BAKWIN, HARRY, Juvenile Delinquency, *J. Pediat.,* Vol. 42, pp. 387–391, March, 1953.

APPENDIX

The Appendix presents sources of information and educational materials on health problems of mothers and children and on health and related services for these groups.

A. Local agencies and organizations

The first resource is one of the local agencies, especially the health department or medical or dental society. The local voluntary health organizations, which are too numerous and varied to list, supply information on the subjects of particular interest to them and make available materials for professional use and for public health education. Many of these are affiliates of national or state organizations and provide pamphlets, films, and other materials prepared by the parent organizations to individuals in the community upon request. Councils of social agencies often have health sections which maintain an inventory of local health resources.

B. State agencies

All states have organizational units in their state departments of health which have responsibility for the broad field of maternal and child health. These are generally known as bureaus of maternal and child health. All states also have units which collect, tabulate, and publish data on vital statistics.

In many states, the unit administering health services for handicapped children is also part of the state department of health, and information on these services can be obtained from the latter. In the other states, health services for handicapped children are administered by the following agencies:[1]

1. Alabama—State Department of Education, Division of Vocational Education, Montgomery
2. Arizona—State Department of Public Welfare, Division for Crippled Children, Phoenix

[1] "Services for Crippled Children," Folder No. 38, Children's Bureau, Washington, D.C., 1952.

3. Arkansas—State Department of Public Welfare, Crippled Children's Division, Little Rock
4. Florida—Crippled Children's Commission, Tallahassee
5. Georgia—State Department of Public Welfare, Crippled Children's Division, Atlanta
6. Illinois—University of Illinois, Division of Services for Crippled Children, Springfield
7. Indiana—State Department of Public Welfare, Services for Crippled Children, Indianapolis
8. Iowa—University of Iowa, Crippled Children's Services, Iowa City
9. Kansas—Crippled Children's Commission, Wichita
10. Michigan—Crippled Children Commission, Lansing
11. Minnesota—State Department of Social Security, Division of Social Welfare, Bureau for Crippled Children, St. Paul
12. Mississippi—State Board of Education, Crippled Children's Services, Jackson
13. Missouri—University of Missouri, State Service for Crippled Children, Columbia
14. Nebraska—State Board of Control, Department of Assistance and Child Welfare, Services for Crippled Children, Lincoln
15. New Mexico—State Department of Public Welfare, Crippled Children's Services, Santa Fe
16. North Dakota—Public Welfare Board of North Dakota, Division of Child Welfare, Bismarck
17. Ohio—State Department of Public Welfare, Division of Social Administration, Services for Crippled Children, Columbus
18. Oklahoma—Commission for Crippled Children, Oklahoma City
19. Oregon—University of Oregon Medical School, Crippled Children's Division, Portland
20. West Virginia—State Department of Public Assistance, Division of Medical Services, Charleston
21. Wisconsin—State Department of Public Instruction, Bureau for Handicapped Children, Crippled Children's Division, Madison

Other services bearing on the health of mothers and children are too widely scattered in different administrative units in the various states to permit individual listing.[2] An inquiry directed to a state governmental agency not concerned with the subject matter of the inquiry will usually be transmitted to the proper agency.

[2] For detailed presentation, see Joseph W. Mountin, Evelyn Flook, and Edward E. Minty, "Distribution of Health Services in the Structure of State Government—1950," Public Health Service Publication No. 184, Washington, D.C.; "Part 2: General Services and Construction of Facilities for State Health Programs," 1952; "Part 3: Personal Health Services Provided by State Government," 1953.

C. National agencies and organizations

The major sources of information in the Federal government are agencies which are part of the Department of Health, Education, and Welfare, Health, Education and Welfare Building, Washington 25, D.C. These agencies, and some of their pertinent publications, follow. They are located in the Health, Education, and Welfare Building unless otherwise indicated.

1. Children's Bureau
   The Child, monthly
   "Chart Book," annually (summary of vital-statistics data)
2. Public Health Service
   Public Health Reports, monthly
3. National Office of Vital Statistics
   Current Mortality Analysis, monthly
   "Monthly Vital Statistics Bulletin"
   "Vital Statistics Special Reports"
   "Vital Statistics of the United States," annually
     (Information in addition to published material may be obtained from
     the National Office of Vital Statistics, in accordance with a tabular
     index in "Vital Statistics of the United States.[3])
4. National Institute of Mental Health, National Institutes of Health,
   Bethesda 14, Md.
   "Patients in Mental Institutions," annual data on institutionalization for
     mental illness, mental deficiency, and epilepsy.
5. Office of Vocational Rehabilitation
   Selected Rehabilitation Abstracts, bimonthly

Some of the leading organizations of professional and technical personnel are

1. American Medical Association, 535 North Dearborn St., Chicago 10,
   Ill.
   Journal of the American Medical Association, weekly
   American Journal of Diseases of Children, monthly
2. American Academy of Pediatrics, 610 Church St., Evanston, Ill.
   Pediatrics, monthly (especially columns "Trends" and "Public Health,
     Nursing and Medical Social Work"); Children's Tumor Registry of
     the American Academy of Pediatrics, 444 East 68 St., New York 2,
     N.Y.
3. American Academy of Obstetrics and Gynecology, 49 East 33 St., New
   York 16, N.Y.
   Obstetrics and Gynecology, monthly
4. American Public Health Association, 1790 Broadway, New York 19,
   N.Y.

[3] See, for example, "Vital Statistics of the United States, 1949," Part I, pp. LXX–LXXI, National Office of Vital Statistics, Washington, D.C., 1951.

American Journal of Public Health, monthly
"Year Book of the American Public Health Association"

5. American Orthopsychiatric Association, 303 Lexington Ave., New York 16, N.Y.
   American Journal of Orthopsychiatry: A Journal of Human Behavior, quarterly

6. American Psychiatric Association, 1270 Sixth Ave., New York 20, N.Y.
   American Journal of Psychiatry, monthly

7. American Psychosomatic Society, 49 East 33 St., New York 16, N.Y.
   Psychosomatic Medicine, bimonthly

8. American School Health Association, Kent State University, Kent, Ohio
   Journal of School Health, monthly, except July and August

9. American Association for Health, Physical Education and Recreation, 1201 Sixteenth St., N.W., Washington 6, D.C.
   Journal of the American Association for Health, Physical Education and Recreation, monthly
   Research Quarterly

10. American Dental Association, 222 East Superior St., Chicago 11, Ill.
    Journal of the American Dental Association, monthly
    Journal of Oral Surgery, quarterly

11. American Society of Dentistry for Children, Mount Royal and Guilford Avenues, Baltimore 2, Md.
    Journal of Dentistry for Children, quarterly

12. American Dental Hygienists' Association, 1735 Eye St., N.W., Washington 6, D.C.
    Journal of the American Dental Hygienists' Association, quarterly

13. American Dietetic Association, 620 North Michigan Ave., Chicago 11, Ill.
    Journal of the American Dietetic Association, monthly

14. American Hospital Association, 18 East Division St., Chicago 10, Ill.
    Hospitals, monthly

15. American Association of Medical Social Workers, 1834 K St., N.W., Washington 5, D.C.
    Medical Social Work, quarterly

16. National League for Nursing, 2 Park Ave., New York 16, N.Y.
    Nursing Outlook, monthly
    "Bulletin of the NLN Department of Public Health Nursing," three times a year

17. American Speech and Hearing Association, c/o Speech and Hearing Clinic, Wayne University, Detroit, Mich.
    Journal of Speech and Hearing Disorders, quarterly

18. American Occupational Therapy Association, 33 West 42 St., New York 36, N.Y.
    American Journal of Occupational Therapy, bimonthly

American Journal of Physical Medicine, bimonthly
"Yearbook of the Occupational Therapy Association"
19. American Physical Therapy Association, 1790 Broadway, New York 19, N.Y.
Physical Therapy Review, monthly
20. International Council for Exceptional Children (the handicapped and gifted), 1201 Sixteenth St., N.W., Washington 6, D.C.
Exceptional Children, eight times a year, October through May
21. National Rehabilitation Association, 1025 Vermont Ave., Washington 5, D.C.
Journal of Rehabilitation, bimonthly
22. Child Welfare League of America (primarily concerned with social aspects of care, especially foster care), 24 West 40th St., New York 18, N.Y.
Child Welfare, monthly

National voluntary health organizations devote much of their budget and energy to the development and distribution of materials relating to health problems for use in local programs. Many of the following provide such materials or will refer the inquiries to possible other sources.

1. National Health Council, 1790 Broadway, New York 19, N.Y.
2. American Cancer Society, 47 Beaver St., New York 4, N.Y.
Cancer, bimonthly
Cancer Current Literature, monthly
Cancer News, quarterly
CA: A Bulletin of Cancer Progress, bimonthly, for the general practitioner
3. American Association on Mental Deficiency, 224 East 28 St., New York 16, N.Y.
American Journal of Mental Deficiency, monthly
4. American Committee on Maternal Welfare, 116 South Michigan Ave., Chicago 3, Ill.
The Mother, quarterly
5. American Diabetes Association, 11 West 42 St., New York 36, N.Y.
A.D.A. Forecast, bimonthly, for diabetics
Diabetes: The Journal of the American Diabetes Association, scientific bimonthly
6. American Hearing Society, 817 Fourteenth St., N.W., Washington 5, D.C.
Hearing News, monthly
7. American Heart Association, 44 East 23 St., New York 10, N.Y.
Circulation, monthly
Modern Concepts of Cardiovascular Diseases, monthly
Circulation—Research, bimonthly

8. Child Study Association of America, 132 East 74 St., New York 21, N.Y.

   Child Study, a quarterly journal of parent education
9. Commission on Chronic Illness, 615 North Wolfe St., Baltimore 5, Md.

   Chronic Illness News Letter, bimonthly
10. Maternity Center Association, 654 Madison Ave., New York 21, N.Y.

    Briefs, monthly
11. National Association for Mental Health, 1790 Broadway, New York 19, N.Y.

    Mental Hygiene, quarterly

    Understanding the Child, quarterly
12. National Epilepsy League, 130 North Wells St., Chicago 6, Ill.
13. National Foundation for Infantile Paralysis, 120 Broadway, New York 5, N.Y.

    National Foundation News, monthly

    "Poliomyelitis Current Literature"
14. National Safety Council, 425 North Michigan Ave., Chicago 11, Ill.

    Accident Facts, annually

    Home Safety Review, monthly, except July and August

    Public Safety, monthly

    National Safety News, monthly

    Safety Education, monthly, except July and August
15. National Society for Crippled Children and Adults, 11 South La Salle St., Chicago 3, Ill.

    The Crippled Child, bimonthly

    "Bulletin on Current Literature," monthly abstracts

    "Bulletin of the National Society for Crippled Children and Adults," monthly
16. National Society for the Prevention of Blindness, 1790 Broadway, New York 19, N.Y.

    Sight-Saving Review, quarterly

    Prevention of Blindness News, intermittent
17. National Tuberculosis Association, 1790 Broadway, New York 19, N.Y.

    American Review of Tuberculosis, monthly

    "Bulletin of the National Tuberculosis Association," monthly
18. Nutrition Foundation, Chrysler Building, New York 17, N.Y.

    Nutrition Reviews, monthly
19. Volta Bureau and Volta Association for the Deaf, 1537 Thirty-fifth St., N.W., Washington 7, D.C.

    Volta Review, monthly, except July and August

The following heterogeneous group of organizations also deserve mention.

1. American Parents Committee, 52 Vanderbilt Ave., New York 17, N.Y.

   "Washington Report on Legislation for Children," occasionally

2. John Tracy Clinic, 806 West Adams Blvd., Los Angeles 7, Calif.
   "Correspondence Course for Parents of Deaf and Hard-of-Hearing Children"
3. Metropolitan Life Insurance Company, 1 Madison Ave., New York 10, N.Y.
   "Statistical Bulletin," monthly
   "Health Bulletin for Teachers," monthly
4. Social Legislation Information Service, 1346 Connecticut Ave., N.W., Washington 6, D.C.
   "Social Legislation Information Bulletin," weekly while Congress is in session, less frequently at other times

LIST OF VISUAL AIDS

The visual materials listed below and on the following pages can be used to implement and supplement the material in this book, particularly when one is speaking to groups of nurses, public health workers, or lay audiences. It is suggested, of course, that a film be reviewed before it is used in order to determine its suitability for a particular group.

Both motion pictures and filmstrips are included in this list of visual materials, and the character of each one is indicated by the self-explanatory abbreviations "MP" and "FS." Immediately following this identification is the name of the producer; and if the distributor is different from the producer, the name of the distributor follows the name of the producer. Abbreviations are used for names of producers and distributors, and these abbreviations are identified in the list of sources at the end of the bibliography. In most instances, the films may be borrowed or rented from local or state 16mm film libraries. (A nationwide list of these local sources is given in "A Directory of 2002 16mm Film Libraries," available for thirty-five cents from the Superintendent of Documents, Washington 25, D.C.) Unless otherwise indicated, the motion pictures are 16mm sound black-and-white films and the filmstrips are 35mm black-and-white and silent.

This bibliography is not inclusive. It is suggested that film users examine the bibliography "Motion Pictures on Child Life," compiled by the U.S. Children's Bureau, Washington and the latest annual edition and quarterly supplements of "Educational Film Guide," a catalogue of some 10,000 films published by the H. W. Wilson Co., New York, N.Y. Both references are available in most libraries. The American Medical Association periodically issues lists of sources of motion pictures on health subjects.[1]

[1] "Sources of Motion Pictures on Health," Committee on Medical Motion Pictures, American Medical Association, Chicago, 1952.

Adolescent Development (MP series; McGraw). Series of five films and correlated filmstrips portraying the interests, problems, and activities of teen-age boys and girls. The titles and running times of the individual films are:

Age of Turmoil (20min)
The Meaning of Adolescence (16min)
Meeting the Needs of Adolescents (19min)
Physical Aspects of Puberty (19min)
Social–Sex Attitudes in Adolescence (22min)

Ages and Stages (MP series; CNFB/McGraw). Series of films, three at present completed, portraying typical behavior patterns of children. The first film is a survey of the important developments during the first 15 years and the other two films, as their titles indicate, focus upon particular ages and stages. The titles and running times of the three films are:

He Acts His Age (13min color or black and white)
The Terrible Twos and Trusting Threes (20min color or black and white)
The Frustrating Fours and Fascinating Fives (22min color or black and white)

And Now To Live (MP; Spastic Fd; 21min). Problems of cerebral palsy and the activities of the training center of the Spastic Children's Foundation.

Angry Boy (MP; MHFB/IFB; 33min). Story of a boy caught stealing at school and the emotional disturbances which are the basic cause of his wrongdoing and are uncovered through psychiatric care.

Breakdown (MP; CNFB/McGraw; 40min). Story of a young woman's schizophrenic breakdown, treatment, and recovery.

Care of the Newborn Baby (MP; USOE/UWF; 31min). Nurse's functions and duties in teaching parents to care for new born babies; what the nurse can do in the home, clinic, and hospital; and how to hold, dress, bathe, and feed a baby. (Correlated filmstrips, same title, 93 frames, also available.)

Child Development (MP series; EBF). Series of 11-minute motion pictures based upon the research of Dr. Arnold Gesell at the Yale Clinic of Child Development. Titles of the individual films are:

Baby's Day at Twelve Weeks
Behavior Day at 48 Weeks
Behavior Patterns at One Year
Early Social Behavior
From Creeping to Walking
Growth of Infant Behavior: Early Stages
Growth of Infant Behavior: Later Stages
Learning and Growth
Life Begins
Posture and Locomotion
Thirty-six Weeks Behavior Day

Child Development (MP series; McGraw). Series of five motion pictures and correlated filmstrips dealing with various phases of child development. Titles of the individual films and their running times are:

Child Care and Development (17min)
Children's Emotions (22min)
Heredity and Pre-Natal Development (21min)
Principles of Development (17min)
Social Development (16min)

Children Growing Up with Others (MP; BIS/UWF; 30min). Illustrates stages in the growth of children showing by example their constant adaptation to the world around them.

Children Learning by Experience (MP; BIS/UWF; 40min). Explains and illustrates how children want to learn and do learn, directly and indirectly, many things by experience.

The Feeling of Hostility (MP; CNFB/McGraw; 27 min). Case history of a young woman, outwardly successful, inwardly unhappy, and of the psychological factors underlying her behavior.

The Feeling of Rejection (MP; CNFB/McGraw; 23min). Case history of a neurotic young woman and of the psychological background of her headaches, fatigue, and dizzy spells.

Feelings of Depression (MP; CNFB/McGraw; 30min). Case history of a hard-working businessman in his early thirties who suffers period of despondency, and of the psychological background of his behavior.

Good Speech for Gary (MP; USC/McGraw; 22min color or black and white). How modern teaching methods help children in the primary grades to overcome speech defects.

Human Growth (MP; Brown Trust; 19min color). Traces the changes in human growth, male and female, from birth to adulthood. Setting of film is in a seventh-grade class and its study of the problem of human growth and development.

Human Reproduction (MP; McGraw; 20 min). Describes by the use of models and animation the male and female reproductive systems and the process of normal human birth. Correlated filmstrip, same title, 30 frames, also available.

Learning to Understand Children. Part 1: A Diagnostic Approach (MP; McGraw; 21min). Diagnostic technique used to determine the causes of a girl's (Ada Adams) emotional and social maladjustment in school. Correlated filmstrip, same title, 37 frames, also available.

Learning to Understand Children. Part 2: A Remedial Program (MP; McGraw; 23min). The remedial program worked out for Ada Adams by her teachers in cooperation with parents and social and health workers. Correlated filmstrip, same title, 34 frames, also available.

Life with Baby (MP; MOT/McGraw; 18min). Pictorial summary of the Gesell studies at Yale and of the physical and mental growth of children from age 1 to age 6.

The Lonely Night (MP; MHFB/IFB; 60min). Story of a girl's emotional disturbances and how psychiatric treatment helped her overcome fear and self-destructiveness. Indicates, as contrast, a way of life that may help prevent emotional disturbances requiring psychiatric care. (Sponsored by Mental Health Authorities of Calif., Conn., Del., Ill., Md., Nev., and R.I.)

Medical Certification of the Causes of Death (FS; USPHS; 59 frames). Explains the importance of accurate cause-of-death certification, and the considerations which govern the selection and ranking of causes entered on death certificates.

Over-Dependency (MP; CNFB/McGraw; 32min). Case study of the effects of a too-dependent childhood upon the personality of a young man.

Performance Testing (MP; Minn U; 30min silent). Use of the manikin, sequin form board, Knox cube, diamond, and memory tests with children of various chronological and mental ages.

Preface to a Life (MP; USPHS; 29min). Parental influences on a child's developing personality illustrated by a series of episodes showing the effects of an overly solicitous mother and an overly demanding father; and, in contrast, the healthy childhood resulting when both parents accept their child as an individual.

Problem Children (MP; Ohio Mental Hygiene/PSC; 20min). Story of two junior high school boys and how their personalities are affected by their relationships in home and school. Illustrates how parents and teachers should work together to provide conditions favorable to the solution of children's problems.

So Much for So Little (MP; USPHS; 11min color). A cartoon film explaining the health hazards threatening a typical American community and the services of a properly staffed local health department.

Your Children's Ears (MP; BIS; 15min). Explains by animated diagrams the physiology of the ear and gives advice to parents on the care of their children's ears.

Your Children's Eyes (MP; BIS; 20min). Explains by animated diagrams the physiology of the eye and gives advice to parents on the care of their children's eyes.

Your Children's Meals. (MP; BIS; 14min). Shows through a series of dramatized incidents how parents can see mealtime from the child's point of view as well as their own.

Your Children's Play (MP; BIS/McGraw; 21min). Shows typical play behavior of children from one to eight years of age and emphasizes the importance of parent understanding and cooperation.

Your Children's Sleep (MP; BIS; 23min). Stresses the importance of sound sleep and advises parents on the ways in which they can ensure it for their children.

Your Children's Teeth (MP; BIS; 14min). Explains the structure of first and second teeth and the parents' responsibility for giving their children a well-balanced diet, teaching them to brush their teeth, and visiting a dentist regularly.

SOURCES OF FILMS LISTED ABOVE

BIS—British Information Services, 30 Rockefeller Plaza, New York 20, N.Y.

Brown Trust—E. C. Brown Trust, 220 S.W. Alder St., Portland 4, Oregon.

CNFB—National Film Board of Canada, 1270 Avenue of the Americas, New York, N.Y.

EBF—Encyclopedia Britannica Films, Inc., Wilmette, Ill.

IFB—International Film Bureau, 57 E. Jackson Blvd., Chicago 4, Ill.

McGraw—McGraw-Hill Book Co., Inc., Text-Film Dept., 330 W. 42d St., New York, N.Y.

MHFB—Mental Health Film Board, 164 E. 38th St., New York 16, N.Y.

Minn U—University of Minnesota, Audio-Visual Education Service, Minneapolis, Minn.

MOT—March of Time, 369 Lexington Ave., New York, N.Y. (Films distributed by McGraw-Hill Book Co., Inc.)

Ohio Mental Hygiene—Ohio Division of Mental Hygiene, State Office Bldg., Columbus, Ohio.

PSC—Pennsylvania State College, Audio-Visual Library, State College, Pa.

Spastic Fd—Spastic Children's Foundation, 1307 W. 105th St., Los Angeles 44, Calif.

USC—University of Southern California, Los Angeles, Calif.

USOE—U.S. Office of Education, Washington 25, D.C.

USPHS—U.S. Public Health Service, Washington 25, D.C.

UWF—United World Films, Inc., 1445 Park Ave., New York 29, N.Y.

AUTHOR INDEX

A

Aaron, J. B., 250
Abbott, L. C., 356
Abramson, H., 271
Adair, F. L., 39, 251
Albrecht, R. M., 177
Aldrich, C. A., 140, 271
Allen, F. H., 151, 368
Amatruda, C. S., 140
Anderson, E. J., 96
Anderson, G., 177
Anderson, G. W., 80, 177, 178, 251
Anderson, O. W., 63
Andrews, F. E., 81
Arey, J. B., 40
Argall, C. I., 273
Armstrong, D. B., 217
Arnstein, M. G., 178
Aron, H. C. S. 178
Ast, D. B., 191
Aufranc, W. H., 178

B

Bachman, G. W., 10
Bade, M., 271
Badger, T. L., 249
Bahlke, A. M., 327
Bain, K., 271, 307
Baird, D., 250
Baker, S. J., 61
Bakwin, H., 290, 368
Bakwin, R. M., 290
Baldwin, R., 355
Barnes, G. R., Jr., 273
Barnett, H. E., 355
Bauer, F. C., 40
Baumgartner, L., 40, 272
Beacham, W. D., 62

Beaven, P. W., 62
Beck, B. M., 368
Beck, M. D., 177
Beecroft, R. K., 134
Beeman, E. A., 177
Beer, J. J., 62
Beigelman, P. M., 177
Beilly, J. S., 250
Bell, J. A., 177
Benda, C. E., 367
Benenson, A. S., 176
Bennett, R. L., 354
Berry, K., 249
Berry, L. H., 368
Bessey, O. A., 207
Betts, W. A., 272
Bevan, A. D., 61
Bibby, B. G., 191
Bierman, J. M., 39, 308
Black, I. S., 290
Bland, E. F., 356
Bloch, H., 272
Bluestone, E. M., 122
Blum, L. H., 326
Boerner, F., 141
Bost, F. C., 289
Bousquet, F. P., Jr., 272
Bowdoin, C. D., 141
Bowlby, J., 368
Bradford, W. L., 176
Bradley, C., 355
Bridge, E. M., 355
Browe, J. H., 207
Bruns, P. D., 273
Buchbinder, L., 271
Buchwald, E., 326
Buck, C. E., 10
Buck, E. W., 367
Bucknall, N., 217
Buell, B., 10

383

SUBJECT INDEX

A